A·N·N·U·A·L E·D·I·T·I·O·N·S

Health
Twentieth Edition

99/00

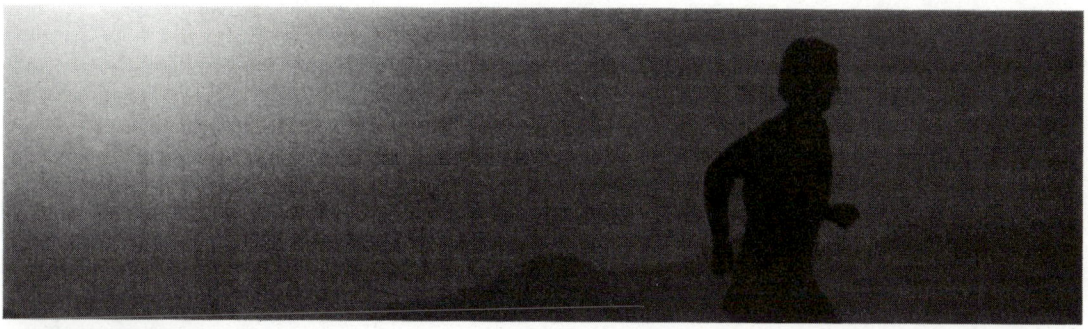

EDITOR

Richard Yarian
Towson University

Richard Yarian is a health educator with extensive training in the area of biomedical health. He received a B.A. in biology from Ball State University. Before leaving Ball State University, he also received both an M.A. and an Ed.S. in the area of health education. He continued his academic training at the University of Maryland where he received a Ph.D. in biomedical health. Following completion of his doctoral program, he became an assistant professor at the University of Maryland and taught courses in the areas of personal health, stress management, drug abuse, medical physiology, and cardiovascular disease.

Dushkin/McGraw-Hill
Sluice Dock, Guilford, Connecticut 06437

Visit us on the Internet
http://www.dushkin.com/annualeditions/

Credits

1. Health Behavior and Decision Making
Facing overview—© 1998 by PhotoDisc, Inc.
2. Stress and Mental Health
Facing overview—Dushkin/McGraw-Hill photo by Cheryl Greenleaf.
3. Nutritional Health
Facing overview—WHO photo.
4. Exercise and Weight Control
Facing overview—© 1998 by PhotoDisc, Inc.
5. Drugs and Health
Facing overview—Couresty of the American Cancer Society.
6. Human Sexuality
Facing overview—Digital Stock photo. 111—Photos by Richard Pierce Photography, Inc. 123—Illustration by Andres Wenngren.
7. Current Killers
Facing overview—© 1998 by PhotoDisc, Inc.
8. America's Health and the Health Care System
Facing overview—© 1998 by PhotoDisc, Inc. 166—Illustration by Philippe Weisbecker.
9. Consumer Health
Facing overview—Dushkin/McGraw-Hill photo.
10. Contemporary Health Hazards
Facing overview—EPA-Documerica photo.

Copyright

Cataloging in Publication Data
Main entry under title: Annual Editions: Health. 1999/2000.
    1. Hygiene—Periodicals. I. Yarian, Richard, comp. II. Title: Health.
ISBN 0–07–039799–6   613'.05   81-643582   ISSN 0278-4653

© 1999 by Dushkin/McGraw-Hill, Guilford, CT 06437, A Division of The McGraw-Hill Companies.

Copyright law prohibits the reproduction, storage, or transmission in any form by any means of any portion of this publication without the express written permission of Dushkin/McGraw-Hill, and of the copyright holder (if different) of the part of the publication to be reproduced. The Guidelines for Classroom Copying endorsed by Congress explicitly state that unauthorized copying may not be used to create, to replace, or to substitute for anthologies, compilations, or collective works.

Annual Editions® is a Registered Trademark of Dushkin/McGraw-Hill, A Division of The McGraw-Hill Companies.

Twentieth Edition

Cover image © 1999 PhotoDisc, Inc.

Printed in the United States of America   1234567890BAHBAH5432109   Printed on Recycled Paper

Editors/Advisory Board

Members of the Advisory Board are instrumental in the final selection of articles for each edition of ANNUAL EDITIONS. Their review of articles for content, level, currentness, and appropriateness provides critical direction to the editor and staff. We think that you will find their careful consideration well reflected in this volume.

EDITOR

Richard Yarian
Towson University

ADVISORY BOARD

Jerry L. Ainsworth
Southern Connecticut State University

Charles R. Baffi
Virginia Polytechnic Institute and State University

David Birch
Indiana University

F. Stephen Bridges
University of West Florida

Donald Brobst
San Jose City College

Annette L. Caruso
Pennsylvania State University Abington

Carlton M. Fancher
Central Michigan University

Anita Farel
University of North Carolina Chapel Hill

Kenneth R. Felker
Edinboro University

Nicholas K. Iammarino
Rice University

Allen Pat Kelley
Essex Community College

Cristine Leadbitter
Northern Arizona University

Judith McLaughlin
Georgia Southern University

M. Jane McMahon
Towson University

Syble M. Oldaker
Clemson University

Judy Peel
North Carolina State University

Glen J. Peterson
Lakewood Community College

Ruth P. Saunders
University of South Carolina

Donna J. Schoenfeld
Rutgers University

Alex Waigandt
University of Missouri Columbia

Roy Wohl
Washburn University

Kenneth Wolf
Anne Arundel Community College

STAFF

EDITORIAL STAFF

Ian A. Nielsen, Publisher
Roberta Monaco, Senior Developmental Editor
Dorothy Fink, Associate Developmental Editor
Addie Raucci, Senior Administrative Editor
Cheryl Greenleaf, Permissions Editor
Joseph Offredi, Permissions/Editorial Assistant
Diane Barker, Proofreader
Lisa Holmes-Doebrick, Program Coordinator

PRODUCTION STAFF

Brenda S. Filley, Production Manager
Charles Vitelli, Designer
Lara M. Johnson, Design/Advertising Coordinator
Laura Levine, Graphics
Mike Campbell, Graphics
Tom Goddard, Graphics
Juliana Arbo, Typesetting Supervisor
Jane Jaegersen, Typesetter
Marie Lazauskas, Word Processor
Kathleen D'Amico, Word Processor
Larry Killian, Copier Coordinator

To the Reader

In publishing ANNUAL EDITIONS we recognize the enormous role played by the magazines, newspapers, and journals of the public press in providing current, first-rate educational information in a broad spectrum of interest areas. Many of these articles are appropriate for students, researchers, and professionals seeking accurate, current material to help bridge the gap between principles and theories and the real world. These articles, however, become more useful for study when those of lasting value are carefully collected, organized, indexed, and reproduced in a low-cost format, which provides easy and permanent access when the material is needed. That is the role played by ANNUAL EDITIONS.

New to ANNUAL EDITIONS is the inclusion of related World Wide Web sites. These sites have been selected by our editorial staff to represent some of the best resources found on the World Wide Web today. Through our carefully developed topic guide, we have linked these Web resources to the articles covered in this ANNUAL EDITIONS reader. We think that you will find this volume useful, and we hope that you will take a moment to visit us on the Web at *http://www.dushkin.com* to tell us what you think.

America is in the midst of a health revolution that is changing the way millions of Americans view their health. Traditionally, most people delegated responsibility for their health to their physicians and hoped that medical science would be able to cure whatever ailed them. This approach to health care emphasized the role of medical technology and funneled billions of dollars into medical research. The net result of all this spending is the most technically advanced and expensive health care system in the world. Unfortunately, health care costs have risen so high that millions of Americans can no longer afford health care, and even among those who can, there is limited accessibility to many of the new technologies because the cost is prohibitive. Despite all the technological advances, the medical community has been unable to reverse the damage associated with society's unhealthy lifestyle. This fact, coupled with rapidly rising health care costs, has prompted millions of individuals to assume a more active role in safeguarding their own health. Evidence of this change in attitude can be seen in the growing interest in nutrition, physical fitness, dietary supplements, and stress management. If we as a nation are to capitalize on this new health consciousness, then we must devote more time and energy to educating Americans in the health sciences so that they will be better able to make informed choices about their health.

Health is such a complex and dynamic subject that it is practically impossible for anyone to stay abreast of all the current research findings. In the past most of us have relied on newspapers, magazines, and television for this information, but today with the widespread use of personal computers and the World Wide Web it is possible to access vast amounts of health information without ever leaving home. Unfortunately, quantity does not necessarily translate into quality and so our task as health educators is twofold: (1) To provide our students with the most current and accurate information currently available on major health issues of our time and (2) to teach our students the skills that will enable them to sort our fact from fiction and become informed consumers. *Annual Editions: Health 99/00* was designed to aid in this task. It presents a sampling of quality articles that represent current thinking on a variety of health issues, and it also serves as a tool for developing critical thinking skills.

The articles in this volume were carefully chosen on the basis of their quality and timeliness. Because this book is revised and updated annually, it contains information that is not currently available in any standard textbook. As such, it serves as a valuable resource for both teachers and students. In an attempt to stay current with the field of health education, this edition of *Annual Editions: Health* has been updated to reflect the most current thinking on a variety of contemporary health issues ranging from selecting effective sunscreens to "date rape." We hope that you find this edition of *Annual Editions: Health* to be a helpful learning tool filled with information presented in a user-friendly format. The content areas presented in this edition generally mirror those that are normally covered in introductory health courses. The 10 topic areas covered are: Health Behavior and Decision Making, Stress and Mental Health, Nutritional Health, Exercise and Weight Control, Drugs and Health, Human Sexuality, Current Killers, America's Health and the Health Care System, Consumer Health, and Contemporary Health Hazards. Because of the interdependence of the various elements that constitute health, the articles selected were written by naturalists, environmentalists, psychologists, economists, sociologists, nutritionists, consumer advocates, and traditional health practitioners. The diversity of these selections provides the reader with a variety of viewpoints regarding health and the complexity of the issues involved. This edition of *Annual Editions: Health* also recommends *World Wide Web* sites that can be used to further explore topics addressed in the articles. These sites are cross-referenced by number in the *topic guide*.

Annual Editions: Health 99/00 is one of the most useful and up-to-date publications currently available in the area of health. Please let us know what you think of it by filling out and returning the postage-paid *article rating form* on the last page of this book. Any anthology can be improved. This one will be—annually.

Richard Yarian

Richard Yarian
Editor

Contents

To the Reader iv
Topic Guide 2
Selected World Wide Web Sites 4

UNIT 1
Health Behavior and Decision Making

Five articles examine how Americans make choices about controlling their health.

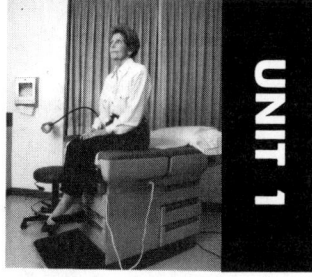

Overview 6

1. **How Does Your Life Measure Up?** Alice Lesch Kelly, *Walking,* March/April 1998. 8
   If you had to choose between length of life and quality of life, which would you choose? Fortunately, good health and a long life generally go hand in hand. Alice Lesch Kelly provides an opportunity to examine your *lifestyle and health behaviors* to see just how well you are doing in your efforts to achieve a long and healthy life.

2. **Why Do Those #&*?@! "Experts" Keep Changing Their Minds?** *University of California at Berkeley Wellness Letter,* February 1996. 14
   Every day it seems that a new discovery is made concerning our health, often contradicting the new finding of just a few weeks past. This article provides the reader with *some sound ways to make informed decisions* when confronted with conflicting evidence.

3. **Yet Another Study—Should You Pay Attention?** *Tufts University Health & Nutrition Letter,* September 1998. 17
   How do you interpret your *risk level* for various illnesses when reading reports of late-breaking news that could affect your health? This article presents four questions to ask yourself to help you make *informed decisions* regarding your *lifestyle choices.*

4. **"Just Do It" Isn't Enough: Change Comes in Stages,** *Tufts University Diet & Nutrition Letter,* September 1996. 19
   James Prochaska, a leading expert on behavior change, describes the *six stages of change* that anyone who wants to achieve lasting success must go through.

5. **Challenging America's Inverted Health Priorities,** Elizabeth M. Whelan, *Priorities,* Volume 8, Number 1, 1996. 22
   Despite the known dangers of tobacco and alcohol use, Americans continue to focus on *minor and often speculative health risks* that account for few deaths and injuries by comparison. Why is this the case? Epidemiologist Elizabeth Whelan urges the participation of scientists and physicians in health debates and the abandonment of *political correctness.*

UNIT 2
Stress and Mental Health

Five selections consider the impact of stress and emotions on mental health.

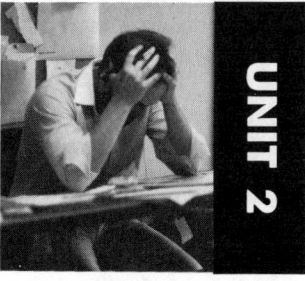

Overview 28

6. **Critical Life Events and the Onset of Illness,** Blair Justice, *Comprehensive Therapy,* Volume 20, Number 4, 1994. 30
   Despite the fact that everyone experiences stress, why is it that not everyone is susceptible to its effects? Blair Justice reasons that the differences are the result of our *sense of support and acceptance,* coupled with our sense of *control over our own lives.*

7. **The Talking Cure for Stress,** Benedict Carey, *Health,* November/December 1996. 37
   First there was the Type A personality, then the Type H personality. Now it seems as though it is neither anger nor hostility that determines if *your personality is predisposing you to premature coronary artery disease.* Rather, it is the intensity with which you react to *negative emotions.*

8. **Using Your Mind to Heal Your Body,** Lori Miller Kase, *American Health for Women,* September 1997. 42
   Most people may not realize that there are *numerous natural stress reducers that can do more for you than drugs,* and without the side effects.

The concepts in bold italics are developed in the article. For further expansion please refer to the Topic Guide and the Index.

9. **Forgiveness,** Ann Japenga, *Health*, May/June 1998. 45
Ann Japenga discusses why **forgiveness is something we need to do to safeguard our own health.**

10. **Bad Mood Rising,** Mary Roach, *Walking*, September/October 1998. 48
Mary Roach takes a humorous look at how and why we get into **bad moods.** She also provides some practical advice on steps to take that can **minimize or manage bad moods.**

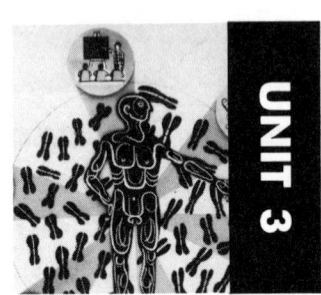

UNIT 3
Nutritional Health

Five articles discuss the effects of diet and nutrition on a person's well-being. Some of the topics addressed are dietary supplements, the importance of fiber, and dietary fat content.

Overview 50

11. **Tall Tales from the Table,** Bill Gottlieb, *Health*, July/August 1998. 52
While **dietary advice** seems to change on a daily basis, some of the most prevalent advice is simply **nutritional myth.** Bill Gottlieb addresses 10 of the most common myths.

12. **The Bitter Truth,** Linda Formichelli, *Walking*, September/October 1998. 55
You know that **vegetables** are good for you and you would like to eat them, but for some reason they just seem to **taste bad.** New findings suggest that the problem may be that you are a "supertaster" and **genetically sensitive to bitterness.**

13. **Are You Getting Enough Fat?** Colleen Pierre, *American Health for Women*, March 1998. 57
Over the past 10 years, Americans have been encouraged to restrict their **dietary fat content.** New findings suggest that the health risks associated with dietary fat may have more to do with the **type** rather than the **amount of fat consumed.**

14. **Bulking Up Fiber's Healthful Reputation,** Ruth Papazian, *FDA Consumer*, July/August 1997. 61
Dietary fiber has been touted for its ability to lower blood cholesterol, prevent certain cancers, correct digestive disorders, and help those with diabetes. How valid are these health claims?

15. **The Vitamin Revolution: B D E,** Harriet A. Washington, *Health*, September 1998. 66
For years nutritionists have held that **nutritional supplements** are not necessary as long as one eats a **balanced diet;** however, recent findings suggest that even a balanced diet may not provide all the nutrients one needs—especially **calcium, vitamins D and E, and the B vitamins.**

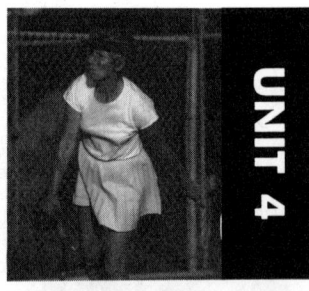

UNIT 4
Exercise and Weight Control

Seven articles examine the influences of exercise and diet on health. Topics discussed include the value of working out, choosing the right exercise, and body weight.

Overview 70

16. **How Fitness Savvy Are You?** *Consumer Reports on Health*, January 1998. 72
Each year millions of American start exercising, only to quit and rejoin the ranks of couch potatoes. Some quit because of injury, some from boredom, and some because they began exercising with misconceptions about what to expect. This article examines **some common myths and misunderstandings regarding exercise.**

17. **How Fit Are You?** *Consumer Reports on Health*, July 1997. 76
Take this test to determine how your aerobic capacity, strength, flexibility, and balance compare to others within your age group. In addition, here are recommendations regarding **exercises you can do** to improve on each of these fitness components.

The concepts in bold italics are developed in the article. For further expansion please refer to the Topic Guide and the Index.

18. **Rebel against a Sedentary Life,** Katherine Griffin, *Health,* April 1997. — **79**
   A recent surgeon general's report on exercise proclaimed that **30 minutes of moderate exercise a day can significantly improve one's health and lengthen one's life.**

19. **The Skinny on Weight Loss,** *Consumer Reports on Health,* February 1998. — **83**
   Every day a new strategy or diet attempts to convince you that there is a simple and easy way to achieve rapid and permanent **weight loss.** This article examines eight **common myths** that can lead to fruitless efforts to lose weight.

20. **The Pressure to Eat,** Kelly Brownell and Bonnie Liebman, *Nutrition Action Healthletter,* July/August 1998. — **86**
   1998 was the first time in our history that **over 50 percent of the population were overweight.** In a nation preoccupied with **avoiding dietary fat,** how could this happen? Kelly Brownell believes that the root cause is **a toxic environment,** defined as easy access to a poor diet that is low in cost, high in calories, good tasting, and heavily promoted.

21. **Does Food Control You?** Winifred Yu, *Walking,* May/June 1998. — **90**
   You're not anorexic or bulimic or a binge eater, but you may have **an obsession regarding your body weight and an unhealthy relationship with food.** This type of **borderline eating disorder** may not be damaging to your physical health, but it is nonetheless limiting the quality of your life.

22. **Binge-Eating That Plagues Adults Now Recognized as a Disorder,** *Environmental Nutrition,* August 1997. — **92**
   "Binge-eating disorder" joins anorexia nervosa and bulimia as serious eating disorders. This essay discusses the scope of the problem, the specific behaviors associated with the condition, and current treatment options.

Overview — 94

23. **The Postmodern Guide to Cold Relief,** Bill Shapiro, *Health,* January/February 1997. — **96**
   By current count, the number of over-the-counter preparations being offered to treat the common cold now number in excess of 2,800. The pros and cons of the major categories of drugs currently available are reviewed here.

24. **Alcohol and Health: Straight Talk on the Medical Headlines,** Charles H. Hennekens, *Health News,* March 31, 1998. — **99**
   Is **alcohol** a life-extending potion or a toxic agent? Dr. Charles Hennekens addresses this question and attempts to sort out the **potential benefits** as well as the **hazards** associated with using alcoholic beverages.

25. **The War over Weed,** Tom Morganthau, *Newsweek,* February 3, 1997. — **101**
   Should **marijuana** be made available for use as a prescription medication to treat selected medical conditions? Tom Morganthau addresses this issue, which has been thrust into the limelight as a result of initiatives passed by legislatures in both California and Arizona.

26. **Will You Pay for Your Past as a Smoker?** *Harvard Health Letter,* June 1998. — **104**
   For the most part, Americans have gotten the message that **smoking is very hazardous to one's health.** In **quitting,** people have **significantly reduced their risk** of developing premature cardiovascular disease and cancer. The bad news is that ex-smokers are still more likely than nonsmokers to develop these diseases.

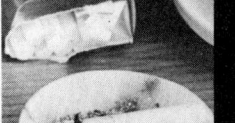

UNIT 5

Drugs and Health

Four articles examine how drugs affect our lives. Subjects discussed include the dangers of tobacco and alcohol, prescription drugs, and of over-the-counter medications.

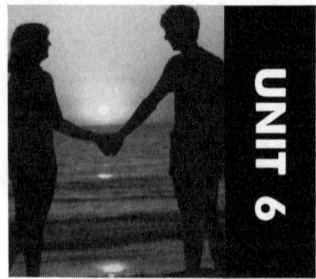

Human Sexuality

Four articles discuss the most recent research on human reproduction and sexuality. The selections consider birth control, STDs, and sexual myths.

Overview 108

27. **Rethinking Birth Control,** Julia Califano, *American Health for Women*, March 1997. 110
    Julia Califano discusses the **contraceptive methods** currently available and evaluates their use according to cost, effectiveness for preventing pregnancy, and drawbacks.

28. **Condoms: Barriers to Bad News,** Tamar Nordenberg, *FDA Consumer*, March/April 1998. 114
    It is generally acknowledged that, besides abstinence, the **male condom** and, to a lesser degree, the female condom are the primary **weapons** we have in the battle **against STDs.** Tamar Nordenberg explains under what circumstances condoms are most likely to fail and what we can do to achieve maximum protection from their use.

29. **America: Awash in STDs,** Gracie S. Hsu, *The World & I*, June 1998. 117
    Americans contract **STDs** at the rate of 12 million new cases each year, and two-thirds of these cases are among **individuals under age 25.** Gracie Hsu discusses the **long-term dangers** of STDs and the difficulties **in combating the spread** of STDs among America's youth.

30. **Your Sexual Landscape,** Beth Howard, *American Health for Women*, April 1997. 122
    How well do you know the **importance of vaginal health**? This area of the female body has been the most neglected in terms of research and medical training, yet this area is as delicately balanced as a "tropical rain forest." Without an understanding of its fragile ecological balance, it is quite easy to disturb that balance and invite infections.

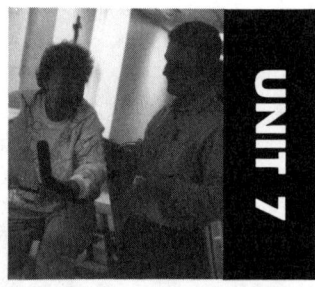

Current Killers

Six selections examine the major causes of death in the Western world. Heart attack, cancer, and AIDS are discussed.

Overview 126

31. **Family History: What You Don't Know Can Kill You,** *Consumer Reports on Health*, September 1996. 128
    Among the risk factors for diseases, one that you cannot change but should be aware of is your **family medical history.** This article describes how some **hereditary conditions** virtually ensure that disease will occur, while others are only **susceptibility** factors.

32. **The Heart Attackers,** Geoffrey Cowley, *Newsweek*, August 11, 1997. 131
    Twenty-five percent of all heart attacks occur in individuals with no known risk factors. Geoffrey Cowley examines some **new risk factors** that are being put to the test.

33. **Heart Disease in Women: Special Symptoms, Special Risks,** *Consumer Reports on Health*, May 1997. 135
    While the total number of deaths due to coronary heart disease (CHD) has dropped by over 50 percent since 1960, the decline for women has been much less dramatic than for men. This essay points out that **differences in diagnostic and preventative approaches** for women have not been explored sufficiently.

34. **Beyond Cholesterol,** Judith Mandelbaum-Schmid, *Health*, July/August 1998. 138
    Americans are urged to reduce their intake of **dietary fat** in an effort to lower serum cholesterol levels. However, new scientific evidence suggests that it is not just one's total cholesterol count that is important but the relative amounts of **various lipid fractions** that may **spell the difference** between a healthy heart and premature coronary artery disease.

The concepts in bold italics are developed in the article. For further expansion please refer to the Topic Guide and the Index.

35. **Strategies for Minimizing Cancer Risk,** Walter C. 142
Willett, Graham A. Colditz, and Nancy E. Mueller, *Scientific American*, September 1996.
In 1996 alone, more than 550,000 Americans died of **cancer.** Approximately 50 percent of these deaths might have been avoided through **primary prevention** and **early detection.**

36. **AIDS, after the 'Cure': Amid Setbacks, Search for** 148
New Hope, Laurie Garrett, *Newsday*, June 14, 1998.
In 1996 **AIDS** researchers revolutionized the treatment of individuals infected with the **HIV virus** by using a new class of drugs known as **protease inhibitors.** Initially these drugs demonstrated considerable promise. However, recent developments suggest that this drug regime may be **too toxic** for many to take and **too weak** to eliminate the virus. Where do we go from here?

Overview 152

37. **Health Unlimited,** Willard Gaylin, *The Wilson Quarterly*, 154
Summer 1996.
No one can dispute the fact that health care costs have risen dramatically over the last 20 years. The most significant factor, according to Willard Gaylin, is that **modern medicine** has expanded its boundaries to include conditions that previously were considered an inevitable **part of the human condition.**

38. **Your Hospital Stay: A Guide to Survival,** *Consumer* 158
Reports on Health, August 1995.
Although America has some of the best health care in the world, recent studies suggest that over 1 million Americans each year are injured due to **preventable mistakes** or the **hazards of hospitalization.** This article explores what you as a patient can do.

39. **Choose Treatments You Believe In,** Peter Jaret, 162
Health, April 1997.
Each year millions of Americans seek out **alternative medical therapies** as a way to cope with their health problems, and most of these patients are pleased with the results. Many in the scientific community believe that what we are witnessing is the power of **the placebo effect** at work.

40. **Alternative Medicine—The Risks of Untested and** 167
Unregulated Remedies, Marcia Angell and Jerome P. Kassirer, *The New England Journal of Medicine*, September 17, 1998.
This editorial takes a critical look at **the standards by which alternative medicine is judged.** The authors—both of whom are physicians—suggest that it is time for the proponents of alternative medicine to be held to the same standards as conventional medicine when it comes to making medical claims.

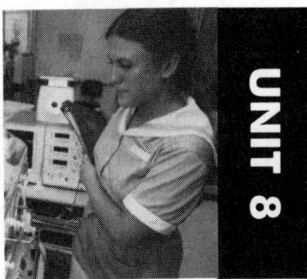

UNIT 8

America's Health and the Health Care System

Four selections discuss the current state of health care in today's society by focusing on self-care, health care costs, and the health care industry.

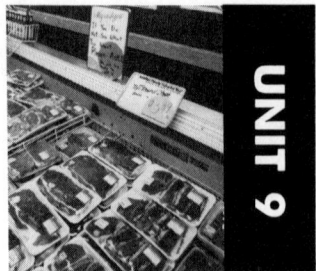

UNIT 9
Consumer Health

Six selections examine how food labeling and food and drug interactions relate to consumer health.

Overview   **170**

41. **How Health Savvy Are You?** *Consumer Reports on Health,* January 1995.   **172**
    Do you pride yourself on staying abreast of health issues? This **quiz** tests your knowledge **of contemporary health issues.**

42. **Nutrition in the News: What the Headlines Don't Tell You,** *Environmental Nutrition,* September 1995.   **177**
    What is a **consumer** to believe? This article discusses why there is so much **conflicting information** in the media, and it provides guidelines to help consumers make sense of it all.

43. **The Switch to OTC: No Prescription, No Protection?** *Consumer Reports on Health,* October 1996.   **179**
    Recently pharmaceutical companies have been successful in getting the FDA to reclassify several prescription medications for sale over the counter. This move has distinct **advantages for manufacturers.** The question is, Does it also **benefit consumers**?

44. **The Doctor Is On,** Katie Hafner, *Newsweek,* May 27, 1996.   **182**
    Last year alone, millions of Americans logged onto the **Internet** in search of information about **medical concerns and health issues.** How good is the information they are getting?

45. **Nature's Pharmacy,** Burkhard Bilger, *Health,* October 1997.   **184**
    Each year consumers spend billions of dollars on supplements in search of better health. Burkhard Bilger looks at the **safety and usefulness** of 10 of the most popular herbs and extracts.

46. **An FDA Guide to Dietary Supplements,** Paula Kurtzweil, *FDA Consumer,* September/October 1998.   **190**
    The "Dietary Supplement Health and Education Act of 1994" gave dietary supplement manufacturers more freedom to market their products and to provide information about their products' benefits. In the wake of all the marketing hype, this article presents the **FDA's recommendations** regarding labeling and the **safe and responsible use of dietary supplements.**

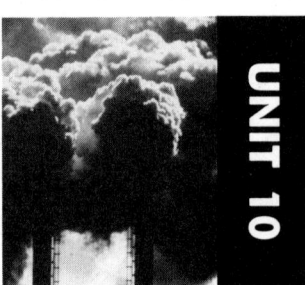

UNIT 10
Contemporary Health Hazards

Six articles examine hazards that affect our health and are encountered in today's world.

Overview   **198**

47. **Quiz: Are You Ready for the Sun?** Cynthia Moekle Pigott, *American Health,* May 1995.   **200**
    Scientific studies linking skin cancer to sunburn have prompted millions of Americans to lather themselves up with **sunscreen lotions.** But do sunscreens really work? This selection tests the reader's knowledge concerning **UV radiation** and provides answers based on the most current information available.

48. **Germ Crazy,** Deborah Franklin, *Health,* May/June 1998.   **202**
    Based on the number of antibacterial products on the market today, some scientists are becoming increasingly concerned that **excessive use of antibacterial products could produce resistant microbes.**

The concepts in bold italics are developed in the article. For further expansion please refer to the Topic Guide and the Index.

49. **The Frog Solution,** Josie Glausiusz, *Discover,* Novmeber 1998. **207**

Scientists are constantly looking for new ways to ***inhibit emerging infectious diseases. Peptide antibiotics,*** the newest antibacterial troops, are found in frogs' skin, honeybees, snakes, pigs' and cows' blood cells, and even in fish, birds, and plants.

50. **Prevent Sexually Transmitted Diseases,** Lauren Picker, *American Health,* October 1995. **211**

While the term ***safe sex*** has primarily been used in discussions concerning ***AIDS,*** it is equally relevant for six other ***sexually transmitted diseases (STDs)*** spreading at a rate of 12 million new cases each year in the United States. Lauren Picker discusses the most common STDs and provides information on their incidence, symptoms, and medical complications.

51. **Irradiation: A Safe Measure for Safer Food,** John Henkel, *FDA Consumer,* May/June 1998. **216**

The FDA has added ***red meat irradiation*** to its long list of foods approved for the process. But not many of these foods can be found on supermarket shelves. Store owners and food producers alike are afraid that consumers will not buy the products, based on misgivings about radiation.

52. **Why Is Date Rape So Hard to Prove?** Sheila Weller, *Health,* July/August 1992. **222**

The National Victim Center estimates that one in every eight women in the United States has been raped, in most cases by someone she knew. Only about 16 percent are reported, and the majority of the ***cases are dropped*** by the prosecution prior to a trial. Sheila Weller examines the issue of ***acquaintance rape*** and discusses why it is so hard to make the charge of rape stick.

Index	**225**
Article Review Form	**228**
Article Rating Form	**229**

The concepts in bold italics are developed in the article. For further expansion please refer to the Topic Guide and the Index.

Topic Guide

This topic guide suggests how the selections and World Wide Web sites found in the next section of this book relate to topics of traditional concern to students and professionals involved with the study of health. It is useful for locating interrelated articles and Web sites for reading and research. The guide is arranged alphabetically according to topic.

The relevant Web sites, which are numbered and annotated on pages 4 and 5, are easily identified by the Web icon (◉) under the topic articles. By linking the articles and the Web sites by topic, this ANNUAL EDITIONS reader becomes a powerful learning and research tool.

TOPIC AREA	TREATED IN	TOPIC AREA	TREATED IN
Alcohol	24. Alcohol and Health 33. Heart Disease in Women 35. Strategies for Minimizing Cancer Risk ◉ *1, 4, 6, 18, 19, 20, 33*		13. Are You Getting Enough Fat? 14. Bulking Up Fiber's Healthful Reputation 32. Heart Attackers 34. Beyond Cholesterol 41. How Health Savvy Are You? ◉ *4, 11, 12, 13, 14*
Alternative Medicine	39. Choose Treatments You Believe In 40. Alternative Medicine 45. Nature's Pharmacy ◉ *30*	Drugs/Drug Addiction	23. Postmodern Guide to Cold Relief 24. Alcohol and Health 25. War over Weed 26. Will You Pay for Your Past as a Smoker? 43. Switch to OTC 45. Nature's Pharmacy ◉ *4, 18, 19, 20*
Cancer	2. Why Do Those #&*?@! "Experts" Keep Changing Their Minds? 5. Challenging America's Inverted Health Priorities 6. Critical Life Events 13. Are You Getting Enough Fat? 14. Bulking Up Fiber's Healthful Reputation 15. Vitamin Revolution 17. How Fit Are You? 24. Alcohol and Health 25. War over Weed 26. Will You Pay for Your Past as a Smoker? 31. Family History 35. Strategies for Minimizing Cancer Risk 41. How Health Savvy Are You? 45. Nature's Pharmacy 47. Quiz: Are You Ready for the Sun? 50. Prevent Sexually Transmitted Diseases ◉ *1, 2, 3, 5, 25, 29, 33*	Environmental/ Health Hazards	5. Challenging America's Inverted Health Priorities 35. Strategies for Minimizing Cancer Risk 47. Quiz: Are You Ready for the Sun? 48. Germ Crazy 49. Frog Solution 50. Prevent Sexually Transmitted Diseases 51. Irradiation ◉ *3, 33*
		Exercise and Fitness	1. How Does Your Life Measure Up? 13. Are You Getting Enough Fat? 16. How Fitness Savvy Are You? 17. How Fit Are You? 18. Rebel against a Sedentary Life 19. Skinny on Weight Loss 33. Heart Disease in Women 34. Beyond Cholesterol 35. Strategies for Minimizing Cancer Risk 41. How Health Savvy Are You? ◉ *4, 15, 16, 17, 31*
Cardiovascular Disease	1. How Does Your Life Measure Up? 6. Critical Life Events 7. Talking Cure for Stress 8. Using Your Mind to Heal 9. Forgiveness 11. Tall Tales from the Table 14. Bulking Up Fiber's Healthful Reputation 15. Vitamin Revolution 16. How Fitness Savvy Are You? 17. How Fit Are You? 18. Rebel against a Sedentary Life 19. Skinny on Weight Loss 24. Alcohol and Health 26. Will You Pay for Your Past as a Smoker? 31. Family History 32. Heart Attackers 33. Heart Disease in Women 34. Beyond Cholesterol 41. How Health Savvy Are You? 45. Nature's Pharmacy ◉ *1, 2, 3, 5, 15, 16, 17, 26, 28, 29, 33*	Genetics	12. Bitter Truth 19. Skinny on Weight Loss 20. Pressure to Eat 31. Family History 34. Beyond Cholesterol 35. Strategies for Minimizing Cancer Risk ◉ *1, 2, 15*
		Health Behavior and Decision Making	1. How Does Your Life Measure Up? 2. Why Do Those #&*?@! "Experts" Keep Changing Their Minds? 3. Yet Another Study—Should You Pay Attention? 4. "Just Do It" Isn't Enough 5. Challenging America's Inverted Health Priorities 29. America Awash in STDs 30. Your Sexual Landscape 31. Family History
Dietary Fat, Fiber	1. How Does Your Life Measure Up? 11. Tall Tales from the Table		

TOPIC AREA	TREATED IN	TOPIC AREA	TREATED IN
Health Behavior and Decision Making (Continued)	35. Strategies for Minimizing Cancer Risk 39. Choose Treatments You Believe In 40. Alternative Medicine 42. Nutrition in the News 44. Doctor Is On 45. Nature's Pharmacy 46. FDA Guide to Dietary Supplements 47. Quiz: Are You Ready for the Sun? ○ **4, 5, 6, 7, 8, 9, 10, 11, 12, 14, 15, 16, 17, 21, 22, 24, 30, 31, 32**		32. Heart Attackers 34. Beyond Cholesterol 35. Strategies for Minimizing Cancer Risk 41. How Health Savvy Are You? 42. Nutrition in the News ○ **11, 12, 13, 14, 30, 31**
		Personality and Disease	6. Critical Life Events 7. Talking Cure for Stress ○ **7, 8, 9, 10**
Health Care Issues	37. Health Unlimited 38. Your Hospital Stay 39. Choose Treatments You Believe In 40. Alternative Medicine ○ **4, 16, 28, 29, 30, 31, 33**	**Sexual Behavior**	28. Condoms: Barriers to Bad News 29. America Awash in STDs 30. Your Sexual Landscape 35. Strategies for Minimizing Cancer Risk 50. Prevent Sexually Transmitted Diseases 52. Why Is Date Rape So Hard to Prove? ○ **21, 22, 23, 24**
Immunity	6. Critical Life Events 36. AIDS, after the "Cure" 45. Nature's Pharmacy 48. Germ Crazy 49. Frog Solution ○ **1, 2, 4, 28, 29, 31**	**Sexually Transmitted Diseases (STDs)/HIV/AIDS**	6. Critical Life Events 27. Rethinking Birth Control 28. Condoms: Barriers to Bad News 29. America Awash in STDs 36. AIDS, after the "Cure" 50. Prevent Sexually Transmitted Diseases ○ **21, 22, 23, 24, 27, 34**
Infectious Illness	23. Postmodern Guide to Cold Relief 28. Condoms: Barriers to Bad News 29. America Awash in STDs 32. Heart Attackers 38. Your Hospital Stay 45. Nature's Pharmacy 48. Germ Crazy 49. Frog Solution 50. Prevent Sexually Transmitted Diseases 51. Irradiation ○ **4, 21, 24, 26, 28, 29, 31, 33**	**Stress**	1. How Does Your Life Measure Up? 6. Critical Life Events 7. Talking Cure for Stress 8. Using Your Mind to Heal 9. Forgiveness 33. Heart Disease in Women ○ **7, 8, 9, 10, 24, 26**
Medical Concerns and Ethics	25. War over Weed 36. AIDS, after the "Cure" 37. Health Unlimited 38. Your Hospital Stay 39. Choose Treatments You Believe In 40. Alternative Medicine 43. Switch to OTC 44. Doctor Is On 45. Nature's Pharmacy 48. Germ Crazy ○ **1, 3, 5, 17, 28, 29, 33**	**Tobacco and Health**	1. How Does Your Life Measure Up? 2. Why Do Those #&*?@! "Experts" Keep Changing Their Minds? 5. Challenging America's Inverted Health Priorities 26. Will You Pay for Your Past as a Smoker? 33. Heart Disease in Women
Mental Health and Depression	6. Critical Life Events 7. Talking Cure for Stress 8. Using Your Mind to Heal 9. Forgiveness 10. Bad Mood Rising 21. Does Food Control You? 45. Nature's Pharmacy ○ **7, 8, 9, 10, 32**	**Vitamins**	15. Vitamin Revolution 32. Heart Attackers 35. Strategies for Minimizing Cancer Risk ○ **11, 12, 13, 14, 17, 31**
Nutrition/ Vitamins	11. Tall Tales from the Table 12. Bitter Truth 13. Are You Getting Enough Fat? 14. Bulking Up Fiber's Healthful Reputation 15. Vitamin Revolution 19. Skinny on Weight Loss	**Weight Control/ Obesity/Other Eating Disorders**	11. Tall Tales from the Table 13. Are You Getting Enough Fat? 14. Bulking Up Fiber's Healthful Reputation 18. Rebel against a Sedentary Life 19. Skinny on Weight Loss 20. Pressure to Eat 21. Does Food Control You? 22. Binge-Eating 33. Heart Disease in Women ○ **15, 16, 17, 24, 26**

Annual Editions: Health

The following World Wide Web sites have been carefully researched and selected to support the articles found in this reader. If you are interested in learning more about specific topics found in this book, these Web sites are a good place to start. The sites are cross-referenced by number and appear in the topic guide on the previous two pages. Also, you can link to these Web sites through our DUSHKIN ONLINE support site at *http://www.dushkin.com/online/*.

The following sites were available at the time of publication. Visit our Web site—we update DUSHKIN ONLINE regularly to reflect any changes.

General Sources

1. U.S. National Institutes of Health (NIH)
http://www.nih.gov
Consult this site for links to extensive health information and scientific resources. Comprised of 24 separate institutes, centers, and divisions, the NIH is one of eight health agencies of the Public Health Service, which, in turn, is part of the U.S. Department of Health and Human Services.

2. U.S. National Library of Medicine
http://www.nlm.nih.gov
This huge site permits a search of a number of databases and electronic information sources such as MEDLINE. You can learn about research projects and programs and peruse the national network of medical libraries here.

3. World Health Organization
http://www.who.ch/Welcome.html
This home page of the World Health Organization will provide links to a wealth of statistical and analytical information about health around the world.

Health Behavior and Decision Making

4. Columbia University's Go Ask Alice!
http://www.goaskalice.columbia.edu/index.html
This interactive site provides discussion and insight into a number of personal issues of interest to college-age people and those younger and older. Many questions about physical and emotional health and well-being are answered.

5. National Institute on Aging (NIA)
http://www.nih.gov/nia/
The NIA, one of the institutes of the U.S. National Institutes of Health, presents this home page to lead you to a variety of resources on health and lifestyle issues on aging.

6. The Society of Behavioral Medicine
http://www.sbmweb.org
This site provides listings of major general health institutes and organizations as well as discipline-specific links and resources in medicine, psychology, and public health.

Stress and Mental Health

7. The Anxiety-Panic Internet Resource
http://www.algy.com/anxiety/panic.html
Information on the symptoms and causes of various anxiety and panic disorders is provided on this site. Links to many related articles are available, and psychopharmacology and other issues are addressed.

8. Dr. Ivan's Depression Central
http://www.psycom.net/depression.central.html
This extensive site describes itself as the "Internet's central clearinghouse for information on all types of depressive disorders and on the most effective treatments," and it lives up to the billing. Students of mental health will turn to this site and its links again and again.

9. National Mental Health Association (NMHA)
http://www.nmha.org/index.html
The NMHA is a citizen volunteer advocacy organization that works to improve the mental health of all individuals. The site provides access to guidelines that individuals can use to reduce stress and improve their lives in small yet tangible ways.

10. University of Sheffield Medical School/Center for Psychotherapeutic Studies
http://www.shef.ac.uk/~psysc/psychotherapy/
Access to *The Online Dictionary of Mental Health* may be gained here. "A global information resource and research tool" covering all of the disciplines contributing to an understanding of mental health is described. The site also provides information about psychotherapy.

Nutritional Health

11. University of Pennsylvania Library
http://www.library.upenn.edu/resources/websitest.html
This vast site is rich in links to information about virtually every subject in health studies. Its extensive population and demography resources address such concerns as family planning and nutrition in various world regions.

12. University of Pennsylvania School of Medicine Nutrition Education and Prevention Program
http://www.med.upenn.edu/~nutrimed/
The aim of the Nutrition Education and Prevention Program is to engage medical students in active learning about nutrition and medicine through interdisciplinary study. This home page provides links to many related Web sites.

13. U.S. Department of Agriculture (USDAI)/Food and Nutrition Information Center (FNIC)
http://www.nal.usda.gov/fnic/
Use this site to find nutrition information provided by various USDA agencies, to find links to food and nutrition resources on the Internet, and to access FNIC publications and databases.

14. Vegetarian Pages
http://www.veg.org/veg/
The Vegetarian Pages are intended to be an independent, definitive Internet guide for vegetarians, vegans, and others.

Exercise and Weight Control

15. American Society of Exercise Physiologists (ASEP)
http://www.css.edu/users/tboone2/asep/toc.htm
The ASEP is devoted to promoting people's health and physical fitness. This extensive site provides links to publications related to exercise and career opportunities in exercise physiology.

16. Health Links
http://www.hslib.washington.edu
Open this site to find links to international health statistics, journals, public health topics, library services, and so on.

17. U.S. Department of Health and Human Services
http://www.os.dhhs.gov
This site has extensive links to information on such topics as the health benefits of exercise, weight control, and prudent lifestyle choices.

Drugs and Health

18. National Institute on Drug Abuse (NIDA)
http://165.112.78.61/
Use this site index for access to NIDA publications and communications, information on drugs of abuse, and links to other related Web sites.

19. University of California at San Francisco/Drug Dependence Research Center (DDRC)
http://itsa.ucsf.edu/~ddrc/about.html
The DDRC studies the pharmacology, physiology, and psychology of drugs in humans. This site provides information on the DDRC's profile of medical marijuana users, its research into the cardiac effects of cocaine, and other topics.

20. University of Chicago
http://uhs.bsd.uchicago.edu/~bhsiung/tips/tips.html
Gain access to a wide variety of information related to psychopharmacology on this site, with its links to specific drug sites and to specific disorders.

Human Sexuality

21. Men's Health
http://www.menshealth.com/new/guide/index.html
This resource guide from Men's Health presents many links, from AIDS/STDs, to back pain, to impotence and infertility, to vasectomy, plus discussions of family issues.

22. Planned Parenthood
http://www.plannedparenthood.org
This home page provides links to information on contraceptives (including outercourse and abstinence) and to discussions of other topics related to sexual health.

23. Sex and Gender
http://www.bioanth.cam.ac.uk/pip4amod3.html
Use the syllabus, lecture titles, and readings noted in this site as a jumping-off point to explore more about sexual differentiation in human cultures as well as the genetics of sexual differentiation and the biology of sex roles in nonhumans.

24. University of Maryland/Women's Studies
http://www.inform.umd.edu/EdRes/Topic/WomensStudies/
This site provides a wealth of resources related to women's physical and emotional well-being: topics such as body image, comfort with sexuality, and relationships.

Current Killers

25. American Cancer Society
http://www.cancer.org/frames.html
Open this site and its various links to learn the concerns and lifestyle advice of the American Cancer Society. It provides information on tobacco and alternative therapies.

26. American Heart Association (AMA)
http://www.amhrt.org
The AMA offers this site to provide the most comprehensive information on heart disease and stroke. The site presents facts on the warning signs of heart disease and stroke, a reference guide, and explanations of diseases and treatments.

27. Body Health Resources Corporation
http://www.thebody.com/cgi-bin/body.cgi
From this site it is possible to access "The Body: A Multimedia AIDS and HIV Information Resource" to learn about treatments, to exchange information in forums, to gain insight from experts, and to help and get help.

America's Health and the Health Care System

28. Agency for Health Care Policy and Research
http://www.ahcpr.gov
The aim of the AHCPR is to improve health care quality through education and research. Open this site to find information on consumer health, U.S. health care policy and trends, clinical research, and managed care.

29. American Medical Association (AMA)
http://www.ama-assn.org
The venerable AMA offers this site for consumers and health practitioners to find up-to-date medical information, peer-reviews resources, discussions of such topics as HIV/AIDS and women's health, examination of issues related to managed care, and important publications.

Consumer Health

30. Alt-MEDMarket
http://alt.medmarket.com/indexes/indexmfr.html
This commercial site bills itself as "the Internet guide to alternative therapies and products." Click on the "Alternative Health E-Mall" for an alternative medicine directory and herbal information center; alternative medicine providers, listed by geographic area and specialty; a listing of articles; and herbs with their corresponding treatments.

31. HealthyWay/Sympatico
http://www1.sympatico.ca/healthyway/
This Canadian site meant for consumers will lead you to many links related to general and reproductive health.

32. Mental Health Net
http://www.cmhc.com/selfhelp.htm
This site and its many links are geared to providing information on mental disorders, with an emphasis on self-help. Aging, dementia and Alzheimer's disease, and topics from cancer to depression are described.

Contemporary Health Hazards

33. Centers for Disease Control and Prevention
http://www.cdc.gov
The CDC offers this page from which you can learn about travelers' health, data and statistics related to disease control and prevention, and general health information.

34. Sexual Assault Information Page
http://www.cs.utk.edu/~bartley/saInfoPage.html
This invaluable site provides links to information and resources on a variety of topics, from child sexual abuse, to date rape, to incest, to secondary victims, to offenders.

We highly recommend that you review our Web site for expanded information and our other product lines. We are continually updating and adding links to our Web site in order to offer you the most usable and useful information that will support and expand the value of your Annual Editions. You can reach us at:
http://www.dushkin.com/annualeditions/.

www.dushkin.com/online/

Unit 1

Unit Selections

1. **How Does Your Life Measure Up?** Alice Lesch Kelly
2. **Why Do Those #&*?@! "Experts" Keep Changing Their Minds?** University of California at Berkeley Wellness Letter
3. **Yet Another Study—Should You Pay Attention?** Tufts University Health & Nutrition Letter
4. **"Just Do It" Isn't Enough: Change Comes in Stages,** Tufts University Diet & Nutrition Letter
5. **Challenging America's Inverted Health Priorities,** Elizabeth M. Whelan

Key Points to Consider

❖ Why do you think that people continue to engage in negative health behaviors when they know that these behaviors will have a negative impact on their health?

❖ What is the difference between clinical or interventional trials, epidemiologic studies, and population-based intervention trials? What are the limitations of each in terms of type of information they yield?

❖ What is the difference between absolute and relative risk as it applies to the likelihood one has of developing a particular health problem? How are these statistics derived?

❖ Explain how the improper use of statistical methods can yield misleading results to an otherwise good research design.

❖ Discuss the six stages of change and the role each serves in bringing about a permanent behavioral change.

❖ Explain the statement: America is a nation fraught with inverted health priorities.

❖ What personal health behaviors would you like to change? What prevents you from making these changes?

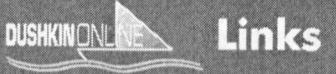 **Links**   www.dushkin.com/online/

4. **Columbia University's Go Ask Alice!**
   http://www.goaskalice.columbia.edu/index.html
5. **National Institute on Aging (NIA)**
   http://www.nih.gov/nia/
6. **The Society of Behavioral Medicine**
   http://www.sbmweb.org

These sites are annotated on pages 4 and 5.

Health Behavior and Decision Making

"That those of us who protect our health daily and those of us who put our health in constant jeopardy have exactly the same mortality: 100 percent. The difference, of course, is the timing." This quote from Elizabeth M. Whelan, Sc.D., M.P.H., reminds us that we must all face the fact that we are going to die sometime. The question that is decided by our behavior is when, and, to a certain extent, how. This book and especially this unit are designed to assist students in the development of cognitive skills and knowledge that when put to use help make the moment of our death come as late as possible in our lives. While we cannot control many of the things that happen to us in our lives, we must all strive to accept personal responsibility for, and make informed decisions about, things that we can control. This is no minor task, but it is one in which the potential reward is life itself.

Perhaps the best way to start this process is by educating ourselves on the relative risks associated with the various behaviors and lifestyle choices we make. To minimize all risk to life and health would be to significantly limit the quality of our lives, and while this might be a choice that some would make, it certainly is not the goal of health education. A more logical approach to risk reduction would be to educate the public on the relative risk associated with various behaviors and lifestyle choices so that they are capable of making informed decisions. While it may seem obvious that certain behaviors, such as smoking, entail a high level of risk, the significance of others such as toxic waste sites and food additives are frequently blown out of proportion to the actual risks involved. The net result of this type of distortion is that many Americans tend to minimize the dangers of known hazards such as tobacco and alcohol and, instead, focus attention on potentially minor health hazards over which they have little or no control. This issue is discussed in detail in the essay "Challenging America's Inverted Health Priorities." "How Does Your Life Measure Up?" by Alice Kelly provides you, the reader, with an opportunity to examine your lifestyle and see just how well you are doing at taking control of those factors that have been found to significantly influence your health and longevity.

Educating the public on relative risk of various health behaviors is only part of the job that health education must tackle in order to assist individuals in making informed choices regarding their health. If the past is any indication of the future, then we must assume that new discoveries in the arena of health will be made, and some of the information that we teach today will become obsolete. The only way to guard against obsolescence is to teach the skills that will enable people to evaluate the validity and significance of new information as it becomes available. Just how important informed decision making is in our daily lives is evidenced by the numerous health-related media announcements and articles that fill our newspapers, magazines, and television broadcasts. Rather than inform and enlighten the public on significant new medical discoveries, many of these announcements do little more than add to the level of confusion. Why is this so? While there is no simple explanation, there appear to be at least two major factors that contribute to the confusion. The first has to do with the primary goals and objectives of the media itself. One only has to scan the headlines on the cover pages of magazines or newspapers to realize that the primary goal of these publications is to entice the potential reader into purchasing their product. How better to capture the readers' attention than to sensationalize and exaggerate scientific discoveries. This is not to blame the media but rather to remind the reader that given the economic realities of the competitive world in which we live, sometimes accuracy and validity take second place to the marketing needs of a publisher.

A second major factor that contributes to confusion and distortions is ignorance on behalf of the American public regarding the criteria on which to judge the quality of scientific information. In the absence of established criteria on which to judge information, how can one be expected to assess its accuracy and validity? If health education's goal is to create informed consumers, then surely it must educate the public regarding the criteria on which to judge the quality of scientific investigations. The articles "Why Do Those #&*?@! 'Experts' Keep Changing Their Minds?" and "Yet Another Study—Should You Pay Attention?" were selected for this unit because they do an excellent job of discussing both the strengths and weaknesses of the scientific methods being used to study health problems.

Let's assume for a minute that the scientific community is in general agreement that certain behaviors clearly promote health while others damage our health. Given this information, are you likely to make adjustments to your lifestyle to comply with the findings? Logic would suggest that of course you would, but experience has taught us that information alone isn't enough to bring about behavioral change in many people. Why is it so difficult to get people to change? Perhaps some individuals do not feel that they are at risk, or perhaps they feel that it is too late in their lives for the changes to have any significant impact on their health. How then is a health educator to assist these individuals in changing their behaviors? "'Just Do It' Isn't Enough: Change Comes in Stages" is an interview with James Prochaska, one of the leading authorities on health promotion and behavioral change. He discusses the stages of change that most people go through when they are successful in making a lasting change in their health behavior. He also suggests strategies that will help with each stage of the process.

While the goal of health education is to promote healthy behaviors that lead to healthy lifestyles, this objective will not be reached unless, or until, the public is armed with the knowledge and skills necessary to make informed decisions regarding their health. Even then, there is no guarantee that the information gleaned will serve to motivate the public into making healthy choices regarding their lifestyle. In a free society such as ours, the choice is, and must remain, up to the individual.

Article 1

Live better, live longer

How Does Your Life Measure Up?

What's more important: How long you live or how well? Here's an eye-opening quiz to help you take stock and an argument for keeping it all in balance.

talk about lucky. When it comes to lifespan, we 1998-ers are luckier than just about any other generation in history. Not only can most of us expect to live a long time, but we have the scientific knowledge to make lifestyle decisions that may stretch our lives even more. ❧ We're lucky when it comes to quality of life, too: Most of us are self-aware enough (or have had enough therapy) to have a pretty good handle on how to make life happy as well as long. ❧ Despite all this, it's good to re-examine our behaviors—and our motives—every now and then. That's where this "Live Better, Live Longer" package comes in. You know what you should be doing to live well and healthfully, but an occasional reminder can't hurt. Take the quiz on the following pages to find out how long, in theory, you can expect to live, and to pinpoint habits that might need changing. Then read our essay, which offers some food for thought on how to make the time you have matter even more. Of course, there are no guarantees that you'll live a long life—or a happy one. But you can stack the odds in your favor. ❧ Now that's lucky.

By Alice Lesch Kelly

1. How Does Your Life Measure Up?

It's an existential irony, a cosmic coincidence: On the day that the "Live Better, Live Longer" Quiz tells me that my squeaky-clean health habits should pave the way for me to live nearly a century, a frightening story in Rolling Stone tells me the world is overdue for a "killer flu" lethal enough to take down even the healthiest of victims in just days and kill millions within months. So let me get this straight: I may live to celebrate a bicentennial of the Civil War, or I could be dead before the next episode of Friends. What do I do with this wildly incongruous information? Optimistically gulp my favorite antioxidant-rich fruit juice and read the Rolling Stone story about Jakob Dylan instead of the one on the flu? (Hey, I should get a point on that life-expectancy quiz just for knowing, at 35, who Jakob Dylan is.) Or do I read the article and give up—start eating, drinking, and making merry now instead of trying to live long enough to lavish my sons' inheritance on a nursing home with a view of the Pacific?

I can't do the hell-in-a-handbasket route—I tried hedonism in college, and I wasn't very good at it; I hated never being able to find my car keys. Instead, I'm sticking with healthful living. But I'll admit that notions like a flu epidemic make me stop and take stock of why I live this way. And the answers surprise even me.

It was something else that pushed me to re-embrace a lifestyle whose cornerstones are getting up early and eschewing pepperoni pizza. I can pinpoint the moment: It coincided with parenthood. Once an avid consumer of the most lurid tabloid tales, I now cannot stomach any newspaper story in which offspring of any age are in danger—a qualifier so wide that it takes me only minutes to get through a newspaper, which is fortunate because my reading time is limited to fleeting moments in the bathroom when I'm not having to explain privacy to a doorknob-dexterous 2-year-old. But when Rolling Stone arrived with the cover line "Killer Flu: The Next Epidemic?" I couldn't resist. Maybe, I thought, Rolling Stone will make it palatable with upbeat quotes from the Spice Girls or hand-washing tips from Barbra Streisand.

It's not just about living a long life: Done right, living healthfully can be a reward in itself.

No such luck. If a killer flu bug comes, there won't be much that we technology-loving humans can do about it. The flu could be so lethal that it may necessitate, according to Rolling Stone, turning the Motel 6 chain into a national network of emergency hospital wards. (I'm sorry, I know this is a serious topic, but does it have to be Motel 6? Can't I die in a Hyatt Regency with a well-stocked honor bar?) Sure, there may be vaccines, but they'll probably be reserved for the president, Pentagon brass, and Michael Jackson. The rest of us are on our own.

And, of course, it's not just a flue that could cheat me out of the next 60 years that the lifespan quiz promises. Dangers lurk everywhere: Drunk drivers, throat-blocking chicken bones, precariously placed penthouse planters.

An active life may not guarantee quantity, but it's highly likely to delivery quality.

So why take such good care of myself? Why eat those five fruits and vegetables every day, why do that 3-mile loop again, why pass up crème brûlée when those sacrifices offer no protection from an unstoppable flu bug or a runaway train?

I figured out the answer as I pondered the flu story. No, smart health choices won't guarantee that I'll live longer than a cheeseburger-eating Marlboro addict. But here's something they do promise: more strength, more energy, and more desire to live fully. If a healthful life were just a prison sentence to serve for 75 years in order to postpone death for a year or two at the very end, I'd opt for the crème brûlée. Rather, I've discovered, living healthfully is a reward in itself, a ticket to experiencing the world in a fuller way now, while I'm young, my children are small, my husband and I can still make each other laugh, and I still enjoy cranking up the volume and singing my lungs out when the Talking Heads play on the radio of the minivan. An active life may not guarantee quantity, but it's highly likely to deliver quality.

So I live heathfully, with an occasional dose of hedonism. I don't replace my walks with doughnut runs—but I do occasionally slow down to take my 2-year-old with me to see if we can beat our personal best, the 45-minute half-mile. I eat well, but when my husband and I manage to lure a dateless babysitter on a Saturday night, we spend a few fat grams and a small fortune at a chic restaurant where the chairs don't turn upside down to hold baby seats.

More important, I try to make sure my strength and energy have an impact in the real world. This is some-

1 ❖ HEALTH BEHAVIOR AND DECISION MAKING

How long will you live? *This quiz will clue you in.*

Score yourself on each question; tally the totals for each section and record them on page 12 to find out your life expectancy.

ENTER YOUR SCORES BELOW

I CORONARY HEART DISEASE (CHD) RISK FACTORS

What is your cholesterol level? (total cholesterol over HDL ratio)

under 160/<3	160–200/3–4	200–220/4–5	220–240/5–6	over 240/>6
+2	+1	-1	-2	-4

Blood pressure (systolic over diastolic)

110/60–80	110–130/60–80	130–150/80–90	150–170/90–100	170/>100
+1	0	-1	-2	-4

Smoking

never	quit	smoke cigar or pipe or close family member smokes	1 pack cigarettes daily	2 or more packs daily
+1	0	-1	-3	-5

Heredity

no family history of CHD	1 close relative over 60 with CHD	2 close relatives over 60 with CHD	1 close relative under 60 with CHD	2 or more relatives under 60 with CHD
+2	0	-1	-2	-4

Body weight (or fat)

5 lbs. below desirable weight (M:<10% fat; F:<16%)	5 lbs. below to 4 lbs. above desirable weight (M:10–15% fat; F:16–22%)	5–20 lbs. overweight (M:15–20% fat; F:22–30%)	20–35 lbs. overweight (M:20–25% fat; F:30–35%)	35 lbs. overweight (M:>25% fat; F:>35%)
+2	+1	0	-2	-3

Age & gender

female under 45 years	female over 45 years	male	stocky male	bald, stocky male
0	-1	-1	-2	-4

Stress

phlegmatic, unhurried, generally happy	ambitious, but generally relaxed	sometimes hard-driving, time-competitive	hard-driving, time-conscious, competitive (Type A)	Type A with repressed hostility
+1	0	0	-1	-3

Physical activity

high intensity, over 30 minutes daily	intermittent, 20–30 minutes 3–5 times/week	moderate, 10–20 minutes 3–5 times/week	light, 10–20 minutes, 1–2 times/week	little or none
+2	+2	+1	0	-2

Total I CHD Factors: _____

II HEALTH HABITS ASSOCIATED WITH GOOD HEALTH AND LONGEVITY

Breakfast

daily	sometimes	none	coffee	coffee and doughnut
+1	0	-1	-2	-3

Regular meals

3 or more	2 daily	not regular	fad diets	starve and stuff
+1	0	-1	-2	-3

Sleep

7–8 hrs.	8–9 hrs.	6–7 hrs.	9 hrs.	6 hrs.
+1	0	0	-1	-2

Alcohol

none	women 3/week	men 1–2 daily	2–6 daily	6 daily
+1	+1	+1	-2	-4

Total II Health Habits: _____

REPRINTED BY PERMISSION FROM B.J. SHARKEY, 1997, *FITNESS AND HEALTH*, FOURTH EDITION (CHAMPAIGN, IL: HUMAN KINETICS PUBLISHERS), 61–65.

1. How Does Your Life Measure Up?

III Medical Factors

Medical exam and screening tests (blood pressure, diabetes, glaucoma)

regular tests, see doctor when necessary	periodic medical exam and selected tests	periodic medical exam	sometimes get tests	no tests or medical exams
+1	+1	0	0	-1

Heart

no history of problems, self or family	some history	rheumatic fever as child, no murmur now	rheumatic fever as child, have murmur	have ECG abnormality and/or angina pectoris
+1	0	-1	-2	-3

Lung (including pneumonia and tuberculosis)

no problem	some past problem	mild asthma or bronchitis	emphysema, severe asthma, or bronchitis	severe lung problems
+1	0	-1	-2	-3

Digestive tract

no problem	occasional diarrhea, loss of appetite	frequent diarrhea or stomach upset	ulcers, colitis, gall bladder, or liver problems	severe gastrointestinal disorders
+1	0	-1	-2	-3

Diabetes

no problem or family history	controlled hypoglycemia (low blood sugar)	hypoglycemia and family history	mild diabetes (diet and exercise)	diabetes (insulin)
+1	0	-1	-2	-3

Drugs

seldom take	minimal but regular use of aspirin or other drugs	heavy use of aspirin or other drugs	regular use of amphetamines, barbiturates, or psychogenic drugs	heavy use of amphetamines, barbiturates, or psychogenic drugs
+1	0	-1	-2	-3

Total III Medical Factors: _____

IV Safety Factors

Driving in car

4,000 mi/year, mostly local	4,000–6,000 mi/year, local and some highway	6,000–8,000 mi/year, local and highway	8,000–10,000 mi/year, highway and some local	10,000 mi/year, mostly highway
+1	0	0	-1	-2

Using seat belt

always	most of time (75%)	on highway only	seldom (25%)	never
+1	0	-1	-2	-3

Risk-taking behavior (motorcycling, skydiving, mountain climbing, flying small plane, etc.)

some with careful preparation	never	occasional	often	try anything for thrills
+1	0	-1	-1	-2

Total IV Safety Factors: _____

V Personal Factors

Diet

lowfat, high complex carbohydrates	balanced, moderate fat	balanced, typical fat	fad diets	starve and stuff
+2	+1	0	-1	-2

Longevity

grandparents lived past 90, parents past 80	grandparents lived past 80, parents past 70	grandparents lived past 70, parents past 60	few relatives lived past 60	few relatives lived past 50
+2	+1	0	-1	-3

Education

postgraduate or master craftsman	college graduate or skilled craftsman	some college or trade school	high school graduate	grade school graduate
+1	+1	0	-1	-2

Job satisfaction

enjoy job, see results, room for advancement	enjoy job, see some results, able to advance	job okay, no results, nowhere to go	dislike job	hate job
+1	+1	0	-1	-2

1 ❖ HEALTH BEHAVIOR AND DECISION MAKING

Love and marriage

happily married	married	unmarried	divorced	extramarital relationship
+2	+1	0	-1	-3

Social

have some close friends	have some friends	have no good friends	stuck with people I don't enjoy	have no friends at all
+1	0	-1	-2	-3

Race

white or Asian	black or Hispanic	American Indian		
0	-1	-2		

Total V Personal Factors: _____

VI PSYCHOLOGICAL FACTORS

Outlook

feel good about present and future	satisfied	unsure about present or future	unhappy in present, don't look forward to future	miserable, rather not get out of bed
+1	0	-1	-2	-3

Depression

no family history of depression	some family history; I feel okay	family history; I am mildly depressed	sometimes I feel life isn't worth living	thoughts of suicide
+1	0	-1	-2	-3

Anxiety

seldom anxious	occasionally anxious	often anxious	always anxious	panic attacks
+1	0	-1	-2	-3

Relaxation

relax or meditate daily	relax often	seldom relax	usually tense	always tense
+1	0	-1	-2	-3

Total VI Psychological Factors: _____

VII FOR WOMEN ONLY

Health care

regular breast and Pap exam	occasional breast and Pap exam	never have exam	treated disorder	untreated cancer
+1	0	-1	-2	-4

Birth control pill

never used	quit 5 years ago	still use, under 30 years of age	use pill and smoke	use pill, smoke, over 35
+1	0	0	-2	-3

Total VII For Women Only: _____

SCORE

To find your personal longevity estimate, tally your score and add your total to the base life expectancy that matches your age. Then go back and see how you can add years to your life by improving behaviors and lifestyle.

		Life Expectancy	
I CHD risk factors total	_____	Nearest age	Base life expectancy
II Health habits total	_____	30	74
		35	74
III Medical factors total	_____	40	75
IV Safety factors total	_____	45	76
V Personal factors total	_____	50	76
		55	77
VI Psychological factors total	_____	60	78
VII For women only total	_____	65	80
		70	82

Grand total _____ **+ Base life expectancy** _____ **= Your longevity estimate:** _____

thing I can do whether I live to be 100 or I meet Kurt Cobain in heaven before the next issue in Rolling Stone hits the mailbox. From that comes courage—the courage to live boldly in a world where humans can be randomly mad and nature can be maddeningly random. From that comes the courage to accept that while I can't control mutating flu strains, I can control the way I treat myself and my family and what I can do to improve quality of life for other people.

If you're in the right frame of mind, walking can help drive you to find the context and commitment to improve your world—a sentiment embraced in the days of Bob Dylan, but relevant still in his son Jakob's day. Walkers know this. The teacher who skips her coffee break to take children on a walk knows it. The tens of thousands of participants who raise millions for breast-cancer research in Race for the Cure walks know it. Making healthful choices can give you the physical strength and emotional clarity you need to live so deliberately, so thoughtfully, and so courageously that in the end you will have lived a full life, whether it was short or long.

That's good enough for me.

> *Living healthfully can give you the courage to think selflessly, to improve the way you treat your family, friends, and the rest of the world.*

Alice Lesch Kelly is WALKING'S *senior editor.*

Why do those #&:*?@! "experts" keep changing their minds?

Let's say that for the last five years you've been paying close attention to health news as reported on TV and in newspapers. Perhaps you learned about antioxidants (notably vitamins E and C and beta carotene), which you can get both from foods and supplements. These antioxidants may help lower the risk of heart disease, cancer, cataracts, and other ills. The scientist who had told you this on the *Today* show was a handsome fellow in a good-looking suit (no rumpled Einstein he). He had led the groundbreaking study that had just appeared in *The Impeccable Journal of Medicine*. Not only was the evidence "very exciting," but he was taking hefty amounts of antioxidant supplements himself. So you started taking the pills. Next thing, you read that a study conducted in Finland showed that not only was beta carotene *not* protective against lung cancer, it actually seemed to increase the risk of getting it. Feeling deceived, you stopped taking your supplements and even gave up your daily carrot. You were tired of carrots anyway.

You may have seen something similar happen with oat bran (good one week, outmoded the next), margarine (you switched to this supposed health food a few years ago, and now it's been tagged as an artery-clogger), DDT and breast cancer (first linked, then not), hot dogs and childhood leukemia (a headline-maker that soon pooped out, since even the researchers had a hard time explaining their findings), and household electricity (cancer again—but by then you had gotten bored). Do these folks just not know what they are talking about?

In fact, the experts don't change their minds as often as it may seem. This newsletter, for example, never told you that margarine was a health food or that oat bran would solve your cholesterol problems. Both these foods were hyped by the media and by manufacturers—but most nutritionists never thought or said there was anything magic about them. A few researchers and journalists eagerly spread the idea that your power line and your electric toaster and clock could give you cancer. Most experts thought all along that the evidence was pretty thin. Headline writers change their minds more often than scientists.

Science is a process, not a product, a work in progress rather than a book of rules. Scientific evidence accumulates bit by bit. This doesn't mean scientists are bumblers (though perhaps a few are), but that they are trying to accumulate enough data to get at the truth, which is always a difficult job. Within the circle of qualified, well-informed scientists, there is bound to be disagreement, too. The same data look different to different people. A good scientist is often his/her own severest critic.

The search for truth in a democracy is also complicated by
- Intense public interest in health
- Hunger for quick solutions
- Journalists trying to make a routine story sound exciting
- Publishers and TV producers looking for audiences
- Scientists looking for fame and grants
- Medical journals thirsting for prestige
- Entrepreneurs thirsting for profits.

It pays to keep your wits about you as you listen, watch, and read.

The search for evidence

In general, there are three ways to look for evidence about health:

- **Basic research** is conducted in a laboratory, involving "test tube" or "in vitro" (within glass) experiments, or experiments with animals such as mice. Such work is vital for many reasons. For one, it can confirm observations or hunches and provide what scientists call plausible mechanisms for a theory. If a link between heart disease and smoking is suspected, laboratory experiments might show how nicotine affects blood vessels.

The beauty of lab research is that it can be tightly controlled. Its limitation is that what happens in a test tube or a laboratory rat may not happen in a free-living human being.

- **Clinical or interventional trials** are founded on observation and treatment of human beings. As with basic research, the "gold standard" clinical trial can and must be rigorously controlled. There'll be an experimental group or groups (receiving a bona-fide drug or treatment) and a control group (receiving a placebo, or dummy, treatment). A valid experiment must also be

Reprinted with permission from University of California at Berkeley Wellness Letter, *February 1996, pp. 4-5. © by Health Letter Associates.*

"blinded," meaning that no subject knows whether he/she is in the experimental or the control group. In a double-blind trial, the researchers don't know either.

But clinical trials have their limitations, too. The researchers must not knowingly endanger human life and health—there are ethics committees these days to make sure of this. Also, selection criteria must be set up. If the research is about heart disease, maybe the researchers will include only men, since middle-aged men are more prone to heart disease than women the same age. Or maybe they'll include only nurses, because nurses can be reliably tracked and are also good reporters. But these groups are not representative of the whole population. It may or may not be possible to generalize the findings. The study that determined aspirin's efficacy against heart attacks, for instance, was a well-designed interventional trial. But, for various reasons, nearly all the participants were middle-aged white men. No one is sure that aspirin works the same way for other people.

■ **Epidemiologic studies.** These generate the most news because so many of them have potential public appeal. An indispensable arm of research, epidemiology looks at the distribution of disease ("epidemics") and risk factors for disease in a human population in an attempt to find disease determinants. Compared with clinical trials or basic research, epidemiology is beset with pitfalls. That's because it deals with people in the real world and with situations that are hard to control.

The two most common types of epidemiologic research are:

Case control studies. Let's say you're studying lung cancer. You select a group of lung cancer patients and match them (by age, gender, and other criteria) with a group of healthy people. You try to identify which factors distinguish the healthy subjects (the "controls") from those who got sick.

Cohort studies. You select a group and question them about their habits, exposures, nutritional intake, and so forth. Then you see how many of your subjects actually develop lung cancer (or whatever you are studying) over the years, and you try to identify the factors associated with lung cancer.

Pitfalls and dead ends

Epidemiologic studies cannot usually prove cause and effect, but can identify associations and risk factors. Furthermore, epidemiology is best at identifying very powerful risk factors—smoking for lung cancer, for example. It is less good at risk assessment when associations are weak—between radon gas in homes and lung cancer, for example.

No matter how well done, any epidemiologic study may be open to criticism. Here are just a few of the problems:

■ People may not reliably report their eating and exercise habits. (How many carrots did you eat each month as an adolescent? How many last month? Few of us could say.) People aware of the benefits of eating vegetables may unconsciously exaggerate their vegetable consumption on a questionnaire. That's known as "recall bias."

■ Hidden variables or "confounders" may cloud results. A study might indicate that eating broccoli reduces the risk of heart disease. But broccoli eaters may be health-conscious and get a lot of exercise. Was it the broccoli or the exercise?

■ Those included in a study may seem to be a randomly selected, unbiased sample and then turn out not to be. For example, searching for a control group in one study, a researcher picked numbers out of the telephone book at random and called his subjects in the daytime. But people who stay home during the day may not be a representative sample. Those at home in the daytime might tend to be very young or very old, ill, or recovering from illness.

Words for the wise

✓ **"May"**: does *not* mean "will."

✓ **"Contributes to," "is linked to," or "is associated with"**: does *not* mean "causes."

✓ **"Proves"**: scientific studies gather evidence in a systematic way, but one study, taken alone, seldom proves anything.

✓ **"Breakthrough"**: this happens only now and then—for example, the discovery of penicillin or the polio vaccine. But today the word is so overworked as to be meaningless.

✓ **"Doubles the risk" or "triples the risk"**: may or may not be meaningful. Do you know what the risk was in the first place? If the risk was 1 in a million, and you double it, that's still only 1 in 500,000. If the risk was 1 in 100 and doubles, that's a big increase.

✓ **"Significant"**: a result is "statistically significant" when the association between two factors has been found to be greater than might occur at random (this is worked out by a mathematical formula). But people often take "significant" to mean "major" or "important."

Some commonsense pointers

✓ **Don't jump to conclusions.** A single study is no reason for changing your health habits. Distinguish between an interesting finding and a broad-based public health recommendation.

✓ **Always look for context.** A good reporter—and a responsible scientist—will always place findings in the context of other research. Yet the typical news report seldom alludes to other scientific work.

✓ **If it was an animal study or some other kind of lab study, be cautious about generalizing.** Years ago lab studies suggested that saccharin caused cancer in rats, but epidemiologic studies later showed it didn't cause cancer in humans.

✓ **Beware of press conferences** and other hype. Scientists, not to mention the editors of medical journals, love to make the front page of major newspapers and hear their studies mentioned on the evening news. The fact that the study in question may have been flawed or inconclusive or old news may not seem worth mentioning. This doesn't mean you shouldn't believe anything. Truth, too, may be accompanied by hype.

✓ **Notice the number of study participants and the study's length.** The smaller the number of subjects and the shorter the time, the greater the possibility that the findings are erroneous.

✓ **Perhaps the most blatantly hyped research of late has been genetic.** But the treatment of human illness by altering human genes is still at a very early stage.

■ Health effects, especially where cancer is concerned, may take 20 years or more to show up. It's not always financially or humanly possible to keep a study running that long.

Reading health news in an imperfect world

And this is only the half of it. Sometimes the flaws lie in the study, sometimes in the way it has been promoted and reported. Science reporters may be deluged with data. Many are expected to cover all science, from physics and astronomy to the health effects of hair dyes. Sometimes health reporters may not even have read the studies in question or may not understand the statistics.

Many medical organizations issue press releases. Some of these are excellent, and some aren't. Some deliberately try to manipulate the press, overstating the case, failing to provide context, and so forth. Researchers, institutions, and corporations often hire public relations people to promote their work. These people may actually know less than the enterprising reporter who calls to interview them.

Finally, people tend to draw their own conclusions, no matter what the article says.

However, the bottom line is pretty good...

None of this means epidemiology doesn't work. *One study may not prove anything, but a body of research, in which evidence accumulates bit by bit, can uncover the truth.* Research into human health has made enormous strides and is still making them. There may be no such thing as a perfect study, but here is only the briefest list of discoveries that came out of epidemiologic research:

■ Smoking is the leading cause of premature death in developed countries.

■ High blood cholesterol is a major cause of coronary artery disease and heart attack.

■ Exercise is important for good health.

■ Good nutrition offers protection against cancer; or, conversely, poor nutrition is a factor in the development of cancer.

■ Obesity is a risk factor for heart disease, cancer, and diabetes.

The list could go on and on. We suggest that you retain a spirit of inquiry and a healthy skepticism, but not lapse into cynicism. *The "flip-flops" you perceive are often not flip-flops at all, except in the mind of some headline writer.*

There is a great deal of good reporting, and it's an interesting challenge to follow health news. You don't believe everything you read or see on TV about politics, business, or foreign relations, so it's no surprise that you shouldn't believe some health news. Luckily, there are many sources for health news—none infallible, but some a lot better than others.

Yet Another Study—Should You Pay Attention?
How to know when to take health research news with a grain of salt

Hot Dogs Cause Cancer? Researchers Say Yes

New warnings revive fears about the danger of eating hot dogs, particularly among children

Study Links Hot Dogs, Cancer

Ingestion by Children Boosts Leukemia Risk, Report Says

SO WENT headlines in the *Los Angeles Times,* the *New York Times,* and the *Washington Post* back in June of 1994. They came on the heels of three studies published simultaneously in a cancer research journal.

One of the studies found that children who eat more than 12 hot dogs a month have nine times the normal risk of developing childhood leukemia. The second suggested that children born to mothers who eat at least one frank a week during pregnancy have double the normal risk of developing brain tumors. The third traced brain tumors in children to *fathers* who ate hot dogs before conception. The risk of leukemia to children born of fathers who consumed hot dogs regularly was 11 times normal.

The problem: the three studies—and most certainly all the media commentary they attracted—were riddled with scientific holes.

To be sure, many of the reports in newspapers and other media outlets did point out weaknesses in the studies. But those weaknesses were strung between unnecessarily alarming headlines and warnings from researchers who, perhaps, had themselves experienced something of a knee-jerk reaction to the research. For instance, the concluding paragraph of the *New York Times* article leaves readers with this quoted advice about frankfurters from the former director of a cancer research center: "Reduce consumption of them as much as you can. They are a source of a possible cancer risk. I would not expose my children to it. It's like secondhand smoking."

Therein lies the difficulty at the heart of the matter. If scientists can't always look at research with a cool eye, how in the world are *you* supposed to? Following, **four questions to ask yourself as you read about study results or hear about them on the news.** They should help you put the latest reports into perspective as you try to make informed decisions about how to improve or maintain your lifestyle habits.

1. *What are the actual numbers as opposed to the relative numbers?* Let's say the hot dog research was airtight and children who eat franks more than a dozen times each month really are nine times (900 percent) more likely to get leukemia than children who eat them less often. The question is, how likely are children to develop leukemia to begin with?

They have a 0.3-in-1,000 chance. If you multiplied that number by nine to get the risk for children who have more than a dozen franks every month, the answer comes to roughly 2.5 in 1,000.

The point here is that even if something is many times more likely to happen under certain circumstances, that doesn't mean its potential influence is great enough to warrant changing the way you live your life.

Adding to the mathematical irrelevance of the findings is that there were only 17 children out of hundreds in the study who ate more than 12 franks each month—much too few to make any declarations about the dangers of hot dogs for the general population.

2. *What type of study was it?* There are three major types of human research—clinical trials, epidemiologic studies, and population-based intervention trials—and each has inherent strengths and limitations.

Clinical trials A clinical trial is an experiment conducted in a controlled setting, often a hospital, where researchers give a group of people treatment—such as a supplement, drug, or diet—and then measure their response. The iron absorption study discussed near the beginning of the News Bite at the top of page 2 in this issue is an example of a clinical trial.

Clinical trials are believed to yield very accurate results that can help establish cause-and-effect relationships between various substances or lifestyle activities and specific health outcomes. However, they tend to be conducted on restricted groups of people that include, for instance, just one age group, sex, or race. That allows the scientists to keep the study environment more "air-tight" so that variations within the population being studied don't confound the results. However, it means the results are not necessarily generalizable to all people. Clinical trials often need to be repeated in different groups with different genetic makeups and lifestyles before a recommendation for the general public can reliably be made.

Epidemiologic studies Epidemiologic studies look at much larger groups of people than clinical trials—up to tens of thousands of subjects. These are not experiments in which researchers control a certain aspect of the subjects' lives but, rather, make *observations* of free-living populations in which they search for relationships between lifestyle or genetic factors and the risk for chronic diseases. Harvard University's Nurses' Health Study, which looks at the lifestyles of some 90,000 women, is an example of epidemiologic research.

Because epidemiologic research is generally conducted on large groups of people, the results tend to be more generalizable to the population at large. However, epidemiology virtually never proves cause and effect; it can only

Did you know... Washing your hands for the 20 seconds recommended by the International Food Safety Council means you should be able to sing "Happy Birthday"

make *associations* on which other researchers might then decide to base a clinical trial to test whether "X" lifestyle actually leads to "Y" condition.

Granted, the more people in the study and the more tightly controlled it is for various lifestyle factors, the higher the chance that there really is something to any association found. But still, one can never automatically assume that an association proves a cause.

To show just how tenuous links brought to light in epidemiologic studies can be, scientists who published research on aspirin and heart disease in the prestigious journal *The Lancet* pointed out that according to one of their findings, people born under the signs of Gemini and Libra are likely to be harmed by taking aspirin rather than helped. If that piece of their research were serious science, the conclusion might be drawn by some that astrological influences directly affect health. The researchers highlighted the association specifically to point out the mistakes that could be made in viewing epidemiologic associations as fact.

Population-Based Intervention Trials

Sort of a cross between an epidemiologic study and a clinical trial, a population-based intervention trial is a project in which large numbers of people live freely rather than in a controlled setting but are given either a treatment or a placebo and then observed to see whether a specific outcome occurs. A study of 29,000 male Finnish smokers that was released a few years ago, in which those who took beta-carotene turned out to be more likely to develop lung cancer than those who didn't, is an example of an intervention trial.

The strength of such studies is that, like epidemiologic research, they can observe thousands of people. The drawback is that they cannot be as well-controlled as clinical trials. Thus, it may not always be the treatment that's having the effect (or the full effect) but something in the subjects' lifestyles that the scientists didn't account for.

3. *Does the study stand alone, or are its results corroborated by other pieces of research?* A single study hardly ever tells the whole story. While the goal of the media is to turn a piece of research into news—or at least to make news sound exciting—the goal of scientists is to add *incrementally* to a body of knowledge. In fact, before a scientist makes a recommendation, there must be supportive evidence from a variety of approaches so that the strengths of all of them combined compensate for the weaknesses in any single one. Clinical and epidemiologic studies are not the only kinds of investigations necessary. There is also research conducted with tissue cultures and with laboratory animals—which often doesn't make the front page or the 6 o'clock news.

Consider the hot dog research. The scientists who conducted it commented that perhaps chemicals in hot dogs called nitrites cause leukemia. One way they could test that theory would be to "contaminate" normal cells in the laboratory with various doses of nitrites and see whether the cells mutated in such a way as to suggest that inside the body, the mutations would develop into leukemia.

They could also feed various doses of hot dogs—or of nitrites themselves—to laboratory animals and see if hot dog-nourished animals developed leukemia at a faster rate than those fed other meats. Cell culture studies and animal studies would also be necessary to help determine why hot dog-eating mothers raised their children's risk of developing brain cancer two-fold while hot dog-eating fathers raised the risk 11-fold. After all, for 9 months, a developing fetus is directly affected by everything its mother eats. Thus, without any clues to a plausible mechanism for how a father's frankfurter consumption could have so much more of an effect than a mother's, the numbers remain in the realm of fluke findings, and the hot dog hypothesis remains just that.

4. *Was the study published in a peer-reviewed journal?* Peer review is the process by which experts in a particular field review a study before it is accepted for publication in order to ensure that it was conducted appropriately. It is their express role to poke holes in the study's design or the researchers' interpretations. Only if they deem the study scientifically "clean" do the publication's editors print it. The journal in which the hot dog-leukemia research was published, *Cancer Causes and Control*, is not peer-reviewed. If it were, the research, riddled as it is with inconsistencies and faulty methodology, probably never would have made it into print.

Mini-Glossary of Research Terms

Placebo-controlled: If a clinical trial or population-based intervention trial is placebo-controlled, that means there is a group similar to the treatment group that is given a mock pill, or placebo. The effect on the placebo group allows researchers to tell whether the actual treatment is having an effect or whether it's just the fact that their subjects are being treated; sometimes just being given a "sugar pill" provides a psychological boost that yields beneficial results.

Double-blind: A double-blind trial is one in which neither the study participants nor the researchers heading the study know who is getting the real treatment and who is getting the placebo until the experiment is over. As a result, the subjects can't knowingly alter their lifestyles during the trial to make the treatment more or less effective, and the researchers are prevented from reading into findings in order to come up with "expected" results.

Prospective study: In a prospective epidemiologic study, scientists look at a group of people at a specific point (or points) in time and then wait to see who gets what diseases before making associations between lifestyle and risk of illness. Harvard's Nurses' Health Study is prospective.

Retrospective study: In a retrospective study, researchers compare people with a disease or other condition to a similar group of people who aren't affected and then look backwards in time to see what differences in their lifestyles might have contributed to the different outcomes in their health status. Some retrospective studies are designed better than others. In the retrospective study that looked at pregnant women's consumption of hot dogs, mothers with teenage children were asked to recall what they ate as many as 14 years ago. (Can you remember what you ate last week?)

---

twice while soaping up. Try it-it takes longer than you think! You should wash from fingernails to forearms in hot, running water.

"Just do it" isn't enough: change comes in stages

The release earlier this summer of the Surgeon General's report entitled *Physical Activity and Health* certainly was well intended. But its advice was far from ground-breaking. Americans had heard it before in countless other official reports: Get some exercise.

Perhaps because more than 60 percent of adults still are not heeding the call to engage in enough physical activity, the report tries to make "enough" sound simpler than ever. Walk, rake leaves, wax your car, wash windows—just do *something*.

Why won't people get off the couch and move their bodies? For that matter, why won't they eat less fat, make a salad, or have fruit for a snack when they know these things are good for them?

James Prochaska, PhD, a psychologist and head of the Health Promotion Partnership at the University of Rhode Island, says it's because change doesn't begin with action. Thus, whenever advice to change starts with the admonition to act—which is most of the time—it can backfire.

Fewer than 20 percent of a population that needs to make a change are prepared for action at any given time, Dr. Prochaska says in his book *Changing for Good* (William Morrow and Company, New York, 1994, $22). "Yet more than 90 percent of behavior change programs are designed with this 20 percent in mind." Everyone else falls through the cracks.

Dr. Prochaska says action is the fourth of 6 stages of change (see box). Apparently, he's onto something. His approach has been used successfully by, among others, the National Cancer Institute to help people stop smoking, by the National Institutes for Alcoholism and Alcohol Abuse to help people stop drinking, and by the Centers for Disease Control and Prevention to curb behavior that leads to HIV infection.

To find out more about the stages of change, we conducted an exclusive interview with Dr. Prochaska.

Q: Don't many people make changes cold turkey? After all, you hear so many people say, "I quit smoking once and for all on January 1st"; or "I woke up one day and said, 'That's it!' and began to exercise."

Dr. Prochaska: We haven't been able to find those folks. Sure, there are people who say that. But if you start to assess them further, you often find that this is not the first time they've taken action. Studies show that on average, New Year's resolutions are made 3 years in a row.

If it is the first time, you have to ask, "What got you doing it at this point?" And you'll see that over time, they have been reevaluating themselves and becoming more aware that their values about healthful living are in conflict with their behavior.

Let's use smoking as an example. People can say exactly when they quit and that it was cold turkey. They can tell you it was sheer willpower. But they may not recognize how their awareness had been increasing, because it's a continuous kind of thing—becoming more and more tuned into the disadvantages of the old behavior and the advantages of change. It's something that happens gradually over time. In other words, they've been going through a couple of the preaction stages of change—contemplation and preparation. And those are stages that, together, could last for years.

Q: You said that some people claim they make a behavior change because of willpower. Is willpower really the crux of it?

Dr. Prochaska: I think it's helpful to think of willpower as equalling commitment. But you have to recognize that commitment alone will not solve the problem. It's an important process, but not the only one.

Think of smokers who enter the hospital for surgery for cardiovascular disease. They may never have made any move to stop—no conscious gathering of information about the dangers of smoking, no self-reevaluation, no thinking about behaviors that can substitute for smoking. But now they're scared, and they make a commitment. What happens is that a year later, 78 percent of them are still smoking. And they lapse back to the precontemplation stage—the first stage of change—where they aren't even thinking about quitting.

Q: Why do they go backwards like that?

Dr. Prochaska: Because they're demoralized. They mistakenly think that because willpower alone didn't get them to stop, they're weak and shouldn't bother to try again. "I can't do it," they say. "I'm not strong enough." They don't recognize that they have to *prepare* to use willpower.

Also, they are not aware that a linear progression through the stages of change, while possible, is rare. Most people lapse at some point. But action followed by relapse is better than no action. People who take action and fail within a month are twice as likely to succeed over the next 6 months as people who don't take any action at all.

But when people don't know that change isn't a smooth process and that willpower isn't the be-all and end-all, they get caught up in self-blame rather than use the experience to help themselves the next time around. And they get defensive. And what makes them even more defensive is other people—loved ones or associates—trying to push them to action. A lot of our defenses build up as a way of not being controlled by the outside world. So if the world is telling us to do something we're not ready to do, one of our reactions is to make sure we don't do it.

Q: What *is* a loved one supposed to do?

Dr. Prochaska: That's a good question, since helping relationships are important in every stage of change. But to avoid being a nag and instead to really do some good, the loved one has to provide the kind of support that matches where the other person is at. Most helpers think the only way to change is to take immediate action. But for somebody in the precontemplation stage, the help, rather than goading, may have to be something less pushy. Like leaving around some articles about the advantages, say, of regular exercise, or of eating more healthfully. A "just for your information" sort of thing.

Q: It seems that when you talk about the various stages of change, you're breaking down the change into small steps so it doesn't appear too overwhelming. But isn't there a point at which you have to take a leap of faith and move forward, even though it feels uncomfortable? Doesn't there have to be some juncture where no matter how well armed you are, you still feel anxious?

Dr. Prochaska: There definitely are points where the norm is going to be anxiety, particularly between the stages of preparation and action. You never know exactly what something is going to feel like until you're doing it. So for most people, there's a bit of "I'm not exactly sure of myself here," or "I feel anxious and uncomfortable about this, but I'm ready to take the step and move forward anyway."

I want to say, though, that historically there has been a lot more anxiety around change than there needs to be. Again, that's because there has been such pressure to go to action, whether or not people have been ready for it. Yet by consciously dealing with change in stages—and we've found that people really do go through change in 6 distinct stages—it's easier to apply appropriate strategies at the appropriate times [see *The 6 stages of change*].

Anxiety also arises because of fear of failure, and it's well-founded because the majority of people do "fail" before they succeed. But if they remind themselves, "Hey, I don't have just one chance. If I don't make it this time, I'm going to use it as a learning experience," it takes the pressure off. It's a way of recognizing that change is a process rather than an event.

Q: What about changes that aren't so cut and dry? With cigarettes or alcoholism, it's an all-or-nothing deal. But with, say, weight loss, the goal isn't to never eat something again. When the goal is less precise, isn't it harder to change the behavior?

Dr. Prochaska: The way around that is to be as specific about behavior change plans as possible. With weight loss, for instance, the ultimate goal is to shed excess pounds. But losing weight is an outcome, not a behavior. What's the specific behavior that's going to get you to that goal? For some people, it's exercising 5 times a week for 30 minutes at a stretch. For others, it's eating 5 servings of vegetables and fruits a day. Most will need a combination of behaviors.

Q: Could people use one set of behavior changes to reach more than one goal? For instance, when people decide to exercise, they're not just moving toward the goal of losing weight. They're also cutting down on their risk for heart disease and other potentially debilitating conditions.

Dr. Prochaska: Absolutely. In fact, looking at it that way increases motivation. There are 2 ways to get more motivated. One is to make a single motive extremely important. The other is to increase the number of motives. That tends to work better. In the case of weight loss, for instance, many people want to shed some extra pounds for the sole purpose of improving their appearance. That might not provide enough impetus in and of itself. But if they take into consideration all the health benefits of losing excess weight—lower blood pressure, more energy, reduced risk of disease—they'll be more inclined to make the necessary behavior changes.

It's the same with exercise. The biggest barrier to regular exercise is "I'm too busy." True, if you think only about the calorie-burning benefit of exercise, "too busy" does have much more sway. But if you recognize all the other benefits—better heart rate, reduced feelings of depression, stronger bones, more flexibility—all of a sudden, you're getting a lot more back for your 30 minutes a day.

Q: Should people set a date for action, or should they just finally decide that "tomorrow is it"?

SPECIAL REPORT

The 6 stages of change

There are 6 stages of change, according to behavioral psychologist James Prochaska, PhD. You need to know which stage you're in to move forward effectively, because each one requires different strategies. Below is a brief description of the stages, with strategies for progressing through them.

1. Precontemplation Precontemplators have no current intention of changing. They often feel a situation is hopeless (perhaps because they've tried to change before without success), and they use denial and defensiveness to keep from going forward. They feel "safe" in precontemplation because they can't "fail" there.

Strategies: Help is needed from others, perhaps in the form of simple observations or, in the case of a problem like alcoholism, confrontation. Such help allows precontemplators to see themselves as others do. Consciousness-raising is important, too. Sometimes it comes from a visit to the doctor or perhaps a stirring life event, such as the birth of a grandchild or a 50th birthday.

2. Contemplation Contemplators accept or realize that they have a problem and begin to think seriously about changing it. *Note:* It's easy to get stuck in the contemplation stage—for years. Traps include the search for absolute certainty (nothing in life is guaranteed); waiting for the magic moment (you need to *make* the moment); and wishful thinking (hoping for different consequences without changing behavior).

Strategies: Contemplators need more consciousness-raising, for example, by reading up on their problem behavior. That allows them to focus on the negatives of their current behavior and to imagine the consequences down the line if they don't do things differently. Emotional arousal, sometimes accomplished by watching a painful movie on the subject (such as *Save the Tiger* in the case of alcoholics), also helps. In addition, "social liberation" can play a big role. For a smoker, social liberation might be eating in the nonsmoking section of a restaurant as a way of experiencing social support for a different way of behaving.

3. Preparation Most people in this stage are planning to take action within a month. They think more about the future than about the past, more about the pros of a new behavior than about the cons of the old one. In other words, they pull themselves in a new direction more than they pull themselves away from an old one.

Strategies: Preparers develop a firm, detailed scheme for action. Many motivate themselves by making their intended change public rather than keeping it to themselves. Social liberation continues to play a role, as does self-reevaluation.

4. Action This is the overt modifying of behavior, and the busiest stage of change. It's also the stage most visible to others.

Strategies: People in the action stage need to apply their sense of commitment to the change. They should also reward themselves, perhaps by buying new clothing after reaching a particular exercise goal or by going out to dinner with money they otherwise would have spent on cigarettes or alcohol. "Countering" is extremely important at this stage—exercising instead of giving in to the desire to eat fatty foods, for instance. Making the environment more change-friendly—say, having cut-up fruit in the house rather than cake and cookies—is crucial, too. Helping relationships with people who support changers' goals and applaud their efforts provide more motivation.

5. Maintenance Often far more difficult to achieve than action, maintenance can last 6 months to a lifetime. Programs that promise easy change usually fail to acknowledge that maintenance is a long, ongoing process. Three common internal challenges to maintenance are overconfidence, daily temptation, and self-blame for lapses.

Strategies: People in maintenance should apply the same strategies as those in the action stage: commitment, reward, countering, modification of the environment, and helping relationships.

6. Termination The problem no longer presents any temptation. The cycle of change is exited. Some experts say termination never occurs, only that maintenance becomes less vigilant over time.

Dr. Prochaska: It's too easy to assume that the next day is going to be the "magic moment." One place people err is "tomorrow and tomorrow and tomorrow." But rarely do they err when they say, "I'm setting this date, and I'm going to go for it."

Q: How far in advance should the date be set?

Dr. Prochaska: If you're already in the preparation stage, a few weeks to a month. And the date doesn't have to be set in December in anticipation of New Year's. As for why you hear so much about people taking action on January 1, it may be that it's seen as an opportunity, if you will. But some people take action on a special birthday, like when they turn 40. Or Labor Day—summer's over; back to work. People tend to have that "new start" feeling in September, that feeling of shifting gears, even years after they have left school. That's why any time in September is excellent—the world is shifting into a new season, and there's a sense of new possibilities.

Challenging America's Inverted Health Priorities

Elizabeth M. Whelan

Elizabeth M. Whelan, Sc.D., M.P.H., co-founder and president of ACSH, is the recipient of the 1996 Ethics Award from the American Institute of Chemists (AIC). The award is given to persons who perform "duties dictated by ethical considerations, in the face of difficulties, for the benefit of the public and/or workers in chemistry and chemical engineering"; who display "leadership in an organization's ethical relationships with the public and/or employees in the field"; and who perform "effective advocacy of organizational and/or governmental policies relating to chemistry that encourage ethical treatment of individuals." Excerpts from her acceptance speech follow:

My organization—my duty—is the American Council on Science and Health. And I accept this award not only for myself but for my colleagues at ACSH—for all those people whose own work and love and, yes, high ethical standards—have made my success possible.

Of the hundreds of people who have been involved in ACSH over the years, I must make special mention of my mentor, Dr. Fredrick J. Stare, founder of the Harvard Department of Nutrition. Dr. Stare and I have worked together for almost two decades now—and together have withstood many attacks, particularly when we have the audacity to state that the American food supply is safe. We were sued for the very act of forming ACSH by the national trade association of health food manufacturers, who accused us of conspiring to undermine their business. But Dr. Stare and I prevailed in court, albeit many years and many thousands of dollars later.

The very public criticism that has been leveled at Dr. Stare and me—remarks meant to discredit and humiliate us—has actually solidified our relationship and strengthened our work.

A second person I would like to acknowledge today is AIC President Dr. Roger Maickel. Roger is an active member of ACSH's board of directors and a tireless fighter in what is always an uphill battle in pursuit of truth. If there is a misleading health claim in the media—about food, pharmaceuticals, the environment—Roger will pursue it until the matter is rectified. Purveyors of health fraud don't stand a chance in his presence.

Our top priority at ACSH is to help Americans distinguish between real and hypothetical health risks—to separate the leading causes of disease and death from the leading causes of unnecessary anxiety. At ACSH we try to ensure that both individual health decisions and public policies are based on sound scientific evidence.

Those of us who protect our health daily and those of us who put our health in constant jeopardy have exactly the same mortality: 100 percent. The difference, of course, is in the timing. I believe that epidemiologists should help people learn how to die young—at a very old age.

Today I will approach the issue of America's inverted health priorities from my vantage point as an epidemiologist—a public health specialist. We epidemiologists have a basic premise, and it

5. Challenging America's Inverted Health Priorities

is also a basic premise of ACSH: That those of us who protect our health daily and those of us who put our health in constant jeopardy have exactly the same mortality: 100 percent. The difference, of course, is in the timing. I believe that epidemiologists should help people learn how to die young—at a very old age. To put that another way: We in public health and epidemiology should be giving people a good shot at avoiding premature disease and death.

Epidemiologists are interested in environmental factors as they relate to premature death. But we have a somewhat different definition of the word "environment" than the average person.

For an epidemiologist, the word "environmental" refers to any and all factors in the causation of disease that are not directly linked to genetic, inherited origins. Environmental factors in disease causation—and by causation here I refer to the concept of increased risk—thus include not only industrial-, air- or foodborne chemicals such as agricultural chemicals, radiation or other products of our technological age but also lifestyle factors. We epidemiologists give high priority to lifestyle factors in the avoidance of early disease and death in the 1990s.

I believe that the purpose—the only purpose—of public health measures, whether carried out at the EPA, at the FDA, in Congress or in the private sector, should be the prevention of premature disease and death. I do not believe that public health efforts should have hidden goals—goals that might include harassing industry, alarming people about nonrisks, banning useful substances or advancing other social and political agendas. The purpose of public health measures should be, quite simply, to protect public health. So what, then, are the leading causes of premature death in 1996?

Each year:

- Two million people die.

- One million people die prematurely (in the sense that these deaths can be postponed) before age 80.

- 500,000 premature deaths—that is, one death in four, or one in two premature deaths—are directly and causally related to the use of tobacco. I cannot emphasize enough how remarkable this number is—and how it so dramatically influences the whole public health scene today.

- 100,000 premature deaths are due to the abuse and misuse of alcohol.

Thus, two causes, tobacco use and alcohol abuse, account for nearly 60 percent of all premature deaths. Smaller but significant numbers of other premature deaths are linked with failure to use lifesaving technology such as seat belts and smoke detectors; with failure to screen for and treat life-threatening diseases, particularly hypertension and treatable malignancies; and with reckless recreation and the abuse of addictive substances. This last category includes those HIV infections that result from IV drug use and unsafe sexual practices.

These causes represent real, documented opportunities for us to make clear progress. They are the modern-day challenges facing epidemiologists and other public health professionals. But what alleged public health risks get the attention of the media, of legislators and of regulatory bodies? Let me give you a few examples:

Each summer for the past few years I have temporarily assumed the role of an "epidemiologist from Mars" who comes to Earth to find out the causes of disease and death. Each year I turn to the leading popular women's magazines as my sources of information—*Ladies' Home Journal*, *Glamour*, *Redbook*, *Self*, *Woman's Day* and the like.

Here's what I have learned: that food additives such as sodium nitrate, BHA and BHT cause cancer; that not eating sufficient carrots and spinach causes strokes; and that eating shark-fin soup combats cancer (sharks never get cancer, they said). Women's magazines have also warned that alarm clocks' electromagnetic fields can cause cancer and that the droppings of pet birds might play a role in the causation of lung cancer. And nearly every magazine takes as a given that pesticide residues in foods are a cancer hazard, particularly to children.

Yet these same wary, seemingly health-conscious magazines are chock full of ads for cigarettes—glamorous, fun, sexy, elegant and—oh, yes—slimming cigarettes.

I now ask you: Are these not inverted health priorities?

I could regale you with many other examples of magazine hype, but I would like to move on to legislation and policies that purport to promote public health.

- There's Superfund, which promises to reduce cancer risk by protecting us from chemical risks at toxic-waste sites, even though the science of epidemiology has never pointed to these sites as a source of risk for cancer, birth defects, miscarriage or any illness.

- There's California's Proposition 65, which requires a warning label—or a ban—on any consumer product containing even a trace level of a chemical that has caused cancer in a laboratory animal. For example, under Proposition 65, Liquid Paper—the familiar "white-out" found in every office—was designated a carcinogen (it contained trace levels of trichlorethylene as a solvent).
- There's the congressionally mandated warning label on saccharin, which says that saccharin causes cancer in animals and may pose a risk to us as well.
- And, perhaps most infamously, there was the substantial publicity given to the agricultural chemical Alar—specifically, to the claim that Alar posed an intolerable cancer risk.

These, then, are examples that underscore my dismay about the inverted health priorities in the United States today. When we at ACSH ask epidemiologists on our scientific advisory board to quantify the contribution of bird droppings, pesticide residues, exposure to chemicals at toxic-waste sites, food additives and the like to premature death, their answer is, "We don't know, but our best guess is zero."

Under a policy of inverted priorities, not only do we pursue public health goals by running rapidly in the wrong direction, but we also push purely hypothetical health issues to center stage and squander our limited public health resources—our time and our financial investment.

What are the implications and the consequences of policies based on these inverted health priorities? I think they are pretty obvious:

Under a policy of inverted priorities, not only do we pursue public health goals by running rapidly in the wrong direction, but we also push purely hypothetical health issues to center stage and squander our limited public health resources—our time and our financial investment.

The mother who worries about Alar in apple sauce may well be the same mother who doesn't worry about putting a helmet on the child perched on the back of her bike or about buckling up her seat belt in the back of a taxi. The father who worries about cellular telephones and electric blankets may be a smoker who doesn't have a working smoke detector at home. The sheer distraction of constantly reading about killer apples and toxic alarm clocks (or whatever happens to be the carcinogen of the week) is at the very least leading to a lack of perspective about what is important and what is not.

But there is at least one other downside risk. As we demand that big Government require American business to protect us from risks that simply do not exist, we all end up paying more for goods and services. A mindless pursuit aimed at controlling hypothetical risks carries an enormous price tag: It not only raises the cost of doing business, but also stifles innovative activity that could dramatically improve the quality of life for all of us.

Why are the public health priorities so inverted in our country? Why are hypothetical health risks given such big play as important causes of disease when mainstream scientists do not see them playing an etiologic role at all? And what are we going to do about it?

These are complex questions. I will briefly outline five reasons why the hyperbole about environment risk prevails and describe some possible, immediate solutions. The five factors I believe are most responsible for our inverted priorities are these:

- first, the highly emotional aspects of health issues;
- second, the enormous political and economic clout of the manufacturers of the leading cause of preventable death—cigarettes;
- third, the failure of most American scientists and physicians to participate in debates about relative health risks;
- fourth, the contamination of the public health profession by an ideologically fueled form of political correctness that chills open dialogue;
- and, finally, the devastating effects of the codification into law of a scientifically baseless, uncritical extrapolation of cancer risks from animal to man.

5. Challenging America's Inverted Health Priorities

First, issues relating to food, the environment and health are highly emotional, highly volatile issues. Psychiatrists tell us that people always fear things they cannot see—things that are unfamiliar, that they do not understand. And people have long projected their fears onto postulated, invisible, hostile agents. Food additives, pesticides and "chemical residues" are ideal targets for such projection.

Psychiatrists also point to a related theme: When it comes to the causes of ill health and other adversity, human beings reject introspection: It's better to blame an outside source—some big, bad industry—than to examine critically one's own lifestyle.

The solution? It must be long term, but we need to make a concerted effort to eliminate the scientific and technological illiteracy now rampant in the United States. We need to advance understanding of the controllable lifestyle factors that contribute to risk and promote the basic toxicological premise that "only the dose makes the poison."

Second, tobacco companies—the manufacturers of the leading cause of death—dominate the print media in this country and exert a tremendous influence on both the print and broadcast media's coverage of health issues.

The tobacco industry spends nearly six billion dollars in advertising and promotion each year. This clearly buys silence and diversion. Surely nothing could make this killer advertiser more content than seeing consumer cancer-prevention efforts focused on "cancer-causing apples" and having the word "carcinogen" used so often it loses all its meaning. Remember: When everything is dangerous, then nothing is.

Over and beyond its influence with the media, the tobacco industry's substantial economic clout—and its deep roots that run throughout corporate America—have served it well. Some day I plan to write a book about the number of times representatives from the food, chemical, pharmaceutical, paper, alcoholic-beverage and every other imaginable industry have made a concerted effort to silence the scientists of the American Council on Science and Health in our attempt to make the dangers of smoking well known.

Cigarette companies have metastasized, if you will, throughout corporate America, buying up everything from General Foods to Miller Beer and from Bulova watches to Saks Fifth Avenue. The number of American corporations that service the cigarette manufacturers—and thus owe them allegiance—is truly staggering. America's health priorities are inverted because the leading cause of death has enough clout to keep the legislative and publicity spotlights off the cigarette—and on the multitude of nonrisks around us.

The solution? We will not be able truly to realign our health priorities until Congress strips the cigarette industry of its privileged legal status and levels the playing field so that the manufacturers of the leading cause of death are forced to scrimmage on the same legal and regulatory turf as the rest of corporate America.

Third, our health priorities are inverted, and nonrisks continue to dominate, because American scientists and physicians essentially remain mute while hyperbole about risk is served up all around them. You might argue that there are few public health professionals who would want to join ranks with the likes of Jane Fonda and Meryl Streep in claiming that trace levels of environmental chemicals cause human disease—but silence is assent. Where are the professionals in toxicology, epidemiology and environmental science when the risks of dioxin, Alar, PCBs and cellular phones are exaggerated? Where are the scientists when their own profession is distorted as laws based on pseudoscience are proposed? Where are the true experts when we need to communicate the reality that we have the safest, most enviable food supply in the world?

Well, I know where they are. They are in their offices, in clinics, in classes and in laboratories. They say they don't want to get involved in what they perceive as a political process. Scientists today are highly specialized, and they feel uncomfortable in public forums. Most of all, scientists dread that four-letter word "safe." Scientists rarely talk in absolutes, yet in the everyday consumer world people need easily understandable concepts of relative risk.

The solution? Get the scientists involved! That is exactly what ACSH is doing. We now have over 250 scientists and physicians as advisors. We are encouraging them to write letters to the editor, to contribute op-ed pieces to major newspapers and to show up in television debates. Our nation's health priorities will remain inverted if the only visible spokesmen on public health issues come from the Chicken Little School of Environmental Hyperbole.

Fourth, our health priorities are inverted because the practice of preventive medicine and public health has become corrupted by a form of politically correct science that abandons the principles of epidemiology and instead advances ideological agendas and social aims. Politically correct science (PCS) is dogmatic and intolerant. Its ideology is anticapitalistic and anti–free enterprise. It sees man, industry and technology as the enemies of nature. It is an ideology that has abandoned science, reason and rationality in favor of intuition, inconsistency and a commitment to goals other than the goal of improved public health. Practitioners of PCS never address real, documented public health threats. Nature, always benign, is the new god; environmentalism and consumerism are the new religions.

The solution? A return to peer-reviewed, mainstream science and a rejection, once and for all, of what is perhaps the darkest side of PCS—the antiquated, destructive view that a growing industrial economy is the enemy of a clean environment and a healthier people. The continued march of PCS undermines our ability to achieve both economic and public health goals.

Now is the time for reason and rationality. It's the time for public health professionals to reclaim their profession—to take it back from Hollywood and the political activists.

Fifth and finally, our nation's health priorities are inverted by our dependence on animal-to-man extrapolation in predicting human cancer risk.

The mouse-is-a-little-man premise dates back to 1958, when Congressman James Delaney of New York proposed a law to ban from the food supply any food additive that caused cancer in any dose in any laboratory animal. The so-called Delaney clause promptly triggered the first major food scare—the great cranberry scare of November 1959. The Delaney clause later prompted the banning of cyclamates, the near banning of saccharin and other media extravaganzas.

The clause originally applied only to additives, but the Delaney concept of mouse to man has now spread to pesticides and to trace levels of environmental chemicals generally. Laws and regulatory definitions relying on rodent data abound at the EPA and elsewhere and are consuming billions upon billions of our limited preventive-medicine dollars—money that could be used on real public health problems.

I am not suggesting that we abandon animal testing, which is critical to biomedical research. I am, however, in favor of at least a little bit of common sense in interpreting these studies and accepting the reality that only the dose makes the poison. As far I know, this common-sense element is totally lacking in the EPA's definition of a "probable human carcinogen" based on one high-dose animal test.

I suggest that we apply the "dose makes the poison" principle to our regulation of pesticides and other environmental chemicals. Obviously, pesticides are inherently toxic: Their job is to kill bugs. We need to encourage agricultural workers to adhere meticulously to occupational protocols that limit workplace exposures. And, just to be extremely conservative about potential toxic levels of pesticides appearing in food, we need to comply with the tolerance levels now set by the EPA. But once that safety protocol is set and met, we should treat minuscule levels of synthetic chemicals in food in the same way that we do low levels of naturally occurring carcinogens and toxins.

For example, we regulate naturally occurring aflatoxin by acknowledging that it is there and monitoring it to ensure it stays within the tolerance levels. Then we stop worrying about it, because trace levels play no known role whatever in the causation of human cancer.

The aflatoxin regulatory approach makes sense. Aflatoxin causes cancer in a full spectrum of animal species and shows a distinct dose-response effect. Aflatoxin is a bad actor, and it is prudent to limit our exposure to it. Note that I said *limit*—not eliminate. Now contrast the common-sense approach for aflatoxin with the regulatory actions and designations made on Alar and saccharin: Consumers were led to believe that the only protection from these chemicals—which in high doses caused cancer in one species—was the exorcist approach: zero tolerable exposure.

I maintain that the fixation on rodent carcinogens—aminotriazole on cranberries in 1959, Alar on apples in 1989 and every pesticide and food additives scare in between—actually CAUSES more premature deaths, both by distracting people from real health risks and by potentially reducing the availability of and increasing the prices of the very fruits and vegetables that protect our health.

At the close of the Rio Summit in 1992, 425 members of the scientific and intellectual community formally objected to the politically correct agenda of those who dominated the conference. Those who objected rejected the theme that man was the enemy and that industry, technology and profits posed a worldwide hazard. They signed what is now known as the Heidelberg Appeal. Over 3,000 scientists have now signed this document.

5. Challenging America's Inverted Health Priorities

The Heidelberg Appeal pledges a dedication to the preservation of the Earth but raises concern about the emergence of what it calls an "irrational ideology" that opposes scientific and industrial progress. The appeal notes that "many essential human activities are carried out . . . by manipulation of hazardous substances. . . . [P]rogress and development have always involved increasing control over hostile forces to the benefit of mankind. The greatest evils which stalk our Earth are ignorance and oppression, not science, technology and industry."

One of my top professional priorities is to encourage our federal and local regulatory agencies to enable the philosophy of the Heidelberg Appeal—to reaffirm the principles of good science and the principles found in worldwide peer-reviewed scientific literature. Our federal and local agencies can do this:

- first, by abandoning all regulatory policies and definitions that designate a chemical as a "probable" or "possible" human carcinogen on the basis of limited animal data;

- second, by incorporating a broad understanding of dose of exposure in determination of potential human risk, thus dismissing concerns about trace levels of chemicals;

- third, by establishing closer ties with prominent academic scientists from universities around the world and by regularly drawing upon their expertise in toxicology, epidemiology and environmental sciences;

- fourth, by obtaining the concurrence and approval of experts on cancer causation at the National Cancer Institute before designating an environmental chemical as a "cancer risk" under conditions of current exposure. Such consultation and verification would avoid baseless cancer scares.

Until we return to mainstream science, our nation's health priorities will continue to be inverted. We must defend peer-reviewed, mainstream science in the public arena. We must stand up for reason and rationality; we all must fight, as I have fought, for the truth. We must stop dogmatic and intolerant politically correct science before it's too late and must reject, once and for all, its darkest side—the view that a growing industrial economy is the enemy of a clean environment and a healthier people. We must not yield to those who would abandon facts in pursuit of the hypothetical—to those who are motivated not out of reason but out of fear and a commitment to goals other than public health.

I will leave you with the wise counsel of a great American—a man who faced and made and stood fast by a harrowing series of life-and-death ethical decisions from which a lesser man might have fled. These words are posted on the door to my office. I see them every day, and every day they give me strength to carry on:

> If I were to try to read, much less answer, all the attacks made on me, this shop might as well be closed for any other business. I do the best I can, and I mean to keep doing so until the end.
>
> If the end brings me out all right, what is said against me won't amount to anything. If the end brings me out wrong, ten angels swearing I was right would make no difference.

The words are Abraham Lincoln's. He fought and won his good fight; let us not shirk in ours.

Unit 2

Unit Selections

6. **Critical Life Events and the Onset of Illness,** Blair Justice
7. **The Talking Cure for Stress,** Benedict Carey
8. **Using Your Mind to Heal Your Body,** Lori Miller Kase
9. **Forgiveness,** Ann Japenga
10. **Bad Mood Rising,** Mary Roach

Key Points to Consider

❖ How have humankind's stressors changed over the last 5,000 years?

❖ What are the major stressors in your life? How do you manage your stress?

❖ Discuss how positive affirmations and feeling a sense of purpose in life can help to reduce stress. How can one gain a sense of purpose and direction by which to live one's life?

❖ If perception is a major component in the stress equation, is there anything one can do to alter one's perception?

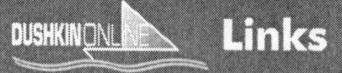 **Links**   www.dushkin.com/online/

7. **The Anxiety-Panic Internet Resource**
   http://www.algy.com/anxiety/panic.html
8. **Dr. Ivan's Depression Central**
   http://www.psycom.net/depression.central.html
9. **National Mental Health Association (NMHA)**
   http://www.nmha.org/index.html
10. **University of Sheffield Medical School/Center for Psychotherapeutic Studies**
    http://www.shef.ac.uk/~psysc/psychotherapy/

These sites are annotated on pages 4 and 5.

Stress and Mental Health

Years of medical research have significantly advanced our knowledge and understanding of the human body to a point where not only can organs be transplanted, but machines can be built to replicate their functions. The one organ that still mystifies and baffles the scientific community, however, is the brain. While more has been learned about this organ in the last 5 years than in all the rest of recorded history, our understanding of this complex organ is still in its infancy. What has been learned, however, has spawned exciting new research and has contributed to the establishment of new disciplines such as psychophysiology and psychoneuroimmunology (PNI).

Traditionally, the medical community has viewed health problems as either physical or mental, treating each type separately. This dichotomy between the psyche (mind) and soma (body) is fading in light of scientific data revealing profound physiological changes associated with mood shifts. The articles "Critical Life Events and the Onset of Illness" and "The Talking Cure for Stress" explore the psychophysiology of emotions and their impact on one's health.

Hans Selye, the father of stress research, described stress as a nonspecific physiological response to anything that challenges the body. Dr. Selye demonstrated that this response could be elicited by both mental and physical stimuli. Some general characteristics of this response include increases in heart rate, muscle tension, blood pressure, blood sugar, blood fats, and blood coagulability. While these responses are adaptive during times of crisis, Dr. Selye found that these same mechanisms could provoke physiological dysfunction if they persisted for prolonged periods of time. These findings clearly suggested that stress could play a crucial role in the etiology of various diseases.

Today researchers are examining the role stress may play in a variety of illnesses. Physical ailments currently believed to be associated with emotional stress include coronary heart disease, hypertension, obesity, diabetes, asthma, tension headaches, migraine headaches, ulcers, cancer, and a generally increased susceptibility to infectious illnesses. If stress is a generalized physiological response, why then are there so many different illnesses associated with it?

While this question has not been conclusively answered, most experts think the explanation may be "the weak organ theory." According to this theory, every individual has one organ system that is most susceptible to the damaging effects of prolonged stress.

Mental illness, which is generally regarded as a major dysfunction of normal thought processes, has no identifiable etiology. One may speculate that this is due to the complex nature of the organ system involved. It may also be that many conditions labeled as mental illnesses are not really illnesses at all, but rather behaviors that society has deemed unacceptable. There is mounting evidence to suggest an organic component to traditional forms of mental illness such as schizophrenia, chronic depression, and manic depression.

The fact that certain mental illnesses tend to occur within families has divided the mental health community into two camps: those who believe there is a genetic factor operating and those who see the family tendency as a learned behavior. In either case, the evidence supports mental illness as another example of the weak organ theory.

For some time now psychologists have known that our thoughts create a mind-set or view through which we see our world and color our perception of it. It would seem reasonable to assume that changing one's view or mind-set could alter one's response to a given stressor. In the article "Critical Life Events and the Onset of Illness," Blair Justice discusses how our perception of an event and not the event itself is the critical factor in establishing the degree to which an event is regarded as stressful. The article "Forgiveness" by Ann Japenga demonstrates how our perception of an event affects not only our behavior and our health but also those around us.

When it comes to perception, there are at least two factors operating. One is the internal dialogue that one carries on with oneself, and the other is one's energy level for coping with stress. "Bad Mood Rising" by Mary Roach addresses the role that our energy level plays in the perceptual process.

Avoiding all stress is not only an impossible task, but an undesirable goal as well. Current thinking on this issue has changed the focus from the elimination of stress to an approach that views stress as an essential component of life and a potential source of health.

While researchers have made significant strides in their understanding of the mechanisms linking stress to physical ailments, they are less clear on the mechanisms involved when it comes to mental illness. Despite this fact, it is a commonly held assertion that perceived stress has a profound impact on one's mental health. While tranquilizers have been the traditional treatment of choice for mental duress, a new branch of medicine termed "behavioral medicine" is utilizing a variety of drug-free techniques to treat such conditions. These techniques are not only drug-free, but they also empower patients to have a sense of control over their stress level. Examples of these techniques include biofeedback, meditation, self-hypnosis, yoga, mental imagery, progressive relaxation, cognitive restructuring, time management training, assertiveness training, goal setting, positive affirmations, exercise, and nutrition counseling. The usefulness of these techniques in treating stress-related disorders is discussed in "Using Your Mind to Heal Your Body."

Although significant gains have been made in our understanding of the relationship between body and mind, much remains to be learned. What *is* known points to perception as the key element in shaping one's response to stressors.

CRITICAL LIFE EVENTS AND THE ONSET OF ILLNESS

Blair Justice, PhD

Professor of Psychology University of Texas School of Public Health, Houston, Texas

■ In 1925, when Hans Selye was a medical student at the ancient German University of Prague and observing his first clinical cases, he asked a question that was considered so naive or pointless that his professor dismissed it as unworthy of reply. The question was: What is the "general syndrome of just being sick?"[1] What young Selye—who over the next 50 years became the world's leading authority on stress and disease—wanted to know was, why do all sick people have certain signs and symptoms in common: fatigue, loss of appetite, aches, pains, and other shared features.

After migrating to Canada and joining the biochemistry department at McGill University in Montreal, Selye began the research that eventually answered, at least in part, his original question. People get sick from "diverse noxious agents,"[2] and the resultant stress on the body produces certain nonspecific effects that sick people share in common. Selye learned that these "noxious" influences may come not only from harmful physical agents (such as viruses, bacteria, excessive cholesterol), but from an individual's appraisal of "noxious" or painful stimuli—how one looks at events in life and the meaning one attaches to them.[3]

After many years of studying the physiological effects on the body of stressors of all kinds—from chemical to emotional—Selye formulated a philosophy of life that he considered essential to health and happiness. Since unfavorable events—failures, rejections, losses—occur in everyone's life avoiding such stressors is impossible. What is important physiologically. Selye noted, is not the event but the person's reaction to it. "It's not what happens that counts; it is how you take it,"[4] he was fond of saying.

Although Selye's own work did not establish this finding, other research, both during his time and since, supports his ideas. These studies carefully document that the level and duration of potentially damaging neurochemicals in the body—such as epinephrine, norephrinephrine and cortisol—are a function of how we appraise life events and circumstances.[5,6] If we interpret a "noxious" experience as meaning it is the end of the world, the heart and immune system, as well as the gastrointestinal system, are placed at increased risk of impairment or compromise.[7,8] If, instead, we view an event as being bad, but not something so bad that we "can't stand it," then the body reacts less intensely. Neurochemicals are elevated just enough to prod us into effective action rather than helpless floundering.

How we react to an event—whether it is an illness, a divorce, a nuclear power plant accident, a pregnancy or childbirth—is strongly influenced by our perceived sense of acceptance and affirmation by others, by our interpersonal relationships and by social circumstances. The emerging science of psychoneuroimmunology (PNI) recognizes the association of such psychosocial factors with changes in biological functioning.

Almost a century and a half ago, Rudolph Virchow recognized that our very resistance to disease is affected by social conditions.[9] This perceptive German pathologist and physician char-

---

*Reprint requests to Blair Justice, PhD, University of Texas School of Public Health, 1200 Herman Pressler, Houston, TX 77030.

acterized medicine as a "social science." He knew that physiological processes are affected profoundly by social factors. Investigating a typhus outbreak in Upper Silesia, Virchow reported that people would not have gotten the disease had they lived in a democratic system and enjoyed more favorable social conditions.[10]

A long-term epidemiological view of mortality and life span across populations suggests that people become more vulnerable to disease when they feel little control over their lives and when they lack nurturing communities and supportive families. Leonard Sagan, in *The Health of Nations*,[11] reports a reduction of mortality and extension of life span when two factors materialize—when community and family supports develop, and a sense of control over one's destiny emerges.

Today we can, at least partially, identify the mechanisms by which psychological and social factors impact biological processes, including the cardiovascular and immune systems. When people have little control in their lives, or when conditions interfere with meeting their basic needs for love or attachment, they become more vulnerable to disease and illness.[12,13] Feeling less in control and unsupported, life events are appraised more negatively giving rise to greater arousal over time of both the sympathetic-adrenal medullary system and hypothalamic-pituitary-adrenal cortical system.[14]

HOW SOCIAL SUPPORT WORKS

After two decades of research, a clearer understanding is emerging of the key features of social support that can help protect people from illness or disease and other effects of excessive stress. Sarason,[15] a pioneer in the field, showed that giving social or tangible "provisions" in the form of information, advice, companionship or money can help a stressed person; however, they are not the critical helping features. The core element, he found, is the person's sense of acceptance, a sense of affirmation and affection he or she feels from others. This is an acquired trait. It becomes part of one's personality and is retained no matter where one goes or what life events are encountered. According to Sarason without a sense of acceptance, a person is vulnerable to illness, disease, and lowered performance.

Marital discord and disruption demonstrate the profound impact that social support can have on health. For example, Somers[16] reports that disruption in a marriage can be the single most powerful sociodemographic predictor of physical and emotional illness. Indeed, poorer immune function has been found in divorced men and women who are lonely and continue to feel drawn to their ex-spouses.[17] Similarly, unhappiness in a marriage, as measured by poor marital quality, is associated with lowered immune functioning.[18] Unhappily married individuals report more illness than either divorced or happily married persons of the same sex, age, and race.[17] These findings suggest that no simple connection can be inferred between an experience, such as being married, and health or illness. Any outcome will be affected by how an individual evaluates his or her experience and reacts to it.

ILLNESS OR DISEASE?

Whether illness or disease emerges from our reaction to life events is an important variable in the new understanding of why—and how—people get sick. Eisenberg,[9] among others, distinguishes between "disease" and "illness." Physicians think in terms of diseases and conceptualize them as abnormalities in the structure and function of individual body organs and tissues. Patients think in terms of how they feel and function as whole human beings, not as separate parts.[19] Eisenberg[9] describes illnesses as "experiences of disvalued changes in states of being and social function." Illness may occur in the absence of disease, just as disease may occur in the absence of illness. The patient is concerned with subjective signs and symptoms that may signal disease. The doctor looks for objective evidence. If none is found, no disease may be present, but an illness may still exist. Nonetheless, disease and illness are equally real to the patient. Whether the evidence is subjective or objective, psychosocial factors influence both the onset and outcome of the problem.

SUPPORT, CONTROL AND HEART ATTACKS

The influence of perceived control and support can be seen in the alternative outcomes of people who experience a heart attack. The critical life event here is myocardial infarction. Both disease and illness are present. The question is: In a group of people with the same tissue pathology receiving equally good treatment, why do some recover much better and faster than others? And, why does illness persist in some patients even when objective measures of pathology show successful treatment of the disease?

One answer involves the patient's opportunity to participate in his or her own treatment. In one study, a group of hospitalized heart attack patients received explanations about the causes, effects and treatment of myocardial infarctions. They learned how they could join in their own treatment.[20] With access to cardiac monitors, they could obtain an EKG tracing whenever they experienced symptoms. They also were taught mild isometric and foot-pedaling exercises which they did under supervision. Compared with a similar group receiving only routine information and no chance to take part in their own recovery, these patients had shorter hospital stays. Whatever greater sense of control and support the first group acquired may have affected how they continued to view their life event. This in turn would impact their cardiovascular system.

Because the cardiovascular system is particularly influenced by strong emotions, which in turn generate stress chemicals, the heart cannot be regarded simply as a mechanical pump if optimal functioning is desired. Payer[10] has observed that "in the United States the heart is viewed as a pump, and the major cause of heart pathology is considered to be due to a physical blockage in the plumbing serving the pump." She adds that "for Germans the heart is not just a pump, but an organ that has a life of its own, one that pulsates in response to a number of stimuli including the emotions."

Research in the United States and elsewhere shows that acute myocardial infarction and angina pectoris—indicating insufficient blood and oxygen supply to the heart muscle—may occur not only because of congested vessels but also because of spasm in coronary arteries, which are not simply inflexible pipes connected to a mechanical pump.[21] Cognitions can give rise to high levels of catecholamines and testosterone. Consequently, they are a key part of the mechanisms underlying arterial spasms and platelet clumping, both of which can lead to myocardial ischemic.[22] Norepinephrine and epinephrine can also stimulate release of thromboxane A2.[23] Both thromboxane A2 and the catecholamines are potent constrictors of smooth arterial muscle and strong stimulators of platelet aggregation.[24]

Given these factors, how well people recover from a heart attack, or whether they ever will ever encounter such a critical event, might therefore depend on their primary care physician's concept of the heart, a pump or an organ with a life of its own, as well as the prescribed treatment or prevention regimen. On patients' part, an increased perception of control and support plays an important role in the effectiveness of both their treatment and prevention programs.

INFLUENCE OF MEANING AND CONFIDING

The effects of trauma, even severe trauma, such as incest or a Holocaust experience, varies according to the meaning ascribed to the event by the survivors and the amount of support they perceive in their lives. Both Frankl[25] and Dimsdale[26] report how survival in concentration camps was deeply affected by whether the prisoner could find meaning in the experience. Even if meaning was expressed in a vow to live in order to seek revenge or to bear testimony, survival was enhanced and a fatal sense of hopelessness and despair averted. The ability to cling to memories of support from loved ones also was a powerful sustaining influence.

More recently, when a Jewish, Russian "refusnik" was released after 10 years of Soviet confinement, he reported that his strength to endure in prison came from knowing that a community of love supported him from the outside.[15] He maintained a strong sense of support even though he was allowed no contact with his family or the outside world for 10 years. As Sarason[15] has indicated, this political prisoner carried in his head a strong feeling that he was accepted, affirmed and loved by those he had left behind. He never doubted that they were thinking of him and working for his release. His sense of support gave him confidence in dealing with his captors. It lowered his anxiety and facilitated positive coping.

Children who recover with the least damage from years of incest or physical abuse are those who find some loving figure in their lives—a teacher, a neighbor or, in adulthood, an understanding spouse—who will listen to them and support them.[27] The most resilient children also perceived some sense of control by turning to God or becoming absorbed in the mastery of a skill.

People who have close ties to others may also benefit from confiding in them during or after a traumatic experience. In a series of recent studies Pennebaker[28] showed that after traumatic events, both psychological and physiological symptoms are relieved by systematically disclosing one's deepest thoughts and feelings either orally or in writing for 15 minutes on each of 4 consecutive days, repeating the cycle as needed. Where there is no one with whom to share painful memories, writing about one's deep feelings can bring significant benefit.[29]

Spiegel et al.[30] found that women with metastatic breast cancer live twice as long if they participate in group therapy, sharing and expressing feelings, and supporting each other in dealing with their disease. Recent studies at UCLA suggest that when people allow themselves to feel and express grief, immune proliferative response increases over time while repression of feelings and depression are associated with a decrease.[31]

PRENATAL INFLUENCES AND CHILDBIRTH

Happy events, as well as traumatic ones, can be critical in one's life. Their effects on health and illness have been well studied. For example, antibody levels are known to fluctuate with mood and happiness, with high mood being associated with high levels and low mood with low levels.[31] Holmes and Rahe,[32] first to demonstrate a correlation between life experiences and illness, argued that adjustment to change, not an event's undesirability, makes an event stressful.[33] Since then, numerous studies have established this. Events that are perceived as undesirable are more strongly correlated with risk of illness than are desirable experiences.[34] Pregnancy and birth are often viewed as happy events, but the mother may not . . . perceive them in this way. Pregnant women who feel that they have little interpersonal support and little control over life's problems may dread having a baby. These women are at higher risk for bearing low-birth weight babies and babies with complications.[35,36,37] Women under equally high stress, measured by the number of changes occurring in their lives, but who have high social support seem to be protected against these problems.[35]

Maternal attitudes toward a pregnancy and having a child have profound effects on the infant, both at birth and later. Studies in the 1970s in Germany, Austria and the United States confirmed that when a baby is unwanted, complications in pregnancy or at birth are more likely to occur.[36,38,39] High levels of catecholamines have been found in the bloodstreams of pregnant women who feel unsupported, without control or are distressed about the prospects of having a baby.[40] Passing the placental barrier, these chemicals impact the embryo and fetus.[41]

This is not the case for women whose pregnancy is welcomed, and who feel supported. What the unborn child reacts to, not only in the mother but in her environment, has increasingly come under investigation. Verny[41] reports that in the 1920s, a German doctor was told by several of his pregnant patients that they felt they should give up going to concerts because their unborn children reacted so stormily to the music. A half century later, research established that from the 25th week on, a fetus will jump in rhythm to the beat of an orchestra drum.[42] Music by both Vivaldi and Mozart seems to calm the unborn, as measured by fetal heart rate and kicking,[43] whereas music by Beethoven and Brahms has the opposite effect. All forms of rock music tend to create internal storms.[43]

SYMPTOMS AFTER NUCLEAR POWER ACCIDENTS

Pregnancy and birth have been the subject of study and speculation since the dawn of humankind. Two new life events equally as profound, however, are so recent that they have become known only in this century—in fact, only in the last decade. One of these new phenomena comes out of today's technology—the creation of nuclear power plants. The other is acquired immune deficiency syndrome (AIDS). The outcomes of people exposed to a nuclear power plant accident or infected with the AIDS virus are influenced by the individual's sense of support and control.

In March 1979 an accident occurred at the Three Mile Island (TMI) nuclear power station near Harrisburg, Pennsylvania. Although the mishap was less disastrous than the later accident at Chernobyl in the former Soviet Union, it took 11 years until the radioactive wreckage was cleared from the site.[44] Damage to the nuclear reactor produced a continued threat of radiation exposure to thousands of people living in the area. Twenty-eight months following the accident, area residents continued to exhibit higher levels of stress than did people in comparison areas who were less affected by the disaster.[45] Psychological, behavioral and biochemical measurements of 103 subjects were taken at intervals of 17 months, 22 months and 28 months after the accident. Residents with the lowest perceived control in their lives experienced the highest somatic distress and depression.[45]

In another study, heightened symptomatology after the accident was associated with a prior history of poorer social support in 312 young mothers living in the TMI area and 161 nuclear power plant workers.[46]

Compared with natural disasters, such as earthquakes, hurricanes or volcanic eruptions, technological disasters seem to have longer-lasting effects on perceived control. The difference, some researchers suggest, may be that technological disasters reflect a *loss* of control while natural disasters are associated with a *lack* of control.[45] People may accept that they lack control over the forces of nature, but believe that they can control technological power. When something goes wrong as in the case of nuclear accidents, the unexpected loss of control can be more profound. In either case, possessing a sense of control and support in one's life generally demonstrates the importance of faith and/or social affirmation for buffering the effects of stress and protecting against illness.[47,48]

PSYCHOSOCIAL EFFECTS, AIDS, AND CANCER

Control and support have an equally significant influence on patients with AIDS, affecting both the onset and course of the disease. Solomon et al. note that "while the prevalent belief among the general public, among persons with AIDS and even the professional community, is that AIDS is invariably fatal, there is a small but growing number of individuals who are alive and well 3, and even 5 years after diagnosis."[49] In Los Angeles, UCLA researchers are studying a group of men who were diagnosed with AIDS as long as 11 years ago.[50] Other investigators are finding that fatalism among those diagnosed with AIDS significantly compromises the immune system and powerfully predicts survival time.[31] Cognitive-behavioral group therapy, in early results, show improvement in immune functioning for HIV-positive persons.[31]

The San Francisco study found that psychological "hardiness" distinguishes long-term AIDS survivors from those who succumb to the disease.[49] "Hardiness" is measured by how much control, commitment and challenge a person reports.[51] Control, on this measure, means the opposite of a helpless-hopeless attitude toward bad events in life. Commitment is the opposite of alienation. People who score high on this dimension find meaning in their work, values and personal relationships. Challenge describes a person's ability to interpret stressful events as changes to be explored and successfully met rather than threats to be dreaded and feared.

Solomon and colleagues also found that one kind of social support seems to distinguish exceptional AIDS survivors who have *Pneumocystitis carinii pneumonia,* a life-threatening complication of AIDS.[49] Those who followed suggestions or took advice from people in their social network lived longer. The San Francisco researchers caution that the number of subjects in their study was small (N=21) and that their results are preliminary. They note, however, that the results are consistent with findings on the effects of control and support in other diseases. For example, Temoshok, Solomon's associate, has reported that a "Type C" coping style is associated with an unfavorable prognosis for cutaneous malignant melanoma.[52] Type C characteristics include being passive, appeasing, helpless and unexpressing of emotion. The San Francisco research group currently is investigating whether Type C in men infected with the AIDS virus is associated with greater risk of developing Kaposi's sarcoma, another serious complication of immune deficiency.

Because the asymptomatic phase of HIV-1 infection can be as long as 10 to 15 years,[53] helping people remain free of symptoms and slowing down the progression of the disease is a matter of top priority. At the Center for the Biopsychosocial Study of AIDS at the University of Miami, researchers report that aerobic exercise training has improved the immunological functioning and psychological health of a group of both HIV-1 seropositive and seronegative men.[54] They note that the exercising not only seems to have direct physiological benefits, but it also results in a greater sense of control. The researchers also are investigating the effects of a program that includes cognitive restructuring, assertiveness training, mental imagery, social support enrichment and progressive muscle relaxation. Preliminary results seem promising, but need further replication.[55]

Similar psychological intervention has been effective in improving affective state and immune function in a group of postsurgical patients with malignant melanoma.[56,57] Thirty-five patients in a 6-week program received stress management, enhancement of problem-solving skills, relaxation training, and group support. Compared to 26 controls, assessment at a 6-month followup showed significant increases in natural killer cells, NK cytotoxic activity, and percent of large granular lymphocytes. The experimental group also showed significantly less depression, fatigue and mood disturbance. They also used significantly more active-behavioral and active-cognitive coping than did the controls.[56,57]

SUMMARY

What can we conclude from these studies? One fact seems certain: there is no simple connection between life events and illness. Whether we get sick from an infection or a negative life experience depends on more than a germ or stress. All disease is multifactorial, and the resources that help protect us have much to do with our sense of support and control over our lives. What happens in our endocrine system and to our immune response is a function of what is going on inside our heads and hearts—the meanings we give to events and the feelings we have about them.

Skeptics have long doubted these tenets.[7,8] However, emerging evidence increasingly dispels these doubts and has replaced them with a biopsychosocial model based on psychoneuroimmunology (PNI). Indeed, Cousins[50] described PNI as "the new science of medicine." To date, more than a dozen academic medical centers in the United States have PNI research programs and the list is growing.

With expanded scientific study of the mind-body connection, people in general will come to recognize that whether they become ill is not always a matter of chance, but to a considerable extent something under their own control.

REFERENCES

1. Selye H: *The Stress of Life.* New York: McGraw-Hill; 1956.
2. Selye H: A syndrome produced by diverse nocuous agents. *Nature* 1936; 138: 32.
3. Selye H: *Selye's Guide to Stress Research.* New York: Van Nostrand Reinhold; 1980.
4. Selye H: *Stress Without Distress.* New York: Signet; 1975.
5. Lazarus RS: *Psychological Stress and the Coping Process.* New York: McGraw-Hill; 1966.
6. Lazarus RS, Launier R: Stress-related transactions between persons and environment. In: Pervin LA & Lewis M ed. *Perspectives in Interactional Psychology.* New York: Plenum; 1978.
7. Justice B: *Who Gets Sick: How Beliefs, Moods and Thoughts Affect Health.* Los Angeles: Tarcher; 1988.
8. Justice B: *Wer Wird Krank?* (A. Pott, trans.). Hamburg, Germany: Goldmann Verlag; 1991.
9. Eisenberg L: Science in medicine: Too much and too limited in scope? In: White KL ed. *The Task of Medicine.* Menlo Park, CA: Henry J. Kaiser Family Foundation; 1988; 290–217.
10. Payer L: *Medicine & culture.* New York: Henry Holt; 1988.
11. Sagan L: *The Health of Nations: True Causes of Sickness and Well-being.* New York: Basic Books; 1987.
12. Leighton AH: *My Name is Legion.* New York: Basic Books; 1959.

13. Leighton AH: Conceptual perspectives. In: Kaplan RN, Wilson AH and Leighton AH ed. *Further Explorations in Social Psychiatry*. New York: Basic Books; 1976.
14. Rodin J: Managing the stress of aging: The role of control and coping. In: Levine B and Holger U ed. *Coping and Health*. New York: Plenum 1979; 171–202.
15. Sarason IG: Sense of social support. Paper presented at the annual meeting of the American Psychological Association, Atlanta, GA; August 1988.
16. Somers AR: Marital Status, Health, and Use of Health Services. *JAMA* 1979; 241: 1818–1822.
17. Kiecolt-Glaser JK, Kennedy S, Malkoff S, Fisher L, Speicher CE, and Glasser R: Marital discord and immunity in males. *Psychosomatic Med* 1988; 50: 213–229.
18. Kiecolt-Glaser JK, Fisher L, Ogrocki P, Stout JC, Speicher EE, and Glaser R: Martial quality, marital disruption, and immune function. *Psychosomatic Med*, 1987; 49: 13–34.
19. Schwartz MA, Wiggins OP: Scientific and humanistic medicine: A theory of clinical methods. In: White KL ed. *The Task of Medicine*. Menlo Park, CA: Henry J. Kaiser Family Foundation; 1988: 137–171.
20. Cromwell RI, Butterfield EC, Brayfield FM, and Curry JJ: *Acute Myocardial Infarction: Reaction and Recovery*. St. Louis: Mosby; 1977.
21. Ornish D: *Stress, Diet and Your Heart*. New York: Signet; 1982.
22. Oliva PB: Pathophysiology of acute infarction. *Annals of Internal Medicine* 1981: 94: 236–250.
23. Hirsch PD, Hillis LD, Campbell WB, Firth BG, and Willerson JT: Release of prostaglandins and thromboxane into the coronary circulation in patients with ischemic heart disease. *NEJM* 1981; 304: 685–691.
24. Moncada S, Vane JR: Arachidonic acid metabolites and the interactions between Platelet and blood vessel walls. *NEJM* 1979; 300: 1142–1149.
25. Frankl VE: *Man's Search for Meaning*. 3rd ed. New York: Simon & Schuster; 1984.
26. Dimsdale JE: The Coping Behavior of Nazi Concentration Camp Survivors. *American Journal of Psychiatry* 1974; 131(7): 792–797.
27. Mrazek FJ, Mrazek DA: Resilience in child maltreatment victims: A conceptual exploration. *Child Abuse & Neglect* 1987; 11: 357–366.
28. Pennebaker J: *Opening Up: The Healing Powers of Confiding*. New York: Morrow; 1990.
29. Pennebaker J: Writing is healing. Presentation at the Hawthorne Training Conference, Houston, TX; March 1990.
30. Spiegel D, Bloom JR, Kraemer HC, Gottheil E: Effect of psychosocial treatment on survival of patients with metastatic breast cancer. *Lancet* 1989; Oct 14: 1888–891.
31. Kemeny M: Mind, emotions and the immune system. Presentation at annual conference of Institute of Noetic Sciences, Arlington, VA; June 1993.
32. Holmes TH, Rahe RH: The social readjustment rating scale. *J of Psychosomatic Res* 1976; 11: 213–218.
33. Holmes TH, Masuda M: Life Change and Illness Susceptibility. In: Dohrenwend BS Dohrewend BF eds. *Stressful Life Events: Their Nature and Effects*. New York: Wiley; 1974: 9–44.
34. Dohrenwend BB, Dohrenwend BP: Life Stress and Illness. In: Dohrenwend BB and Dohrenwend BP eds. *Stressful Life Events and Their Contexts*. New York, Prodist; 1981: 1–27.
35. Nuckolls KB, Cassel J, Kaplan BH: Psychosocial assets, life crisis, and the prognosis of pregnancy. *Am J Epi*, 1972; 95: 431–441.
36. Morris NM, Udry JR, Chase CL: Reduction of low birth weight birth rates by the prevention of unwanted pregnancies. *Am J Public Health* 1973; 3(11): 935–938.
37. Norbeck JS, Tilden VP: Life stress, social support, and emotional disequilibrium in complications of pregnancy: A prospective, multivariate study. *J of Health and Social Behavior* 1983; 24(3) 30–46.
38. Rottman G: Untersuchungen uber Einstellung zur Schwangerschaft und zur fotalen Entwiklung. In: Graber H ed. *Geist und Psyche* Munchen: Kindler Verlag; 1974.
39. Lukesch M: Psychologie Faktoren der Schwangershaft. Unpublished dissertation, University of Salzburg; 1975.
40. Kruse F: Nos souvenirs du corps maternal, *Psychologie Heute* 1978: 56.
41. Verny T, Kelly J: *The Secret Life of the Unborn Child*. New York: Summit Books; 1981.
42. Liley A: The fetus as a personality. *The Australian and New Zealand Journal of Psychiatry* 1972; 6: 99–105.
43. Clements M: Observations on certain aspects of neonatal behavior in response to auditory stimuli. Paper presented at the Fifth International Congress of Psychosomatic Obstetrics and Gynecology, Rome; 1977.
44. Wald M: After the meltdown, lessons from a clean-up. *New York Times* 1990; April 24: B5–B6.
45. Davidson LM, Baum A, Fleming, Gisriel MM: Toxic Exposure and Chronic Stress at Three Mile Island. In Lebovits AH, Baum A, and Singer JE eds. *Advances in Environmental Psychology*. Hillsdale, NJ: Erlbaum, 1986; 6: 35–46.
46. Bromet EV, Schulberg HC: The Three Mile Island Disaster: A Search for high-risk Groups. In Shore JH ed. *Disaster Stress Studies: New Methods and Findings*. Washington, DC: American Psychiatric Press; 1986: 2–19.

47. Levine JS, Schiller PL: Is there a religious factor in health? *J Religion & Health* 1987; 6: 9–36.
48. King DG: Religion and health relationships: A review. *Journal of Religion and Health* 1990; 29(2): 101–112.
49. Solomon GF, Temoshok L, O'Leary A, Zich J: An Intensive Psychoimmunologic study of long-surviving persons with AIDS. *Annals of the New York Academy of Sciences* 1987; 496: 647–655.
50. Cousins N: New dimensions in healing. Presentation at the Tenneco Distinguished Lecture Series, University of Houston, TX; March 1990.
51. Kobasa SCO, Maddi SR, Puccetti and Zola MA: Effectiveness of hardiness, exercise and social support as resources against illness. *J Psychosomatic Res* 1985; 29(5): 525–533.
52. Temoshok L, Heller BW, Sagebiel RW, Blois MS, Sweet DM, DiClemente RJ, and Gold ML: The relations of psychosocial factors to prognostic indicators in cutaneous malignant melanoma. *J Psychosomatic Med* 1985; 29: 139–153.
53. Munoz A, Wang MC, Good R, Detels H, Ginsberg L, Kingsley J, et al.: Estimation of the AIDS-free times after HIV-1 seroconversion. Paper presented at the Fourth Annual Meeting of the International Conference on AIDS, Stockholm, Sweden, June 1988.
54. Antoni MH, Schneiderman N, Fletcher MA, Goldstein DA: Psychoneuroimmunology and HIV-1. *J Consulting and Clinical Psychology* 1990; 58(1): 38–49.
55. Antoni M: Psychosocial stress management and immune functioning in an HIV-1 risk group. Paper presented at the annual meeting of the American Psychological Association, New Orleans, LA; August 1989.
56. Fawzy FW, Cousins N, Fawzy NW, Kemeny ME, Elashoff R, Morton D: A structured psychiatric intervention for cancer patients; I. Changes over time in methods of coping and affective disturbance. *Arch Gen Psychiatry* 1990; 47: 720–725.
57. Fawzy FI, Kemeny ME, Fawzy NW, Elashoff R, Morton D, Cousins N, et al.: A structured psychiatric intervention for cancer patients; II. Changes over time in immunological measures. *Arch Gen Psychiatry* 1990; 47: 729–735.

The Talking Cure for Stress

By Benedict Carey

It's not working less or simplifying your life. The real stress solution, new research suggests, is finding out what you're afraid of.

FLIGHTS ARE DELAYED, some savage Hurricane Hilda is spinning along the coast, and the airport lounge in Raleigh-Durham is a mess of elbows, bad breath, and strangers vying for pay phones and tickets. An ambassador class passenger is click-clicking his gold card on the counter for service. An executive in Chanel and pearls is foul-mouthing her cell phone. There are a pair of lipsticked Southern ladies wearing frightened smiles, an art history type in a Bowdoin sweatshirt coldly stabbing her laptop, and an edgy herd of ESPN males hovering around the bar. A lone Maryknoll sister holds her ground like a figurine, glaring damnation upon the whole congregation.

This is stress, by any definition, and if you believe the experts, it's eventually going to kill one or two of these poor souls. That is, the physiological response to such tense situations (and a continual assault of milder ones) will, over time, speed the bruising and hardening of arteries until plaque builds up, a clot springs loose, and *zap*—heart

The timorous Southern ladies with the frightened smiles may be just as much at risk for heart disease as the pushy, foul-mouthed executive in pearls.

attack. But which people are most likely to succumb?

Mr. Goldcard is a good guess, as is the woman in Chanel. They appear to be classic Type As, the pushy, ambitious characters first described by San Francisco cardiologists Meyer Friedman and Ray Rosenman in the early 1960s as being at risk for heart disease. But even as *Type A personality* was becoming part of our vernacular in the seventies and eighties, the concept was falling apart in scientific circles as a reliable predictor of heart disease.

What about the ill-tempered art historian from Bowdoin? Or the unforgiving Sister Penelope? They may be better bets, if only because they're both radiating some disgust for humanity. In the past decade Duke University researchers Redford Williams and John Barefoot have shown that people who come across as hostile on standardized questionnaires seem to suffer more heart attacks, earlier, than those who appear more easygoing. Nevertheless, this so-called Type H theory has fared only slightly better than its Type A counterpart.

This isn't to say that pushy or spiteful characters aren't endangering their hearts; many of them surely are. But recent research from the heart rehabilitation clinic of James Blumenthal, also at Duke, suggests it's not anger or hostility per se that puts a person at risk, but the tendency to experience almost *any* negative emotion more intensely than other people. And that includes less overtly stressful ones like fear, disappointment, anxiety, or frustration. Blumenthal calls such people "high responders," and they're just as likely to be the timorous Southern ladies with the frightened smiles as the executive in pearls who's swearing like a stevedore.

The trouble with all this fine-tuning of the "heart disease personality" is that it hasn't offered a way out. It's all well and good to discover that your tendency to overreact to unpleasant experiences may be putting you at risk of heart disease—not to mention insomnia, depression, fatigue, and other stress-related ills. But is there anything you can do to change your risk profile? Common sense suggests that learning better ways of managing your emotions could help, but believe it or not, little research has actually shown that to be the case.

That's Blumenthal's mission. Over the past seven years he's been conducting a study to see whether it's possible for "high responders" to step back, reflect on why they react as they do, work on changing their emotional habits—and lower their risk of heart disease in the process. So far, the results have been encouraging.

G<small>RACE MATTHEWS</small> is a mild-mannered, almost timid woman who couldn't sustain scalding, Type H hostility for more than a few minutes. Most of her adult life, she lived in the sort of traditional family arrangement that can be a cardiovascular blessing. He ran the grocery store, she looked after the kids, they all went to church, and for a while life had a June-and-Ward-Cleaver simplicity. Only in this case Ward strayed, and his long-running affair was common knowledge to everyone but his wife. In 1984 Matthews had a heart attack, followed by a triple bypass. Her marriage failed a few years later, turning its domestic curator further inward, to empty afternoons at home and exhausting bouts of anxiety and depression. The first sign that Matthews's emotional life might be fueling her heart trouble turned up after she volunteered for Blumenthal's study and showed up in his lab for an odd and unnerving procedure called mental stress testing.

For raw aggravation, embarrassment, and pure silliness, mental stress testing rivals bad performance art. Yet it does seem to finger the truly unsuspecting. Picture this scene: Arriving in the clinic, Matthews seats herself in a vaulted room. Two white-coated women fasten electrodes to her chest (neglecting to mention whether the wires can deliver electric shocks), then ask her to give a three-minute disputation on one of three questions: Should abortion be outlawed? Should public schools have to designate prayer periods? Should smoking be banned in public places? She has all of 30 seconds to prepare.

"I heated right up," Matthews says. "I picked the abortion question, and I feel very strongly against it."

Then comes the math: Add one large integer to another, and divide by a third, and there's no paper or pencil, and the two women are saying, "Hurry, hurry," like a couple of bond traders afraid of losing their inside advantage. Finally the strangest game of all: Matthews holds a metal pointer and, while watching her hand in a mirror, traces an engraved Star of David on an electrified plate. The plate snaps like a poodle when the pointer touches the star's edges. There's no electric shock, but the snapping certainly jangles the nerves.

The truth is, everyone goes a little warm in the temples performing these tasks. But only when heart rate and blood pressure leap far above average does someone rate as a "high responder." During stressful situations, this person's body is more likely than a nonresponder's to produce excessive levels of fight-or-flight hormones like cortisol and norepinephrine. These chemicals are critical to your survival if a saber-toothed tiger is flushing you out of the tall grass or some heavy-browed clan rival is giving you the stare-down. They interrupt digestion, put sensory nerves on full alert, squeeze the arteries, and churn the heart, moving blood into the muscles. Yet if every new situation or petty hassle touches off this battlefield response, researchers say, it's only a matter of time before indigestion and insomnia become chronic; precious arteries become pocked, worn, and clogged; and the master pump strains under the load.

Blumenthal's team can actually see some of this happening, using nuclear imaging technology to view the heart while patients squirm and sweat. As the arteries tighten, for example, the heart sometimes gasps for more blood, and one of its chambers may fall out of rhythm with the others—a momentary condition called ischemia that tells you the heart is headed for trouble.

"I saw the pictures of my heart, and it was going crazy," says Robert Whalin, a gregarious, semiretired salesman who ended up in Blumenthal's study after he had a triple bypass in 1989. "All my life I was doing that to myself, pushing the accelerator."

To be sure, elation or sexual excitement also gooses the heart, and there's no reason why that muscle should know the difference between an unpleasant revving and a pleasant one. But while studies have also linked positive arousal to heart strain, Blumenthal is convinced it's the disagreeable feelings that do most of the damage. In a recent study of 100 patients, he found that high responders are two to three times more likely to suffer heart attacks or need surgery than their more tranquil peers. "It seems the negative emotions more readily put people in danger," he says, "and the people who experience those emotions most deeply are not necessarily the high hostile personalities or the classic Type As."

Indeed, they range from cautious Grace Matthews to the exuberant Bob Whalin to Alvin Schultzberg, a publishing consultant in the Durham area, who's opinionated but not explosive, thoughtful but hardly retiring. While Matthews has verged on depression, and Whalin reveled in a flamboyant, almost desperate ambition, Schultzberg's only indulgence is an abiding perfectionism in his work. He's hard on himself, and he doubts that anyone else has the commitment and discipline to work at his level. "I could vividly imagine all the terrible things that would happen if something didn't go right," he remembers. "Deadlines would be missed, the quality of my work wouldn't be good, my reputation would suffer, and I'd fail somehow." His heart failed instead,

Commonsense Lessons Behind the Self-Help Clichés

Many people who react strongly to mental stress are falling prey to what therapists call cognitive distortions—self-destructive habits of thinking that can transform meaningless episodes into plagues of anxiety. Cognitive therapy works by helping people identify these patterns in themselves and substitute forgiving alternatives.

ALL-OR-NOTHING THINKING

An assignment is either done to perfection or badly botched. The boss is either an amazing genius or a total fool. *My God, I yelled at my kids. I must be an awful parent.*

The fact is, Mozart had days when the harpsichord clanged, and General Washington lost more than a few battles. Remind yourself that no single episode defines a person, and a sole flaw rarely characterizes an entire project.

DISCOUNTING THE POSITIVE

Many people possess the unadmirable ability to find guile in every act of kindness, bad luck in every stroke of good. Every compliment is considered insincere, every success a fluke. *They wouldn't be telling me they liked my new haircut if I hadn't just gained ten pounds.*

Who cares? These days compliments are as rare as acts of chivalry, and they're more often genuine than not. Lap them up.

ASSUMING THE WORST

You know what others are thinking and how things will turn out—and none of it's good. No matter what they say, you sense that friends are annoyed with you, coworkers are unimpressed, and perfect strangers are making fun. And, of course, you're absolutely sure it's going to rain during your upcoming vacation in Hawaii.

Therapists recommend adopting a kind of forced optimism. Despite what you might infer from their faces and gestures, people are usually more generous-spirited than you think. And why not plan for sun? At least you'll be in a better mood when you get there, and your family won't hate you for having been such a grouch.

OVERGENERALIZING

A close cousin to all-or-nothing thinking, this is the habit of identifying every turn for the worse as part of a dark pattern of failure. A missed promotion or a rejected invitation for a date will be followed by more of the same, because all situations are alike.

Try to evaluate each event independently. Perhaps the guy is involved in a messy breakup—or he just doesn't go for blonds. On the other hand, if you're passed over for a promotion three times in a row, find out what you may be doing wrong instead of throwing up your hands in despair.

PERSONALIZING

A primary source of guilt, this is the tendency to assume responsibility for events that are genuinely beyond your control. Say a colleague cuts off a conversation in mid-sentence. Or someone on the bus is glaring your way. Or a friend walked right by this morning without saying hello. You ask, What did I do wrong?

The answer, say counselors: nothing. If you really did sour a deal or say something awful, most people will let you know. —B.C.

landing Schultzberg in the hospital in 1989 for angioplasty, a procedure for clearing out blocked arteries.

With patients like these, each in the grip of a different negative emotion, Blumenthal saw the task ahead clearly. "It was logical to see whether we could give them tools to moderate their intense sensations," he says. For that, he turned to group therapy.

WHEN FRIEDMAN and Rosenman introduced the idea of the Type A personality in the 1960s, most therapists still used their couches. They wanted to know how often your mother comforted you, whether your father was absent or abusive, how you fared on the playground. To soothe mental distress, they believed, you had to understand its source. Today, although this approach is still practiced widely, something called cognitive-behavioral therapy is on the rise. Cognitive therapists don't care what happened in the sandbox. They are interested only in altering the way you interpret emotional challenges (that's the cognitive part), thus enabling you to change what you do in response (the behavioral).

Blumenthal's stress management trial is a model of this method. In early 1989 he recruited 107 subjects from Durham and surrounding areas. All were otherwise healthy people who'd had either a heart attack or some type of surgery for heart disease sometime in late middle age. Blumenthal split them into three squads: 33, including Matthews, Whalin, and Schultzberg, gathered for counseling in groups of eight or nine once a week for 16 weeks; 34 participated in an exercise program three times a week for 16 weeks; and 40 composed a control group that was monitored but given no therapy of any kind.

In the cognitive therapy group, counselors began by outlining the symptoms of severe stress, including chest pain, insomnia, fatigue, trembling, a tendency to smoke or drink more, and (everyone's favorite) "an overwhelming urge to cry or run and hide." "When people see this list," says Mike Babyak, a Duke psychologist who conducts therapy sessions for Blumenthal's current heart patients, "they realize right away how stressed they have been. Members of the group start talking, they begin to believe in it, and we're on our way."

The program proceeded, in effect, by coaxing its students to stroll beside themselves and study the person they had become. They were told to keep a diary, detailing all the times during the day when they felt pent up or anxious and explaining why. This may be the most important part of the program, says Babyak, because it forces people to be aware of what pushes their buttons.

The next trick was to break the emotional routine. This is the smell-the-roses phase of counseling, when patients are advised to remove their watches, play with a dog, eat more slowly, walk more slowly, chat with the grocer or the neighbor, and, for the truly fearless, verbalize their worries to someone close. "Obviously, not everyone can do all these things," says Blumenthal, "but just trying a few is all we ask."

Finally the students began to relearn some commonsense lessons whose value has been buried in self-help cliché—ideas that should help them unwire their fight-or-flight response to stressful situations. Such as:

ALL INDICATIONS TO THE CONTRARY, THE WORLD IS NOT ABOUT TO COLLAPSE. Many heart patients have the sort of paralyzing pessimism that forecasts disaster based on the flimsiest of evidence. As in, "I had an extra slice of peach pie, so I'll never stick to a diet." Or, "She criticized my report, so she must think I'm incompetent."

Schultzberg says that in his case this fear of failure often masquerades as realism. "I'm a doubter, someone who focuses on the dark side of things to prepare myself for what could go wrong. I always thought I was using those negatives to make a positive, but now I'm not sure it always worked out that way."

NOTHING PERSONAL, BUT PEOPLE DON'T ALWAYS BEHAVE THE WAY YOU EXPECT THEM TO BEHAVE. Children dye their hair green, lifelong Democrats vote for Perot, good Christians forget to write thank-you notes. These are not meant as insults and shouldn't be taken that way. "I'll give you an example," says Whalin. "My 35-year-old son didn't show up for my last birthday party. He said he would, he lives nearby, he had no reason not to come. Well, there was a time when that would have made me climb the walls. But this time I didn't. Now I know that my expectations aren't always met, so I called him later, we talked and decided to get together the next weekend."

THOUGH YOU MAY FIND THE COMPANY AWKWARD AT FIRST, SPEND SOME TIME WITH YOURSELF. This is a matter of taking a half hour, usually before bed, to detach yourself from the hold of the day's events. Some people listen to relaxation tapes, others meditate, and still others put Gregorian chants on the headphones and transport themselves to a mountain stream, an empty beach, a quiet London pub. "I know this stuff sounds very soft, very New Age, and that's a shame because it really does work," says Schultzberg. "After seven years this is the part of the course I enjoy most. I spend some time each night relaxing, just floating, and nothing touches me."

EVEN IF YOU COME CLEAN WITH FATHER NOONAN EVERY WEEK, FIND A FRIEND WHO WILL LISTEN TO YOUR TROUBLES. "All that time in the marriage I didn't really have anyone who knew me or cared much about me," says

Blumenthal doesn't pretend that his therapy is anything more than glorified good sense or that it will turn anyone into the Dalai Lama.

7. Talking Cure for Stress

This is the first glimmer of direct evidence that counseling alone—without changes in diet and exercise—can reduce the risk of heart attack.

Matthews. "I had friends through church, but they knew about my husband's affair and didn't bother to tell me. I understand why they didn't. But back then I just felt like a fool, like I was worthless, and that no one was interested in me."

Indeed, this kind of emotional isolation is what some psychologists now think lies at the core of all type As and Hs, as well as more low-key types, like Matthews, who develop heart disease because they're depressed, anxious, or frightened.

"A person may be extremely hostile, feel terrible rage," explains Blumenthal. "But if he's got a friend who sees it and can say, 'Hey, what's going on? Don't get so upset about it,' that can make all the difference."

As it happens, according to Jonathan Schedler, a research psychologist affiliated with Harvard University, the test that researchers used to identify Type H personalities essentially measures something he calls interpersonal warmth.

"It has to do with whether you see the important people in your life as benevolent or malevolent, whether they offer nourishment or frustration," says Schedler. "The fact is, humans are emotionally frail. We need real support from other people, and those who don't acknowledge it are going to feel besieged."

MOST DOCTORS HAVE never much cared for the idea that emotions affect the risk of disease. Human beings are a confused, contradictory, goofy species, alternately hostile and kind, responsible and reckless, solitary and social—hard to classify as Type A or H or anything else. Moreover, doctors say, it's a small step from believing that personality impinges on health to blaming yourself for getting sick or, worse, blaming yourself for failing to unclog arteries or shrink a tumor through positive thinking. We can eat right, shun cigarettes, and exercise daily, and still many illnesses—like most emotions—will simply happen to us.

Nonetheless, Matthews, Whalin, and Schultzberg should give skeptics some second thoughts: These three, like most of the others who received Blumenthal's stress counseling, have remained remarkably healthy. In the past seven years most of the original 33 have suffered no heart attacks and needed no further surgery for heart disease. Though still preliminary (the data has yet to be published), Blumenthal's study offers the first glimmer of direct evidence that counseling alone—without changes in diet and exercise—can reduce the risk of heart attack.

Blumenthal doesn't pretend that his therapy is anything more than glorified good sense or that it will turn anyone into the Dalai Lama. Whalin remains the fierce, theatrical character he was before the counseling, Schultzberg is still the philosopher-consultant who suspects he's one of the few who know how the world wags, and Matthews remains the unassuming traditionalist. But all have become fairly tolerant observers of themselves; each has identified his or her weak emotional limb and attempted to brace it. Matthews found her first confidante in Blumenthal's study group and now has several good friends through the local women's Republican club; Schultzberg husbands his Olympian standards, aiming for excellence rather than perfection, as he puts it; and Robert Whalin has become his own oral historian, a Studs Terkel chronicling the Whalin Years.

"Tell-ya-story," he says. He's talking loud, pulling on his white Hemingway beard, pacing around his living room as if in front of a large audience. "I used to spend a lot of time in airport bars. I traveled a lot, I drank a lot, and once in a while I'd be sitting next to some guy who'd start telling me his problems. He was having troubles with his boss, misunderstandings with his wife, couldn't talk to his daughter, whatever. And I'd lean over and say, 'Listen. I've got something magic in my wallet. I can't tell you whether it's black magic or white magic, but it will change your life.'"

He laughs, drops into an easy chair. "It was a dime! Back in those days you could make a phone call with a dime. And I'd say, 'Call that person—the wife or boss or whoever it was—and tell them what you're telling me.' But the point is, it was all an act. I didn't really care what happened to those people. I just wanted them to say, 'Gee, what a great guy!'"

Needless to say, Whalin never used the dime himself. Lounging deep in his easy chair, he tries to imagine what he'd say to his former self, the airport-bar therapist who almost died of heart disease years ago. After nearly five minutes, he sits up and addresses the far wall, on which hangs a picture of his wife, Eva, with their three young children. "Today I'm not one person. All my life I was one person; the primary person in the world was me. Now I'm multiple people—wife, kids, friends—and everything I do affects them. I never believed that before. I would have had a better life if I'd known it back then. I would have been happier, made others around me happier. I would have had more of all that."

One day last August Eva Whalin came home from the hospital where she works and said to him, "There was a man lying on a stretcher all by himself. No one was tending to him. And I asked myself, 'What would Bob do if he were here? He'd go talk to him.'"

"So that's what she did," says Whalin, grinning like an acquitted criminal. "That's the first time anyone has ever told a story like that about me."

Benedict Carey is a staff writer.

Using Your Mind to Heal Your Body

Meditation, yoga and biofeedback: These **natural stress reducers** can **do more for your heart** than drugs and surgery, without the side effects

BY LORI MILLER KASE

THERE'S NO QUESTION ABOUT IT: Your state of mind affects your health. And that includes your heart. Every day, it seems, the evidence becomes more compelling: Letting go of negative feelings like stress, anger and depression helps your body, while holding on to them hurts it. Take the case of Patricia Chapman. For years this Silicon Valley professional ran on adrenaline, juggling a pressure-filled job at a high-tech company with two children and a hectic social life. "I had such a perfection complex, but I couldn't be perfect at anything," recalls Chapman, now 54. "I was always in a hurry."

In 1989 Chapman was diagnosed with cardiac arrhythmia, an irregular heartbeat. Three years later, her heart was beating an extra 250 times every hour. By the end of 1993—a stressful year in which Chapman divorced and went through a restructuring at work—she had 700 extra heartbeats per hour. Then, in the midst of one of her hour-long commutes, she suffered a ventricular tachycardia, a life-threatening form of arrhythmia, that landed her in the hospital.

Most experts would agree that Chapman's state of mind contributed to her poor physical condition. "Psychological well-being can have a big impact on your risk of cardiovascular disease, not to mention your recovery from heart attack and heart surgery," says Richard R. Heuser, M.D., director of the cardiac catheterization laboratory at Columbia Medical Center in Phoenix, AZ.

Hostile types, for example, have been found to develop coronary artery disease at four to five times the rate of their mild-mannered counterparts. Chronic worriers face an increased risk of sudden cardiac death, and depression is emerging as a major risk factor for heart disease (see "The Depression Connection"). This means big trouble for women, who are twice as likely as men to experience anxiety and depression.

How Emotions Harm the Heart

Scientists are beginning to understand how negative emotions do their damage. For example, acute stress sets off a rush of adrenaline and other hormones that cause the heart to beat faster and blood pressure to surge, while signaling cells to dump fat into the bloodstream for quick energy.

Repeated blood pressure surges can damage the arterial linings, which can lead to ischemia or a blockage of the coronary artery (coronary thrombosis). Fat in the bloodstream that isn't burned by muscles gets converted into cholesterol and can end up as plaque in the coronary arteries.

In a study at the Institute of HeartMath in Boulder Creek, CA, researchers found that anger and anxiety can cause the heart's rhythms to become desynchronized. That increases the risk of arrhythmia, which, in its most dangerous form, can prevent the heart from pumping enough blood to the brain and other vital organs.

Of course, everyone gets angry and feels anxious from time to time. The question is, when do such emotions become dangerous? "When you experience them routinely during the day," says Redford Williams, M.D., director of the Behavioral Medicine Research

8. Using Your Mind to Heal Your Body

Model of Health

Supermodel **Cheryl Tiegs** wasn't just posing for our photo shoot at Canyon Ranch Health Resort in Tucson, AZ: She's living proof that maintaining a healthy body and mind is the ticket to lifelong good looks. At 50 Tiegs is raising a six-year-old son, Zach, and designing women's eyewear, hosiery and watches, yet still manages to find time for fitness. Every day.

"My latest passion is yoga," she says. "I take a 1½-hour class three times a week. It's a really hard workout. I feel stronger, more flexible and more centered. I also weight train, hike and play tennis." To keep her energy up, Tiegs relies on a protein-packed diet, along with half a Balance bar at 4 p.m. and at bedtime. "I also take vitamins and drink tons of water."

Though Tiegs was blessed with great genes, she does rely on a few good beauty products. Her favorites include Lorac lipstick in Farrah (a pale pink), Bob Kelly cream rouge in Natural and Maybelline Great Lash mascara in Very Black. But her best-kept beauty secret is meditation. "I meditate for half an hour every day," she says. "I go into my room, close the door, turn off the phone, light a scented candle and breathe deeply. It calms me down instantly."

Center at Duke University in Durham, NC, and author of *Anger Kills* (see "How Hostile Are You?").

Calming the Mind

Teaching heart disease patients to unwind is a new goal at progressive cardiac rehabilitation programs. At Duke University's Center for Living, patients learn anger-control and relaxation techniques. At the Cleveland Clinic in Ohio, patients use biofeedback. And those who go on retreats with the Preventive Medicine Research Institute in Sausalito, CA, learn yoga.

Most doctors aren't suggesting that mind-body approaches to heart disease replace conventional treatments, but rather that they fill in where medication and surgery fall short. After all, drugs for high cholesterol and blood pressure don't resolve underlying problems. Even the effects of angioplasty and heart surgery last for only a limited period of time.

Four Ways to Manipulate Your Mind-Set

A number of studies have shown that practicing mind-body techniques improves heart health in a variety of ways, from lowering blood pressure to reducing arrhythmia. Added bonus: There are no dangerous or unpleasant side effects.

Meditation

What it is: Transcendental meditation is an ancient Indian practice that involves learning a special sound, or mantra, to achieve a state of "restful alertness." Researchers have shown that TM can elicit a variety of beneficial changes including a slowing of heart and breathing rates. Herbert Benson, M.D., founding president of the Mind/Body Medical Institute at the Beth Israel Deaconess Medical Center in Boston, calls this set of changes the "relaxation response" and has developed a simple way to achieve it.

How to do it: (1) Sit quietly in a comfortable position. (2) Close your eyes. (3) Relax all your muscles, beginning with your feet and slowly moving up to your face. (4) Breathe through your nose. As you slowly exhale, say the word "one" silently. (5) Continue for 10 to 20 minutes. (6) Put distracting thoughts out of your mind and don't worry about whether you achieve a deep level of relaxation.

Effectiveness: Dr. Benson has shown that patients with hypertension who practiced achieving the relaxation response significantly reduced blood pressure levels and required fewer medications over a three-year period, while those with cardiac arrhythmias experienced fewer of them. Overall, patients had fewer symptoms of anxiety, depression and hostility.

Savvy Sources: *The Relaxation Response* by Herbert Benson, M.D., and *Minding the Body, Mending the Mind* by Joan Borysenko, M.D. You can also order audiotapes ($10 each) from Dr. Benson's institute by writing to the Division of Behavioral Medicine, Beth Israel Deaconess Medical Center, 110 Francis St., Boston, MA 02215, or by calling 617-632-9530.

Biofeedback

What it is: Biofeedback uses electronic equipment that monitors a patient's physiological functions and translates them into sounds or video images. A trainer then teaches the patient to control these functions with conscious thought, often using relaxation techniques.

How to do it: Patients are connected via sensors on their fingers or forehead or by blood pressure cuffs to equipment that displays signs of bodily stress, such as rapid heart rate. Often the training part takes just a few days.

Effectiveness: According to the Association for Applied Psychophysiology and Biofeedback in Wheat Ridge, CO, biofeedback can reduce blood pressure in up to 80% of patients.

Savvy Sources: You can request a free brochure about biofeedback, plus a list of certified practitioners, by sending an SASE to the Association for Applied Psychophysiology and Biofeed-

---

The Depression Connection

Anxiety and hostility aren't the only dangerous emotions. New research indicates that depression is also a hazard to your heart. The latest study, published in the journal *Circulation*, found that people who had been diagnosed with depression 13 years earlier were four times as likely to suffer a heart attack as those who weren't depressed.

What's more, some evidence suggests that you don't have to be clinically depressed to be at risk. A study of 730 Danish men and women found that being chronically blue (that is, having some symptoms of depression but not enough to be diagnosed with the disorder) boosts the likelihood of heart attack.

Several factors seem to underlie the connection. Depressed people have more rapid heart rates, higher levels of stress hormones, and heart rhythms that don't adjust well to changes in physical activity. They also appear to have stickier platelets, so their blood may clot more easily, putting them at greater risk for blocked blood vessels and heart attacks.

But there may be other contributing factors: Compared with nondepressed people, the depressed are less likely to curb unhealthy habits like smoking and drinking or to practice healthy ones like eating well and exercising.

2 ❖ STRESS AND MENTAL HEALTH

How Hostile Are You?

Three aspects of hostility can harm your health: anger, aggression and cynicism. Ask yourself the following questions to gauge whether negative emotions are putting your heart at risk. Place a check next to all that apply to you.

ANGER:
- ☐ When you're stuck in a traffic jam, do you quickly start to feel irritated and annoyed?
- ☐ When someone treats you unfairly, are you apt to think about it for hours?
- ☐ When you remember something that made you mad, do you feel angry all over again?

AGGRESSION:
- ☐ If a friend or coworker disagrees with you, are you likely to get into an argument about it?
- ☐ Do you often use profanity when you are arguing with a friend or relative?
- ☐ If another driver butts in front of you in traffic, do you flash your lights and honk your horn?

CYNICISM:
- ☐ In the express line at the store, do you check whether anyone has too many items?
- ☐ When you're a passenger in a car, do you try to stay alert for obstacles ahead?
- ☐ If there's an important job to be done, do you prefer to do it yourself?

Three checks or fewer, hostility probably isn't a big problem for you; between four and six, you may be putting your heart at risk; seven or more and your hostility is in the danger zone. It's time to start practicing those mind-body techniques or talking to your doctor or therapist to find out how you can help yourself.

Adapted from Anger Kills by Redford Williams, M.D., and Patricia Williams, Ph.D.

Cognitive Restructuring

What it is: Rooted in the belief that stress arises from negative thinking patterns, cognitive restructuring involves substituting positive thoughts for negative ones.

How to do it: Every time a negative thought enters your mind and you begin to feel angry or stressed, think about something positive—specifically, something or someone you appreciate. "This can neutralize your physiologic response to stress and change your heart rhythm," says Rollin McCraty, M.D., research director of HeartMath.

Effectiveness: In a recent study done at the Mount Zion Medical Center in San Francisco, heart patients who practiced cognitive restructuring for 14 months reduced the number of daily episodes of ischemia by half.

Savvy Sources: *Cognitive Therapy and the Emotional Disorders* by Aaron T. Beck, M.D., *The Wellness Book* by Herbert Benson, M.D. and Eileen M. Stuart, R.N., *Feeling Good: The New Mood Therapy* by David D. Burns, and *Freeze-Frame* by Doc Lew Childre.

Lori Miller Kase is a Simsbury, CT, writer specializing in health.

---

back, 10200 West 44th Ave., Suite 304, Wheat Ridge, CO 80033-2840.

Yoga

What it is: Some experts say this 3,000-year-old Indian practice is the earliest known mind-body system designed to heighten awareness and promote healing. There are many types of yoga, but most involve deep breathing and a sequence of poses that encourage flexibility, strength and balance.

How to do it: Beginners will benefit from classes, where a teacher can offer guidance. You can also try out some basic poses on your own. The Sivananda Yoga Vedanta Center, based in Val Morin, Quebec, recommends beginning with the Standing Forward Bend: With your legs together, center the weight of your body on the balls of your feet. Inhale deeply as you stretch both arms straight up over your head. Feel as though your entire body is extending upward. Hold for one to two minutes. Then exhale, stretching down toward the floor. Grab the backs of your legs and breathe gently, holding the position for at least 10 seconds; feel your hips stretching upward. Rise slowly and shake out your arms and legs.

Effectiveness: Several studies have shown that regular practice of hatha yoga, one of the gentler types of yoga, can reduce blood pressure, slow heart rate and elicit the relaxation response.

Savvy Sources: *Yoga for Women* by Paddy O'Brien, *Yoga Mind & Body* by the Sivananda Yoga Vedanta Center, and the *Yoga Journal* (available on newsstands or by calling 800-I-DO-YOGA). You can also order videos from the journal.

Taking the Natural Approach

The following centers offer mind-body programs for patients with heart disease:

- **The Behavioral Medicine Program,** Columbia-Presbyterian Medical Center, 622 West 168th St., Box 427, New York, NY 10032; 212-305-9985
- **Cardiac Rehabilitation Program** Attn: Faye Fitzgerald, Henry Ford Hospital, 2799 West Grand Blvd., Detroit, MI 48202; 313-972-1919
- **The Center for Living,** Duke University Medical Center, 1300 Morreene Rd., Durham, NC 27710; 919-660-6600
- **The Center for Mind-Body Medicine,** 5225 Connecticut Ave. NW, Suite 414, Washington, DC 20015; 202-966-7338
- **The Mind/Body Medical Institute,** Beth Israel Deaconess Medical Center, 110 Francis St., Boston, MA 02215; 617-632-9530
- **The Preventive Medicine Research Institute,** 900 Bridgeway, Sausalito, CA 94965; 415-332-2525

Forgiveness

Imagine your seven-year-old child was kidnapped by a stranger in the middle of the night. Now imagine forgiving the man who did it.

By Ann Japenga

FOR MOST AMERICANS SETTLED EAST OF THE MISSISSIPPI, SOONER OR later the time comes to pack the brood in the jalopy and go see what's out west. For the Jaeger family of Detroit, the call came in 1973. Bill Jaeger, a die designer for the auto industry, saved his paychecks and hoarded days off. He bought a new GMC van, and his slim blond wife, Marietta, sewed curtains for the windows.

They set out for their first-ever camping trip on a June morning, van stuffed full of kids, borrowed tents, and sleeping bags. The couple's five children pressed to the windows and drank in the sights: Badlands National Park, Mt. Rushmore, the Black Hills. At every rest stop seven-year-old Susie—the gangly, dark-haired youngest child—practiced cartwheels. Then it was everyone back in the van. Marietta would make a quick head count, and they were off again.

On June 23 they reached their destination: Missouri Headwaters State Monument, near Three Forks, Montana. Here, where the Gallatin, Jefferson, and Madison rivers converge to form the Missouri, the clan set up camp beside a river rumbling with snowmelt.

Even bedtime held new thrills for the kids. Four of them had a tent all to themselves, an arrangement that lent itself to secret nighttime conversations. On the third night Susie and 13-year-old Heidi awoke at about two and whispered awhile before dropping back to sleep. A few hours later Heidi was roused by a cold breeze on her shoulders. Groggy, she groped to locate the source. Her hand brushed grass where there should have been canvas. Suddenly fully awake, she found a hole sliced in the side of the tent. Two of the sleeping bags beside her were still occupied, but Susie was gone. Quickly the alarm spread, and the campground lit up. Searchers found Susie's two stuffed lambs on the grass outside the tent.

The next few heart-stopping hours blurred into days and then weeks as the sheriff was notified, then the FBI. Military crews with tracking dogs combed haystacks and outbuildings, Boy Scouts hacked at the underbrush with machetes, search planes droned overhead, and boats patrolled the river.

Marietta, the parent who usually took charge in crises, managed for a time to keep her composure, reassuring the kids and communicating with authorities and the press.

It was the boats that finally undid her. Two weeks into the ordeal—the family was still living in the campground, now guarded by an FBI command post—she spent an entire day watching as a search boat inched its way down the Madison. Each time the craft halted, the men on board would reel in a net, examine its contents, and let it out again. At every stop the young mother feared that her daughter's body would be the haul.

As anger and panic rose in Marietta, her stomach roiled and a heavy weight seemed to press against her chest. She fought her feelings, terrified that they would become uncontrollable.

But that night everything she'd been holding in boiled into a murderous rage. When she crawled into her sleeping bag, she turned to her husband and said that even if the kidnapper returned Susie unharmed, she would happily kill him with her bare hands.

She lay awake all night. Whenever a car pulled into the campground, she wondered if it was the kidnapper bringing Susie back—or just another tourist snapping pictures of the now-famous tent where the child was abducted. Each time a car drove away, the ensuing silence intensified both her anger and the heaviness in her chest.

Then, near dawn, she heard a voice. Some might call it her conscience; others would say it was the echo of a strict Catholic upbringing. What Marietta heard was God telling her, "I don't want you to feel this way." The admonition resonated: As a child she'd been taught to love her enemies and pray for those who hurt her.

As she pondered the message, the weight of her chest seemed to lift and her stomach relaxed. She fell into the first deep sleep she'd had since Susie vanished.

The next morning nothing had really changed. She still wanted to murder the monster who'd snatched her little girl. But she'd opened the door just a crack to the possibility that revenge wasn't the best course.

This is how forgiveness often starts: not with a rush of compassion but with a weary willingness to try.

That day and the next and the next brought no solid leads. Five weeks after Susie's abduction, the Jaegers reluctantly rolled up their sleeping bags and piloted the van homeward, Marietta now counting four heads after every rest stop instead of five.

Back in their squat cinder-block bungalow on the outskirts of Detroit, Bill sank into silent brooding and began packing a gun wherever he went.

For her part, Marietta recalled the flicker of revelation she'd had by the river. And she remembered relatives who'd died embittered over ancient affronts. The conclusion was obvious: Hatred of the magnitude she was feeling got people nowhere.

She decided that the best thing she could do for herself was to try to forgive. So she would have to make a concerted effort to transform her loathing for the kidnapper into something approaching understanding.

Her project was on her mind as soon as she awoke every day and began preparing breakfast for her family. But the focused effort came on weekday afternoons, in the lull after lunch, when Marietta retreated to her tiny bedroom and sat on the edge of the bed.

For inspiration, she remembered when she was a high school freshman and a nun assailed her in front of the class, saying she had plagiarized a paper. Though humiliated by the false accusation, Marietta believed that retaliation was wrong. So she told herself that the nun was a worthy person at heart and that she must have been hurt to lash out so unfairly at a child.

Contemplating that episode now, Marietta reminded herself that even if he hadn't acted like one, the kidnapper was still a member of the human race and so had intrinsic worth. In the eyes of the God Marietta believed in, the kidnapper was as precious as Susie. The thought was hard to swallow. At this point the exercise was purely mechanical.

To bring about a change of heart, Marietta resolved not to talk about the kidnapper in subhuman terms, no matter how great the temptation. She didn't have to pretend to like him or that he hadn't committed a detestable wrong. But she would have to watch her language.

Everyone from the police to her friends and family spoke of the criminal in invective. Marietta's own parish priest told her, "I hope they fry the son of a bitch." On several occasions Marietta asked acquaintances to please tone down their talk. She sympathized but let them know she was working in a different direction.

In another strategy, Marietta found a way to apply the classic precept "Pray for your enemies." She tried to think of one good thing to wish on the kidnapper. It grated. It was so much easier to want him to hurt as badly as her family did.

A practical hitch was that she knew nothing about him, except that he probably lived in the West. She didn't know his name and had to call him "the man who has Susie." How about wishing "the man who has Susie" clear skies, then? Even criminals must appreciate a fine day. She could try wishing him that.

At first every conjured image rankled and seemed disloyal to Susie. How could Marietta picture good things happening to the man who stole her baby?

Her work became even harder each time a development in the case rekindled her rage, as when a man claiming to have Susie called authorities and talked about ransom, but hung up before he could be identified.

Marietta's wishes came more easily, though, as the weeks passed. One day the kidnapper would find a valued object he'd lost—courtesy of Marietta. In keeping with the western theme, she visualized him catching a prize fish.

In time Marietta recognized the practical wisdom in what she was doing: If the kidnapper had Susie, she wanted her child's temporary caretaker to be content, not miserable and vindictive. If he no longer had Susie—which Marietta realized was a possibility—she wanted him to come forth and confess. This too, Marietta thought, was more likely if the man was not feeling tormented.

So every weekday afternoon she sent Susie's kidnapper wishes for blue skies and dappled trout, until the kids came home from school.

THE RELIEF Marietta Jaeger felt when she focused on compassion for the man who wronged her was more than an imaginary salve. Some of the biggest names in mind-body medicine—Dean Ornish, Carl Simonton, and Bernie Siegel among them—are convinced that forgiveness is essential to physical and emotional well-being. Joan Borysenko, a cancer cell biologist and a pioneer in studying how emotions affect the body, goes so far as to say that forgiveness is the mind's most powerful healing tool.

At Harvard Medical School in the 1980s, Borysenko operated one of the country's first mind-body clinics. Patients suffering from all manner of stubborn illnesses found their way to her, ready to spend ten weeks trying therapies like meditation and yoga.

One such patient, whom Borysenko calls George, was a Jewish man who suffered from bleeding ulcers and insomnia. In getting to know George, she found he had cut off contact with his daughter Rachel because she'd married a non-Jew against his wishes. When George practiced meditation, his mind, rather than quieting down, raged at Rachel.

After seeing many patients like George, Borysenko had an epiphany. "I realized that when people are filled with resentments, that amounts to chronic stress," she says. "When you have a stress-related illness and you're subjecting yourself to constant stress, it's very difficult to heal."

So she began teaching people to forgive. But first she had to correct some misconceptions. Forgiveness, she told her patients, is not a shortcut around anger; it's a way to move on once anger has subsided and to avoid getting mired in resentment. Nor does forgiveness require inviting a wrongdoer back into your life.

Instead, the operative words are *give* and *gift*. You are giving a gift of acceptance to someone, whether that person deserves it or not. Doing this runs counter to instinct, Borysenko says, but the effort mends minds and eases pain.

When George started working to recall the things he once loved about his daughter, his symptoms lessened. In fact, Borysenko says that every patient at the clinic who could move away from resentment improved both mentally and physically.

Though the scientific study of forgiveness is still in its infancy, findings so far confirm the benefits Borysenko and others have observed. In a study at the University of Northern Iowa, psychologist Suzanne Freedman worked with 12 incest survivors. After 14 months only the six who'd been taught forgiveness techniques had become less depressed and anxious. Similar studies—of college students with negligent parents, elderly people harboring old grudges, and men angry at their partners for having an abortion—show that those who forgive have lower levels of anxiety, higher self-esteem, and better emotional health than those who don't.

"I'm continually surprised by the strong results we get," says Robert Enright, a psychologist at the University of Wisconsin at Madison who studies forgiveness. "There's something to this that people ought to know about."

A 1990 Taiwanese study by Enright and Tina Huang was the first to suggest that the forgiveness-health link goes beyond emotional healing. Among a group of women struggling to forgive hurts such as betrayal by a friend or coworker, those who were able to get rid of their grudges showed fewer spikes in blood pressure when they retold their stories.

Forgiveness as a means to emotional recovery makes intuitive sense. But why should letting go of bitterness improve physical health? One answer lies in the plentiful research showing hostility to be a major risk factor for coronary artery disease.

The crushing weight Marietta Jaeger felt in her chest reflects what was presumably happening in her body as her fury grew. Adrenaline sped into her bloodstream, raising her pulse and blood pressure. Her arteries narrowed, and the blood surged through her heart.

Such short bursts of rage are unlikely to harm a healthy young heart like Marietta's. But if Marietta were to stoke her anger again and again over the course of months or years, the pounding blood could erode minuscule portions of her coronary artery walls. Platelets in her blood would clump to fill the abrasions. Over time plaque could accumulate in the damaged areas, leading to coronary artery disease.

As yet no one has studied what happens in the arteries when people release their rancor. But it's reasonable to assume, Borysenko says, that forgiveness, by providing an antidote to anger, may interrupt the heart-damaging process.

ONE YEAR TO THE MINUTE after Susie was snatched from her tent, and nearly a year after Marietta began the laborious process of trying to forgive, the Jaegers' phone rang in the middle of the night.

Marietta sprinted toward the kitchen in the dark and banged her toes on a stool the kids had left in the way. Hopping forward on her good foot, she switched on the tape recorder attached to the phone by the FBI, then grabbed the receiver.

"Is this Susie's mom?" the caller asked. "I'm the guy that took her from you."

Marietta's voice came through the wires so relaxed it was as if she was accustomed to chatting with kidnappers every night at this hour. She didn't gasp, weep, threaten, beg, or scream.

The man said that he'd read a newspaper interview in which Marietta said she wished she could talk to the kidnapper. Now, by the tone of his voice, Marietta could tell he was calling to taunt her for the notion. But he hadn't counted on the homework she had been doing every day after lunch.

When she heard the man's voice, mocking though it was, she realized something had genuinely shifted in her. She was still desperate for word of Susie, but her efforts at the edge of her bed had allowed her to see this man as something other than evil personified. Yes, he had done something vile. As a result, her child was in dire trouble. Yet the man was someone else's beloved child, and he too was in trouble. The compassion she felt for him came through in her voice.

She asked evenly whether Susie was alive and whether he had hurt her. The caller assured her that Susie was fine and that he'd only hurt her "a little" that first night when he had to choke her to keep her from crying out.

Why did he choose the Jaegers' tent? He said he had crouched outside and listened to Heidi and Susie whispering late that night. Then he waited two hours until they were sound asleep before slitting the side of the tent.

As he talked Marietta could hear the clicks of the FBI tracer on the line; she knew the caller must be hearing the interference, too. But every time he became anxious and said he had to hang up, Marietta gently drew him in again.

"Can we have her back?" Marietta asked.
"I'm kind of in an awkward position to do that," he said. "I've gotten used to her."
"Why did you take her?"
He stammered for a moment, then said, "I've always wanted a little girl of my own." Click. Click. Click.

The caller was weakening, responding to Marietta's concerned tone by staying on the line far longer than was safe for him. But what finally brought down his defenses was when she asked with total sincerity, "What can we do to help you?"

There was a brief silence. Marietta realized the kidnapper was crying. "I wish I knew the answer to that," he said.

The conversation, miraculously, lasted more than an hour, but the tracer malfunctioned and located the caller in Sarasota, Florida: a dead end. Then the FBI matched a voiceprint of the anniversary call with a call to a suspect in a murder case in the same region: David Meirhofer, a popular baby-sitter living in the small town of Manhattan, Montana.

On the strength of that evidence, the FBI took out a search warrant for an abandoned ranch near Meirhofer's home. More than 1,000 bone fragments discovered at the site were shipped to the Smithsonian for analysis. The lab work showed one fragment to be the backbone of a young girl.

When Meirhofer was arrested, he confessed that he had murdered Susie Jaeger about a week after kidnapping her. He also admitted to having killed a teenage girl and two young boys. Marietta's ability to forgive had almost certainly saved lives. Meirhofer was a suspect in other unsolved murders and had attempted still another abduction from a Girl Scout camp before he was caught.

Hours after his confession Meirhofer committed suicide. He was buried near Three Forks, not far from the place where the Jaegers had Susie's remains laid to rest.

In the years that followed, Bill Jaeger continued to seethe over the family's agonizing loss. He developed bleeding ulcers and heart problems, and in 1987 he collapsed on the kitchen floor, dead of a heart attack at 56.

His wife, on the other hand, held to the course she'd embarked on beside the Missouri headwaters. Today a grandmother of seven, Marietta emanates energy and goodwill as she travels around the country giving workshops on forgiveness. People come to her with grievances large and small; she tries to show them how the steps she followed can help them.

"If anyone thinks forgiveness is for wimps, they haven't tried it," she tells audiences. "It takes daily, diligent discipline."

Her listeners protest that surely she must still get mad—say, on Susie's birthday? "No," she says. "I still grieve and I will always grieve at the horrible things Susie had to endure. But she's not in that place of suffering now, and I have absolutely no anger or hatred toward David."

In recent years Marietta has befriended Meirhofer's mother, 71-year-old Eleanor Huckert. Several years ago Marietta made a return trip to Montana, and she and Huckert went together to visit the graves of their children.

Afterward the two mothers sat at the Huckerts' dining room table, sipping coffee and thumbing through old scrapbooks. There was David on the front porch—a rosy-cheeked little boy, scrubbed and eager to set out for his first day of school. There were Mother's Day cards and other tokens of affection from a son Huckert described as doting.

As she studied the smiling boy in the snapshot, Marietta felt that her struggle to invest the faceless criminal with humanity was complete. More important, Marietta realized that her homework had been worthwhile.

"If you remain vindictive, you give the offender another victim," she says. "Anger, hatred, and resentment would have taken my life as surely as Susie's life was taken."

Ann Japenga is a contributing editor.

Bad Mood Rising

Without notice or an obvious reason, a bad mood can eclipse even the sunniest of personalities

By Mary Roach

I am NOT in a bad mood. Just because the guy at the pharmacy had the nerve to tell me my plan doesn't cover birth control pills when I've got a pamphlet RIGHT HERE saying that it does, just because the dry cleaner wants $18 to clean a simple white dress, just because the back steps smell like cat pee and taxes are unjust and my jeans don't fit right does NOT mean I'm in a bad mood. Does it?

Hard to say. A bad mood arrives unannounced. Like garlic breath or spinach between the teeth, you don't know it's there till someone else point it out. And you don't blame mood for how you're feeling, you blame the world. You feel you're justified in your rage, that anyone would be raging if they were having the sort of morning you're having.

When in fact you're having a perfectly ordinary morning. The pharmacist was right: The coverage starts at the end of the month. The white dress is, after all, a wedding dress. The back steps have always smelled like cat pee, and no one's jeans since the dawn of time have ever fit them right. The only thing that's different this morning, for whatever reason, is that you're viewing the world through the ugly, crooked spectacles of ill humor, through rattlesnake venom and rust and clotted milk.

Luckily for me, I have a mood barometer in my kitchen. It's a 6-inch chrome rod that looks like a faucet

When I hear myself blaming faulty kitchen appliances for the downfall of society, I know it's time to figure out what's really going on.

handle, which, in fact, it is. My faucet gives the impression of being infinitely adjustable, yet it dispenses only two temperatures: scalding and cold. Most days, it is what it is: a minor annoyance. But if I'm in a bad mood, it is the very incarnation of shoddy craftsmanship and capitalist greed, of spousal procrastination and what's wrong with the world. When I hear myself blaming faulty kitchen appliances for the downfall of civilized society, I know it's time to figure out what's really going on.

Which shouldn't be all that hard. I write about health for a living. I know about all manner of physiological and psychological phenomena that affect a person's mood. It could be simply the time of day. Our most vulnerable times are said to be 4 p.m. and 9 p.m. to 11 p.m., says psychologist Robert E. Thayer, Ph.D., author of *The Origin of Everyday Moods* (see box "Anatomy of a Bad Mood"). Skipping meals can put you in a funk, as can a bad night's sleep. Sometimes it's hormones. Sometimes it's too much time alone in the office; studies show a strong link between social activity and mood. It could even be the weather: There are studies that link rainstorms—more specifically, the negative ions they create—to good moods, and warm dry winds to bad ones.

So I think about what might be causing my funk. More often than not, I'm forced to conclude that I am simply a moody person. Which makes me think about how pathetic I am for falling prey to my moods and not rising above them. My own lacking character takes its place alongside the pharmacist and the neighbor's cat and capitalist greed, and I end up feeling even worse.

It's a downward spiral. A bad mood poisons the rest of your character. It KOs your joie de vivre, deep-sixes your Sealy Posturpedic morning. It's all you

Anatomy of a Bad Mood

IT'S TRUE THAT EVERYTHING FROM PMS TO WEATHER TO LACK OF EXERCISE can cause a bad mood. But on a day-to-day basis, our moods can be attributed to a much simpler equation: a combination of our energy and tension levels. So claims Robert E. Thayer, Ph.D., professor of psychology at California State University at Long Beach and author of *The Origin of Everyday Moods* (Oxford Press, 1997).

In his book, Thayer describes the connection between the two. The first factor, our circadian rhythm, is a natural cycle of energy that goes something like this: Our energy levels tend to rise steadily from the time we awake until they reach their highest levels, around noon or 1 p.m.; they drop in the midafternoon to late afternoon, reach a subpeak in the early evening, and decline until sleep. A low energy level is generally associated with a negative mood; a high energy level, with a better mood.

But it's only when a low energy time coincides with what Thayer calls a "tense-tired" state—a mixture of fatigue with nervousness, tension, or anxiety—that you have the recipe for a truly foul mood. Case in point: Thayer did an experiment in which participants rated their energy and tension levels at five specific times each day for 10 days. Each subject had a personal problem that was bothering him or her, and each was asked to rate how serious the problem appeared at those times. What did he find? Problems were rated as more serious later in the day and when the person was in a tense-tired mood.

So how does this info help the perpetually perturbed? By charting your rhythm, you can manage your funks, says Thayer. Start by rating your energy level on a five-point scale (from "extremely" to "not at all") every hour during waking hours for three days. By doing so, you'll find your high- and low-energy times, enabling you to schedule activities around them. For instance, you can steer clear of heated situations during low-energy times so they don't appear worse. —*Victoria Parker*

---

can do to sit upright on the couch. You don't feel like doing anything. How can you? You're too busy reviewing the things that are wrong with the world, all the ways you have been mistreated and misunderstood in the past. For as long as it lasts, a bad mood is a fulltime job. So you don't do the dishes. You don't write a thank you note to your aunt and uncle who sent you a garden tablecloth for a wedding present when you don't even have a garden table, let alone a garden or even a backyard, thank you very much. Soon you feel guilty and lazy on top of grouchy, pissy, and exasperated. Self-loathing sets in, followed by self-pity, tears, another nap.

There is, of course, a simple and effective cure for the soured mood, and that's a walk. Indeed, it is the easiest thing in the world to walk away from a foul mood. A study by Thayer showed that the energizing effects of a 10-minute walk are still noticeable an hour later. In fact, I should get up right now and go for a walk. But unfortunately, I can't. I've lost my sunglasses, and it's too bright out there, and all the squinting I do has already given me wrinkles on my brow, and did I mention how much the dry cleaner wants to clean one simple little satin dress . . .

Mary Roach is a freelance writer living in San Francisco

Unit 3

Unit Selections

11. **Tall Tales from the Table,** Bill Gottlieb
12. **The Bitter Truth,** Linda Formichelli
13. **Are You Getting Enough Fat?** Colleen Pierre
14. **Bulking Up Fiber's Healthful Reputation,** Ruth Papazian
15. **The Vitamin Revolution: B D E,** Harriet A. Washington

Key Points to Consider

- Given the controversies that abound in the area of nutrition, what guidelines should an individual use to make dietary decisions?

- What advice would you give to someone regarding the issue of reducing dietary fat?

- What advice would you give someone who is considering making significant dietary changes?

- What dietary changes could you make to improve your diet? What is keeping you from making those changes?

- How would you advise someone who was considering using dietary supplements?

- What recommendations would you give regarding the inclusion of dietary fiber in one's diet?

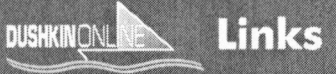 **Links** www.dushkin.com/online/

11. **University of Pennsylvania Library**
    http://www.library.upenn.edu/resources/websitest.html
12. **University of Pennsylvania School of Medicine Nutrition Education and Prevention Program**
    http://www.med.upenn.edu/~nutrimed/
13. **U.S. Department of Agriculture (USDAI)/Food and Nutrition Information Center (FNIC)**
    http://www.nal.usda.gov/fnic/
14. **Vegetarian Pages**
    http://www.veg.org/veg/

These sites are annotated on pages 4 and 5.

Nutritional Health

Compared to the sciences of biology, chemistry, and physics, nutritional science is still in its infancy and many unanswered questions remain. This unit will provide the most current information available on topics ranging from common nutritional myths and fallacies to a discussion on why some people hate the taste of vegetables.

For years, the majority of Americans paid little attention to nutrition, other than to eat three meals a day and, perhaps, take a vitamin supplement. While this dietary style was generally adequate for the prevention of major nutritional deficiencies, medical evidence began to accumulate linking the American diet to a variety of chronic illnesses. The most ominous link between diet and disease involves dietary fat and coronary heart disease. Current recommendations suggest that the types of fats consumed may play a much greater role in disease processes than the total amount of fat consumed. "Are You Getting Enough Fat?" examines this issue and suggests that we may actually be healthier if we increased our intake of both monounsaturated fats (olive and canola oils) and omega-3 fatty acids (fish oil). Evidence is mounting that we have overreacted to the dietary fat issue.

One of the most obvious manifestations of our fat phobia is the high consumer demand for reduced-fat snack foods. The food industry has responded to this demand by introducing low-fat versions of many of the most popular snack foods. Many of these low-fat versions may have just about as many calories as the original products. Our aversion to fat has become so pervasive that we have come to equate the healthfulness of foods based on fat content alone. A prime example of this way of thinking is our attitude regarding nuts. While nuts are high in fat, researchers have found that the types of fats they contain (monounsaturated) may actually reduce LDL (Low Density Lipoproteins) and help to reduce one's risk of heart disease. Although nuts are relatively high in calories, researchers have found that people who tend to snack on nuts feel more satisfied and are less likely to overeat later. "Tall Tales from the Table" addresses this issue regarding nuts and nine other common misconceptions that people have regarding foods.

While fats have increasingly come under fire as a source of health problems, carbohydrates have been given high ratings for health. Nutritionists generally agree that Americans should eat more complex carbohydrates, particularly those that come from fruits, vegetables, whole grains, and cereals. Carbohydrates in this form are a good source of vitamins, minerals, and fiber.

While there may be several factors that influence our eating patterns, one in particular stands out and that is our sense of taste. Recent studies have found that many vegetables have a slightly bitter taste and some individuals are particularly sensitive to this taste. "The Bitter Truth" examines the issue of taste sensitivity and suggests ways in which vegetables can be prepared to mask or reduce the bitter taste.

Over the past few years, dietary fiber has become a hot issue in dietary circles. Several studies reported that individuals who had been eating high-fiber diets demonstrated a lower incidence of colon cancer and lower blood cholesterol levels. While individuals who ate high-fiber diets did have lower rates of both colon cancer and cardiovascular disease, these health benefits could also be explained by the fact that these individuals would naturally eat less foods high in dietary fat. Another variable is the fact that most of the foods that are high in dietary fiber are also high in other important nutrients, including the much-touted antioxidant vitamins. "Bulking Up Fiber's Healthful Reputation" examines the claimed benefits of a high-fiber diet.

The use of dietary supplements is another highly controversial topic. Today, approximately 33 percent of Americans take some form of dietary supplement regularly. The National Academy of Sciences (NAS) provides the consumer with Recommended Daily Allowances (RDAs) of vitamins. Critics contend that RDAs should be raised to levels that would maximize health rather than merely prevent deficiencies. Over the last couple of years, vegetables that include broccoli, brussels sprouts, cabbage, and cauliflower have received publicity because they appear to contain potent anticancer compounds. The net result of all the hype and publicity is a new megavitamin craze in which supplement makers are claiming to pack several servings worth of these vegetables in a single pill. Most experts agree that the best route to good nutrition is eating a well-balanced diet, but evidence is mounting that this alone may not guarantee that you are getting enough of certain vitamins to achieve optimal health. "The Vitamin Revolution: B D E" discusses why a balanced diet alone may not provide you with enough of these vitamins.

Article 11

TALL Tales from the TABLE

BY **BILL GOTTLIEB**

IN ANCIENT NORSE MYTHOLOGY Ymir the four-mouthed giant got his daily servings of dairy foods directly from the four udders of Audhumla the cow; she, meanwhile, ate nothing but frost. In modern America your friends and relatives put their faith in myths about food that are every bit as far-fetched. Anyone who swallows these ten whoppers is risking health problems as varied as food poisoning, colon cancer, osteoporosis, and heart disease, not to mention a waist bigger than Ymir's. Are you clinging to outdated doctrines?

1
Store-Bought Salad Mix Doesn't Need to be Washed

SORRY. Innocent-looking greens have been known to harbor *Escherichia coli* 0157:H7, a bacterium with a seriously bad attitude. Eat something tainted with this E. coli strain, and you'll be grateful to live to regret it. Children, elderly people, and anyone with a weak immune system can die from the infection. For the rest of us, symptoms commonly include at least a week of abdominal cramps and severe diarrhea.

Undercooked hamburger has been to blame in most cases, but that's changing. "Fresh vegetables are becoming an increasingly important source," says Fritz Käferstein of the World Health Organization. Case in point: In July 1995, 70 people in western Montana got sick after eating E. coli–contaminated lettuce. Two months later lettuce laced with the same bug infected 30 people at a Boy Scout retreat in Maine. More recently a batch of organic mixed greens grown in California sickened 61 people in Illinois, Connecticut, and New York.

How can you be safe? Look for prepackaged greens with a national brand name, such as Fresh Express, Salad Time, Dole Classic Salads, and Ready Pac Produce. "These products do not have to be washed again to remove E. coli," says Sandra Bastin, a food and nutrition specialist at the University of Kentucky in Lexington. "They have been washed thoroughly and expertly by the food manufacturer—far better than you could do at home."

If there's no big name on the product, you do need to wash it—in cold running water. Don't be fooled by words like *fresh, natural,* and *organic*. The California greens responsible for the recent

What you don't know about

outbreak were grown organically.

Also check the "use by" date on the package. "The produce may look okay after that date," says Sue Snider, a food and nutrition specialist at the University of Delaware, "but I would be very cautious about using it." That's because a bacterial time bomb may be ticking away on some produce. Many bugs are harmless in small amounts but can multiply—and cause food poisoning—after the stamped date.

2 Sweets Are a Good Pick-Me-Up

NO SUCH LUCK. People will swear that a candy bar or piece of chocolate instantly gives them an energy lift, albeit one that's inevitably followed by a crash. It's folklore. "Neither the rise nor the fall happens," says Kristine Clark, director of sports nutrition at Penn State University. Most sweets contain not only carbohydrates, which the body can use quickly, but also fat and protein, which slow the carbs' absorption. "What you get is a slow rise in blood sugar," says Clark.

What about a can of cola or a glass of juice? If you haven't eaten all day and your blood sugar is extremely low, that more-or-less straight dose of sugar can give you a boost. But such rock-bottom blood sugar is rare, says Ann Grandjean, director of the International Center for Sports Nutrition in Omaha, Nebraska. If you're sure the need is real, Clark says, pop jelly beans or hard candies, or grab a glucose polymer sports gel.

The real key to sustained energy in work or play, however, is eating well at every meal, day in and day out. "I exercise every day," says Clark, "and I never eat or drink anything with calories during my workout because my overall diet meets my energy needs."

3 Many People Shouldn't Eat Dairy Foods

NOTHING DOING. It's true that dairy products contain a sugar called lactose and that about 75 percent of the people on earth don't make enough lactase, the enzyme that breaks down this sugar. The resulting condition, called lactose intolerance, is signaled by bloating, cramping, gas, and even diarrhea.

But no one has to suffer from lactose intolerance, says Dennis Savaiano, a professor of foods and nutrition and dean of Purdue University's school of consumer and family sciences. You can easily train your intestines to deal comfortably with dairy, he says. How? Gradually introduce milk into your diet. Drink a third to a half cup with each meal for one week, then bump it up to two cups the next week. In his research Savaiano found this painless two-week adjustment turned "maldigesters"—people who were supposedly lactose intolerant—into "digesters." From then on they could eat as much or as little dairy as they wanted.

There are other ways to make your digestive tract more receptive to milk. Eat yogurt. The fermentation that turns milk into yogurt generates lactase; eating yogurt ups the amount of lactose your body can digest. (Most frozen yogurt won't do the trick, however.) Or drink nonfat chocolate milk; the cocoa slows digestion so intestinal bacteria have more time to break down the lactose.

Savaiano says any maldigester who follows these tips will extinguish her symptoms. And it's worth trying. Avoiding dairy foods is a particularly bad idea for women, who need plenty of calcium to protect their bones from osteoporosis. If you try Savaiano's method and still have digestive problems, you may have irritable bowel syndrome or some other condition, and should see your doctor.

4 Beef Is Bad for Your Heart

NOT SO FAST. For years ranchers and food scientists have been working to breed leaner cattle. And they've succeeded. Today the leanest cuts—top round, eye of round, round steak, sirloin, flank steak, tip roast, porterhouse, T-bone, and tenderloin—can pack as little artery-clogging saturated fat as chicken and turkey. This better beef still delivers five crucial B vitamins, including B-12, which you can't get from plants. Plus, it's loaded with zinc and iron.

So go ahead and enjoy lean beef (burgers are too fatty to qualify). Nutrition specialist Bastin says a few times a week is fine. Just keep each serving under three ounces, a portion about the size of your palm or a deck of cards.

5 Nuts Have Too Much Fat to Be a Healthy Snack

OH YEAH? Tell that to the 26 people studied by Gene Spiller, director of the Health Research and Studies Center in Los Altos, California. When he added three ounces of almonds to their daily diet, their fat intake rose from 67 to 90 grams a day, with 37 percent of their total calories from fat—higher than the recommended 30 percent. But their average LDL cholesterol—the kind linked to heart disease—fell from 154 to 133, reducing their odds of a fatal heart attack by 10 percent. Other studies have confirmed these findings.

Spiller attributes the drop in LDL cholesterol to the almonds' heart-protecting monounsaturated fat. Peanuts, hazelnuts, pistachios, macadamias, cashews, and pine nuts are also rich in monounsaturates. A handful or two a day (up to an ounce) can help. And the extra fat won't mean extra pounds, Spiller says. Munching nuts as a morning or afternoon snack helps people feel satisfied—and less inclined to overeat later.

6 The Lower the Fat, the Healthier the Diet

NOT SO. If you eat a very low fat diet—getting less than 20 percent of your calories from fat—you can set off health problems, says John Foreyt, director of the nutrition research clinic at Baylor College of Medicine in Houston. Fat-stripped diets are typically loaded with starches and refined sugars. Overdosing on these carbohydrates can raise your level of triglycerides, a blood fat linked to heart disease and stroke.

The best idea, says Foreyt, is to aim for balance, variety, and moderation. Get about 50 percent of your calories from carbohydrates in fruits, vegetables, and whole grains; about 20 percent from protein in lean meats, poultry, and fish; and not more than 30 percent from fat.

That said, some people with diagnosed heart disease have actually seen their narrowed arteries reopen after they adopted vegetarian diets with as little as 10 percent of daily calories from fat. But such meal plans can be tough to follow (even olive oil on salads is banned), and many experts remain worried that high triglycerides will result.

7. Brown Bread Is Always a Smarter Choice Than White

AS IF. A lot of brown bread sold in supermarkets is nothing more than white bread with a fake tan. "Brown bread can look like whole wheat bread because caramel coloring is added to it. But it isn't whole wheat," says Joan Salge Blake, an assistant professor at Boston University's Sargent College of Health Sciences.

What is it? Well, it's been made with either white flour (from which the wheat kernel's bran, germ, and husk have been removed) or so-called wheat flour (75 percent white, 25 percent whole wheat).

How can you know the true colors of a loaf on the shelf? Read the label. Whole wheat should be the first ingredient and only type of flour in the bread.

Why favor whole wheat? In a word, fiber. That's roughage, or the indigestible part of food that can help prevent or treat a range of ills: digestive problems, diabetes, obesity, even colon cancer. A slice of whole wheat bread delivers about two grams of fiber; a slice of white bread, maybe a gram. That means two slices of whole wheat toast in the morning and a sandwich made with whole wheat bread at lunch would give you eight grams of fiber—more than a third of the recommended daily minimum.

8. Giving In to Cravings Is a Sure Way to Gain Weight

THINK AGAIN. For many people *resisting* what they want is the problem, says Kelly Brownell, a psychologist at Yale University and a leading expert on weight loss. This type of person adopts a rigid diet, swearing off the "bad" foods she craves.

But that rigidity makes self-control even more difficult, and the dieter inevitably eats the forbidden treats—and feels guilty and ashamed. Those negative feelings trigger more eating. The person then tries even harder not to give in, and the dismal cycle continues.

The solution if you're stuck in this pattern, says Brownell, is to enjoy the foods you crave in moderation. Don't force yourself to choose between no ice cream and the entire quart; have a small scoop or so. Rather than the whole box of cookies, eat one or two. By allowing yourself the treat, you won't feel restricted, and you'll find it much easier to stick with your eating plan.

For other people, however, sampling foods that are high in fat and sugar, like ice cream, or high in fat and salt, like potato chips, always leads them to eat more and more.

There's hope even then, Brownell says. "If your weight-control psychology is positive rather than negative—if your goal is to eat healthfully rather than depriving yourself of foods you love—you'll have the best chance of losing weight and keeping it off."

9. Bottled Water Is Safer Than Tap Water

IT MERELY SEEMS THAT WAY. In fact, when it comes to purity, tap water may be a better bet. Municipal water supplies are tested every day for disease-causing microbes and chemical contaminants. Bottled water, which is regulated by the Food and Drug Administration rather than the Environmental Protection Agency, may or may not be tested, ever.

Besides, many people who drink water from bottles *are* drinking tap water. According to the American Dietetic Association, 85 percent of bottled water is municipal water. That's right: Some bottlers take city water, filter out any local taste and odor, slap a price on it, and let you spring for it. What's more, a lot of bottled water has no fluoride, an additive that impedes tooth decay.

But isn't bottled water safer because it's free of chlorine? Don't chlorination and its by-products raise cancer risk?

While it's true that the antibacterial chemical is added to virtually all municipal water supplies, you can quit worrying, says Bruce Ames, a molecular and cell biologist at the University of California at Berkeley and a leading expert on cancer-causing substances. "The amounts in tap water appear far too small." You get far more potential carcinogens in a cup of coffee, he says, and no one's uncovered any evidence that coffee causes cancer. "I drink tap water," Ames says. "You can really help prevent cancer by not smoking and by eating a diet rich in cell-protecting fruits and vegetables."

10. Everyone Should Eat Three Square Meals a Day

IT AIN'T NECESSARILY SO. Three midsize meals a day suit most people. But five or six little ones—what nutritionists are calling mini-meals—may be a better plan for many others, says Evette Hackman, an associate professor of food and nutrition at Seattle Pacific University.

Someone trying to lose weight might find that eating smaller, more frequent meals keeps her from overindulging at lunch and dinner. Small meals every few hours may help a person with diabetes control her blood sugar levels. They can also help keep heartburn at bay.

What would a typical day's mini-meals look like? For breakfast you might have a glass of fruit juice and a low-fat muffin with low-fat cream cheese (total: 300 calories). For your midmorning snack, a slice of bread with peanut butter and a piece of fruit (another 300). For lunch, a bowl of soup and a turkey sandwich on whole wheat bread (400). In the afternoon, a handful of sliced vegetables and some crackers with a low-fat dip (300).

For dinner you could have three ounces of lean meat, a side dish of broccoli, a small serving of pasta with tomato sauce, and a small salad (400). An evening snack could be one cup of nonfat yogurt with fresh fruit (300). Grand total: 2,000 calories, about what's right for an active 135-pound woman.

Bill Gottlieb is coauthor of The Doctors Book of Preventive Home Remedies, *which will be published by Rodale Press later this year.*

The Bitter Truth

Find out if you're a supertaster—someone whose taste buds say yuck to vegetables. If that's you, here are ways to get your RDA.

By Linda Formichelli

For as long as I can remember, the point has been driven home to me: "Eat your vegetables. They're good for you." Just how good is becoming more and more apparent, what with all the studies and news reports showing how they protect us against everything from cancer to heart attacks. I know that vegetables are our friends. So why do I find them so vile?

There, I've said it, for bitter or worse. But I'm not alone in my feelings. Vegetable haters are everywhere... our numbers are legion. No matter how much we hear about veggies' disease-fighting power, we just can't overcome our dislike enough to take advantage of all the nutritional benefits they deliver.

People who don't like vegetables are often dismissed as picky eaters. And if you are one, you know what I mean. "Not liking vegetables has really been a burden," says Kate de Fuccio, a graduate student at the University of Michigan. "People will literally tease me. It becomes a control issue where they think they can 'fix' me and try to force vegetables on me."

But there may be more to a dislike of veggies than being picky. Recent research has uncovered a group of people called supertasters who are genetically sensitive to bitterness. Like color-seeing people in a color-blind world, veggie haters may actually taste flavors that veggie lovers don't.

Until the late 1970s, taste researchers grouped people as "tasters" or "nontasters," depending on their ability to taste a chemical called phenylthiocarbamide. Then Linda Bartoshuk, Ph.D., a taste researcher at the Yale University School of Medicine, began to test people for sensitivity to a similar chemical, called 6-n-propylthiouracil. Her research revealed a subset of tasters who were particularly sensitive to the bitter flavor. She dubbed such people "supertasters." About 25% of the population are supertasters, 25% nontasters, and the rest regular tasters. Almost two-thirds of supertasters are women, and Asians and African-Americans tend to be more sensitive than Caucasians.

> **Like color-seeing people in a color-blind world, veggie haters may actually taste flavors that veggie lovers don't.**

As luck would have it, the compounds that give vegetables their health benefits also happen to be—you guessed it—bitter. Does this mean that supertasters' acute sensitivity cause them to shun veggies? To find out, Adam Drewnowski, Ph.D., director of the nutrition program at the University of Michigan at Ann Arbor, tested subjects using the bitter grapefruit. He found that supertasters tend more than tasters and nontasters not to like grapefruit because of the bitter cancer-preventive agent naringin. "The results showed that supertaster status does alter preferences," says Drewnowski.

Veggies may be bitter, but their benefits are sweet. According to The American Dietetic Association, vegetables contain compounds that help prevent and reduce cancer and heart disease,

3 ❖ NUTRITIONAL HEALTH

and fiber that speeds toxins through the digestive tract before they can do harm. The compounds that make veggies cancer-fighting powerhouses are called phytochemicals. "We think there are thousands of phytochemicals, but only a fraction of them have been discovered," says Melanie Polk, R.D., director of nutrition education at the American Institute for Cancer Research. Vegetables contain so many still-undiscovered phytochemicals that no food supplement or vitamin can take the place of a variety of fresh fruits and vegetables in the diet.

But don't let the bitter taste of veggies keep you from your five a day. We talked with nutritionists and taste researchers to find out what you can do to take the bitter edge off of your veggies.

Sometimes fat is good. Especially if it helps you eat more veggies. According to Paul Breslin, Ph.D., an assistant member at the Monell Chemical Senses Center in Philadelphia, some bitter compounds are lipophilic, meaning they readily dissolve in fat. So it's possible that putting a little fat in the form of a cheese sauce or creamy salad dressing on vegetables will suppress the bitter taste.

Sprinkle them with sugar. Last year the British Cancer Research Campaign, in conjunction with a major frozen-food chain, launched a new line of flavored foods—including chocolate-covered vegetables—in hopes of getting kids to eat their greens. Granted, chocolate-dipped greens may be going a bit too far, but the idea behind it is valid. If you find veggies too bitter, try going the Mary Poppins route and look for recipes that call for a spoonful of sugar.

Shake on some salt. Ever notice how your favorite chocolate recipe contains salt, or how salted cantaloupe tastes sweeter? Breslin says that salt blocks bitter flavors (such as the naturally sharp flavor of chocolate) and acts as a filter that lets more desirable flavors shine through. Lightly dusting your veggies with salt may make them more palatable.

Heat them up. If the bitterness of raw vegetables makes you skimp on greens, try microwaving, steaming, or stir-frying them instead. The process of heating them up helps dull the bite. "Chinese people tend to be sensitive to bitterness, but they eat a lot of vegetables," says Drewnowski. "How? They stir-fry them."

Hide them away. Maybe Mom had the right idea hiding veggies in the meatloaf. If you really can't stomach the taste of vegetables, the best thing might be to mask their flavor with other foods. "You can chop vegetables up really small and hide them in other things, such as a casserole or an omelet," suggests Polk. "Or try pureeing vegetables in a soup. The flavors meld very nicely, and you won't taste the vegetables as much."

Other ideas that take advantage of this principle: Try zucchini or carrot bread, grate carrots into hamburgers or tomato sauce, or toss bits of chopped vegetables into macaroni or potato salad from the deli.

You've tried all these suggestions, but still can't bear veggies? Take heart. As vegetables' popularity grows, more types of veggies are becoming available in the local supermarket—some of which may be more palatable than others. If you don't like the tangy green bell pepper, you can try its sweeter red, yellow, or orange counterparts. Have you ever tried celeriac? Or salsify? You may find yourself pleasantly surprised.

Whatever you do, don't give up on the health benefits of veggies for good. As we grow older, our sense of taste tends to become duller—no wonder kids are the most passionate veggie haters of all. So the vegetable you found bitter a few years ago might be a palate-pleaser today. "Please pass the brussels sprouts." It could happen.

Linda Formichelli is a freelance writer who lives in Attleboro, Mass.

The Supertaster Test

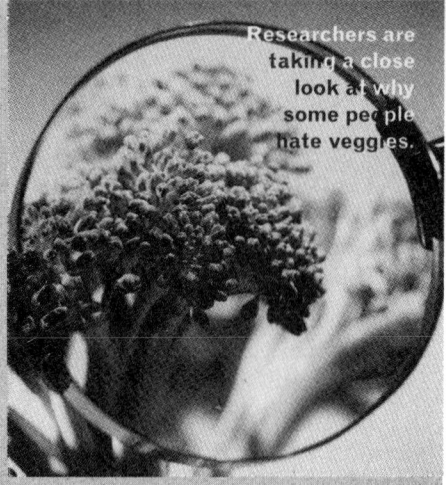

Researchers are taking a close look at why some people hate veggies.

THIS TEST SOUNDS STRANGE, but it works. Put a gummed reinforcer ring (the kind you use on loose-leaf paper) on your tongue with one edge touching in the middle of your tongue and the other edge touching the side. Use a cotton swab to dab blue food coloring in the center of the ring. Remove the ring and, using a magnifying glass, count the pink circles on the blue background. These rings are called fungiform papillae, and they correspond to the number of taste buds. If there are more than 30 circles in the ring, you're a supertaster; between five and 10, you're a nontaster; and anywhere in between, you're a regular taster. —*L.F.*

Supertaster Sauce

WITH ITS HEADY INDIAN SPICES and sweetness, this dressing can cut the bitterness in vegetables. Drizzle on steamed broccoli, cauliflower, brussels sprouts, or carrots.

- ¼ cup olive oil
- ¼ cup pineapple juice
- 2 Tbs. plain nonfat yogurt
- 1½ tsp. curry powder
- ½ tsp. dry mustard
- ¼ tsp. salt
- ⅛ tsp. cayenne pepper

In a small bowl, combine all the ingredients and whisk until emulsified. Makes ½ cup, enough to lightly coat 4 cups chopped vegetables (4 to 6 servings). —*Camela Zarcone*

Are You Getting Enough Fat?

Eating a little fat will make you feel a lot fuller.

AFTER A DECADE IN WHICH EVERYONE FRETTED OVER FAT GRAMS, NEW RESEARCH SHOWS THAT SOME TYPES OF THE MUCH MALIGNED STUFF CAN PROTECT AGAINST HEART DISEASE, CANCER AND STROKE. AND A LITTLE OF THIS FORMERLY FORBIDDEN PLEASURE GOES A LONG WAY

BY COLLEEN PIERRE, R.D.

In my nutrition counseling office, I see a constant parade of women trying to cut most of the fat from their diet. Many think 10 or 20 grams of fat a day is plenty; a few won't tolerate a single gram. They're proud of themselves and their "healthy" diets. When I break the news that they need to eat *more* fat, they turn pale. They are terrified of fat and don't know how to manage it in their diet without managing it right out.

Sound familiar? The American Dietetic Association's 1997 trends survey shows that 13% of adults believe they should eliminate all fat. About 60% of people surveyed by the Washington-based Food Marketing Institute ranked fat as their greatest nutritional concern, compared with 16% just a decade ago. Think about it: We discuss fat over dinner ("How many grams do you think this piece of chicken has?"), scour the supermarket for the latest lowfat creations (we spent $18 billion on these foods in 1996) and devour lowfat cookbooks and diet plans (many large bookstores stock over 100 of them). "We've created a fat-phobic society," says Angela Guarda, M.D., director of the eating and weight disorders program at Johns Hopkins University School of Medicine in Baltimore.

Dr. Guarda and other researchers say fat fear is backfiring. A growing number of women are eating too little fat to maintain healthy body functions such as vitamin absorption and fertility. And most of us are also missing out on the benefits of certain types of fat. That's right: Scientists are discovering that not only is fat essential, but some types may also be *protective* against common diseases. A sampling of the research:

♦ *New England Journal of Medicine* Although fats from butter, margarine and fatty meats can raise heart disease risk, a diet rich in monounsaturated fats, like those found in olive and canola oils, can significantly lower it.

♦ *Journal of the American Medical Association* A diet rich in monounsaturated fat may reduce stroke risk.

♦ *Archives of Internal Medicine* A study of 61,000 Swedish women showed that those with the highest intakes of monounsaturated fat reduced their risk of breast cancer by half. Polyunsaturated fat (the type found in large quantities in margarine, corn, soybean and sunflower oil) increased cancer risk, although more research is needed to confirm the relationship. Surprisingly, saturated fat had no effect.

♦ *New England Journal of Medicine* Eating at least 3½ ounces of fish a day lowers your heart attack risk 10%.

♦ *Journal of Nutrition* Preliminary studies show that the type of fat in dairy products delivers a compound that may reduce cancer risk.

♦ *Journal of Medicine and Science in Sports and Exercise* Runners who increased their fat intake from 16% to 42% of calories didn't gain weight, and they lowered their risk of heart disease. In related studies, runners on higher-fat diets improved endurance, muscle strength and immune system function.

As a result of these and other studies, a group of leading nutrition researchers recently met at Tufts University in Boston to review the current recommendation to limit fat to 30% of calories—no more than 60

3 ❖ NUTRITIONAL HEALTH

Pistachio pleasures: These crunchy treats are chock-full of heart-smart fat and pack about 165 calories per ounce.

grams a day on an 1,800-calorie-a-day diet. Read on for the issues the experts addressed and to see whether you would benefit from more fat in your diet or you need to reconsider the types of fat you eat. One promise: You can get the tempting taste of fat into your meals without hurting your heart or your waistline.

FAT'S HATS

The function of fat goes way beyond making food taste good (although it does a fine job of that). Fat, along with carbohydrates and protein, the two other components in most foods, delivers energy to your body. Of the three, the fat molecule slows digestion the most, providing your body with a more constant energy supply so you're less likely to feel hungry between meals.

Try this experiment: One day for breakfast have a cup of your favorite cereal with half a cup of skim milk, a cup of orange juice and a banana (for a total of 360 calories and two grams of fat). Note when you start to feel hungry again. The next day eat half as much cereal, use 1% milk instead of skim, cut back to ¾ cup of orange juice and add two tablespoons of almonds (358 calories and nine grams of fat, total). Again, see when you get hungry. Even though both meals have about the same number of calories, the second breakfast will keep you satisfied longer.

Besides staving off hunger, fat coats every nerve and is the major part of every cell membrane. It helps your body absorb vitamins A, D, E and K, nutrients essential to better vision, stronger bones, a healthy heart and quick blood clotting, respectively. And cholesterol, found in foods that contain fat, is the raw material for

Fat: The Good, Bad and Ugly

Even though many women look at the total fat content on nutrition labels, they don't bother to see what type of fat the food contains. That's too bad, because while some kinds of fat wreak havoc on our hearts, other types can protect us. Check out this chart of fats, listed from best to worst. One caveat: All fats are high in calories, so you should keep an eye on your total calories to avoid gaining weight.

TYPE	RISK	REWARDS	RECOMMENDATION
Monounsaturated fat Olive and canola oils, olives, avocados and most nuts, including almonds, filberts, macadamias, peanuts, pecans, cashews and pistachios	None	Lowers heart disease risk by lowering total and LDL (bad) cholesterol without lowering HDL (good) cholesterol. Eat mostly this type of fat. Try to use olive or canola oil instead of other vegetable oils	butter or margarine.
Omega-3 fatty acid High-fat fish (salmon, herring, anchovies, sardines), dark green leafy vegetables, and soybean and canola oils	None	Reduces stroke and heart disease risk; lowers total and LDL cholesterol and raises HDL cholesterol.	Eat fish a few times a week; just don't fry it.
Polyunsaturated fat Vegetable oils (sunflower, safflower, corn and soybean), sunflower seeds and some nuts (walnuts, Brazil nuts, pine nuts)	In excess, lowers HDL cholesterol and may promote plaque buildup and cancer risks.	Reduces total and LDL cholesterol.	Limit the amount to 10% of total calories.
Saturated fat High-fat meats such as ground beef, high-fat dairy foods and tropical oils such as coconut oil	In excess, raises heart disease risks by increasing total and LDL cholesterol, creating artery-blocking plaque.	Improves food flavor; may reduce stroke risk.	Limit the amount to 8% of total calories.
Trans fats Margarine, especially in stick form, and crisp processed foods such as cookies, crackers and chips	Increases heart disease risk by increasing LDL and decreasing HDL cholesterol.	None	Avoid foods with hydrogenated oil listed in ingredients.

building hormones that control fertility. So there's no question you need fat—for your heart, for your bones, for your babies. The big debate is how much?

Guacamole returns! Dip into an avocado, a fruit rich in monounsaturated fat, which doesn't raise LDL (bad) cholesterol.

FATTY FOOD, FAT PEOPLE?

Before figuring out your optimum fat intake, you should know that not every bit of the fat you eat goes from lips to hips, says Dr. Guarda. The relationship between fat and weight gain is indirect at best. A single gram of fat has nine calories, while the same amounts of protein and carbohydrates have four calories each. As a result, people who eat a lot of fatty foods are consuming a lot of calories and are often overweight. So when you cut the amount of fat in your diet, theoretically you should also be shaving calories. For instance, reducing your fat intake by 20 grams should save you about 180 calories (20 grams multiplied by nine calories per gram).

But there are two snags in this premise. For acceptable taste, food manufacturers often add sugar to their lowfat products, so the regular and lowfat versions of many processed foods such as cookies have about the same amount of calories. And women who severely restrict the amount of fat in their diets tend to make up for the calorie savings by eating more food.

In a study published in the *International Journal of Obesity,* researchers monitored participants' lunches for about a month. When given food labeled "lowfat," the participants ate more and consumed more calories than when they were given a meal labeled "high-fat." "Women perceive lowfat foods as a license to eat more," says Alice H. Lichtenstein, D.Sc. (doctor of science), an associate professor of nutrition at Tufts.

Another reason some women overeat on a lowfat diet is that they're hungry all the time, says Margo Denke, M.D., an associate professor of internal medicine at the University of Texas Southwestern Medical Center in Dallas and one of the researchers participating in the Tufts meeting. "I recommend a little more protein and fat to some of the women I counsel, because it prevents them from needing so many calories to feel full," says Dr. Denke. The main message: To lose weight, you need to mind calories and portion sizes, not just fat grams. "Women who eat an 1,800-calorie diet with 35 grams of fat won't lose more weight than those who eat an 1,800-calorie diet with 50 grams of fat. A calorie is a calorie," says Dr. Denke.

Olive oil tour: Like wine, each brand of olive oil offers a unique taste experience. Just don't go overboard, because each tablespoon has about 120 calories.

THE ISSUE AT HEART

Fat doesn't contribute to weight gain as long as you control your overall calorie intake, but it does impact heart disease. Dozens of studies have linked a diet high in saturated fat (the type in butter, fatty meats and high-fat dairy products) with a greater chance of developing heart problems. Those studies led the American Heart Association (AHA) in Dallas to recommend that Americans adopt a diet containing 30% or fewer calories from total fat.

Although some researchers still support the AHA's recommendation because it has significantly lowered the average amount of saturated fat in the American diet, and because nearly all high-fat foods (even olive oil) have at least a little saturated fat, a growing number of nutrition experts fear it may have been too simplistic. "Some scientists thought the public was too simpleminded to understand that all fats aren't the same and that they should restrict just saturated fat, not all fat," says Walter Willett, M.D., chairman of the nutrition department at the Harvard School of Public Health. "As a result, many women aren't consuming the types of fat that are healthy for their heart."

The Good-Fat Diet

A diet rich in monounsaturated fat seems to protect against heart disease. So follow this plan for a day, and adjust your regular menu to this style of eating.

BREAKFAST

1 cup wheat-based cereal topped with 3 dried apricots, 2 tbsp. almonds, 2 tbsp. pecans, 1 tbsp. toasted wheat germ

1 cup skim milk

1 medium banana

LUNCH

2 slices whole wheat bread topped with 2 tbsp. natural peanut butter

1 cup plain yogurt with ⅓ cup raspberries or blueberries

1 cup sliced raw sweet red peppers

1 medium orange

DINNER

3 oz. broiled salmon fillet

1 cup cooked brown rice with 1 tsp. butter

1 slice whole wheat bread with 1 tsp. butter

1 cup cooked spinach with dash nutmeg and 1 tbsp. toasted pine nuts

1 large salad with 1 oz. feta cheese, 3 small ripe olives and 2 tbsp. dry-roasted sunflower seeds

Nutrition information:
2,024 calories; 76 g fat (34% of calories from total fat, 7% of calories from saturated fat, 15% of calories from monounsaturated fat, 9% of calories from polyunsaturated fat).

3 ❖ NUTRITIONAL HEALTH

Figuring Fat Grams

To calculate the number of fat grams you can eat, multiply the number of calories you consume daily (say 1,800) by the percentage of calories from fat you'd like your diet to contain (30%, or, 3) and divide by nine (60 grams is the answer in this example). Or just check out this cheat sheet:

CALORIES	% OF CALORIES FROM FAT	TOTAL FAT (GRAMS)
1,500	20	33
1,500	25	42
1,500	30	50
1,500	35	58
1,800	20	40
1,800	25	50
1,800	30	60
1,800	35	70
2,000	20	44
2,000	25	56
2,000	30	67
2,000	35	78

Dozens of studies have shown that a diet rich in monounsaturated fat works to lower cholesterol levels and heart disease risk. Dr. Willett's most recent exploration on the subject, published last November in the *New England Journal of Medicine,* analyzed the diets of more than 80,000 women aged 34 to 59 for 14 years. During that time, nearly 1,000 of the women developed heart disease. Dr. Willett and his colleagues showed that women were likeliest to have heart disease if they had a low intake of monounsaturated fat and a high intake of saturated fat and trans fat (the kind in most margarines and processed snack foods).

The numbers are astounding: If a woman replaced about half of the saturated fat in her diet with carbohydrates from foods such as bread and pasta, researchers figure she'd reduce her heart disease risk about 15%. But if a woman substituted monounsaturated fat for half of the saturated fat in her diet, she'd drop her chance of developing heart disease about 40%. And if she also replaced half of her trans fat intake with monounsaturated fat, she'd reduce her risk of heart disease 50%. "Women are doing the right thing for their hearts by eating less red meat, butter and high-fat dairy products," says Dr. Willett. "But instead of replacing those foods with margarine, pasta and bread, they'd get *more* benefit from eating nuts and olive and canola oils, because these foods will give them the maximum protection against heart disease."

ONE FAT INTAKE DOESN'T FIT ALL

Fortunately, there's not much debate about the *minimum* amount of fat required to maintain body functions such as fertility and vitamin absorption. Nearly every major medical organization recommends that both men and women get no less than 15% of calories from fat (about 25 to 30 grams for a 1,500- to 1,800-calorie-a-day eating plan).

Most researchers agree that saturated fat and trans fats are trouble. Less than one-third of your total fat intake should come from saturated fat. And you should avoid trans fats as much as possible. (To figure out how these recommendations can fit into a meal, see "The Good-Fat Diet.") What's a lot murkier—and far more individualized than scientists once thought—is the optimum amount of *total fat* needed to protect against disease.

Ronald Krauss, M.D., head of the AHA nutrition committee, says a low-fat diet can reduce your level of LDL (bad) cholesterol. But even Dr. Krauss concedes that "the range of individual response is wide. It varies from a 5% to 20% reduction."

So the amount of total fat that's best for you seems to depend on your genetic makeup and a host of other factors. Researchers say to consider:

♦ *Exercise.* The more you work out, the more fat you need, says Peter J. Horvath, Ph.D., an associate professor of nutrition at the University of Buffalo in New York. His studies show that while inactive women don't need more than 25% of calories from fat, the very active (such as marathoners) could eat 50% of calories from fat. If you exercise a few times a week for 45 minutes at a clip, you could probably use 30% to 35% of calories from fat. But if you decide to train for a 10K, for instance, up your fat intake a bit to improve your endurance and strength, says Dr. Horvath.

♦ *Diabetes or insulin resistance.* Since a high-carbohydrate diet may produce surges in blood sugar, many dietitians favor an eating plan that has about 35% of calories from fat, 50% from carbohydrates and 15% from protein, says Ann Coulston, R.D., a senior research dietician at Stanford University Medical Center. Just watch your calories carefully, because weight gain worsens these conditions (dropping a few pounds, of course, helps them).

♦ *High cholesterol.* While the AHA still endorses a diet with 15% to 30% of calories coming from fat, such a plan lowers levels of good cholesterol in many people, a major risk factor for heart disease. So some scientists suggest a diet that has 30% to 35% of calories from fat, with most of the fat coming from monounsaturated sources. See what your doctor thinks, and get your cholesterol checked a few months after changing your diet. Then adjust your diet if needed.

Medical groups probably won't endorse diets with more than 30% of calories from fat anytime soon, but many Americans can get up to 35% of their calories from fat, as long as it's mostly monounsaturated and they watch calories, says Dr. Willett. "Not only would eating more nuts and olive oil improve the taste of your meals," he adds, "but it would do a world of good for your heart."

Crunch fest: Almonds and many other types of nuts are rich in vitamin E, a nutrient that guards against heart disease.

Bulking Up Fiber's Healthful Reputation

by Ruth Papazian

More Benefits Of 'Roughage' Are Discovered

PHOTOGRAPHS BY NORMAN WATKINS

Because it causes gas, bloating, and other uncomfortable side effects, fiber may be the Rodney Dangerfield of food constituents. But with more and more research showing that a high-fiber diet may help prevent cancer, heart disease, and other serious ailments, roughage has started to get some respect.

The problem is that most Americans don't get enough fiber to realize its potential benefits. The typical American eats only about 11 grams of fiber a day, according to the American Dietetic Association. Health experts recommend a minimum of 20 to 30 grams of fiber a day for most people.

The Food and Drug Administration has recognized fiber's importance by requiring it to be listed on the Nutrition Facts panel of food labels along with other key nutrients and calories. And, based on scientific evidence, the agency has approved four claims related to fiber intake and lowered risk of heart disease and cancer.

The most recent claim, approved in January 1997, allows food companies to state on product labels that foods with soluble fiber from whole oats may reduce heart disease risk when eaten as part of a diet low in saturated fat and cholesterol. Foods covered include rolled oats, oat bran, and whole-oat flour.

FDA concluded that the beta-glucan soluble fiber of whole oats is the primary component responsible for lowering total and LDL (low-density lipoprotein), or "bad," blood cholesterol in diets including these foods at appropriate levels. This conclusion is based on a scientific review showing a link between the soluble fiber in whole-oat foods and a reduction in coronary heart disease risk.

The other three claims, allowed since 1993, are:

3 ❖ NUTRITIONAL HEALTH

Diets low in saturated fat and cholesterol and high in fiber are associated with a reduced risk of certain cancers, diabetes, digestive disorders, and heart disease.

- Diets low in fat and rich in fiber-containing grain products, fruits, and vegetables may reduce the risk of some types of cancer.
- Diets low in saturated fat and cholesterol and rich in fruits, vegetables, and grain products that contain fiber, particularly soluble fiber, may reduce the risk of coronary heart disease.
- Diets low in fat and rich in fruits and vegetables, which are low-fat foods and may contain fiber or vitamin A (as beta-carotene) and vitamin C, may reduce the risk of some cancers.

Found only in plant foods, such as whole grains, fruits, vegetables, beans, nuts, and seeds, fiber is composed of complex carbohydrates. Some fibers are soluble in water and others are insoluble. Most plant foods contain some of each kind.

Some foods containing high levels of soluble fiber are dried beans, oats, barley, and some fruits, notably apples and citrus, and vegetables, such as potatoes. Foods high in insoluble fiber are wheat bran, whole grains, cereals, seeds, and the skins of many fruits and vegetables.

Fiber's Health Benefits

What can fiber do for you? Numerous epidemiologic (population-based) studies have found that diets low in saturated fat and cholesterol and high in fiber are associated with a reduced risk of certain cancers, diabetes, digestive disorders, and heart disease. However, since high-fiber foods may also contain antioxidant vitamins, phytochemicals, and other substances that may offer protection against these diseases, researchers can't say for certain that fiber alone is responsible for the reduced health risks they observe, notes Joyce Saltsman, a nutritionist with FDA's Office of Food Labeling. "Moreover, no one knows whether one specific type of fiber is more beneficial than another since fiber-rich foods tend to contain various types," she adds.

Recent findings on the health effects of fiber show it may play a role in:

- **Cancer:** Epidemiologic studies have consistently noted an association between low total fat and high fiber intakes and reduced incidence of colon cancer. A 1992 study by researchers at Harvard Medical School found that men who consumed 12 grams of fiber a day were twice as likely to develop precancerous colon changes as men whose daily fiber intake was about 30 grams. The exact mechanism for reducing the risk is not known, but scientists theorize that insoluble fiber adds bulk to stool, which in turn dilutes carcinogens and speeds their transit through the lower intestines and out of the body.

The evidence that a high-fiber diet can protect against breast cancer is equivocal. Researchers analyzing data from the Nurses' Health Study, which tracked 89,494 women for eight years, concluded in 1992 that fiber intake has no influence on breast cancer risk in middle-aged women. Previously, a review and analysis of 12 studies found a link between high fiber intake and reduced risk.

In the early stages, some breast tumors are stimulated by excess amounts of estrogen circulating in the bloodstream. Some scientists believe that fiber may hamper the growth of such tumors by binding with estrogen in the intestine. This prevents the excess estrogen from being reabsorbed into the bloodstream.

- **Digestive Disorders:** Because insoluble fiber aids digestion and adds bulk to stool, it hastens passage of fecal material through the gut, thus helping to prevent or alleviate constipation. Fiber also may help reduce the risk of diverticulosis, a condition in which small pouches form in the colon wall (usually from the pressure of straining during bowel movements). People who already have diverticulosis often find that increased fiber consumption can alleviate

The claim above, linking whole oats and a reduced risk of heart disease, is the most recent FDA has allowed for fiber-containing food.

14. Bulking Up Fiber's Healthful Reputation

High-fiber diets may help blunt the effects of smoking and other risk factors for heart disease.

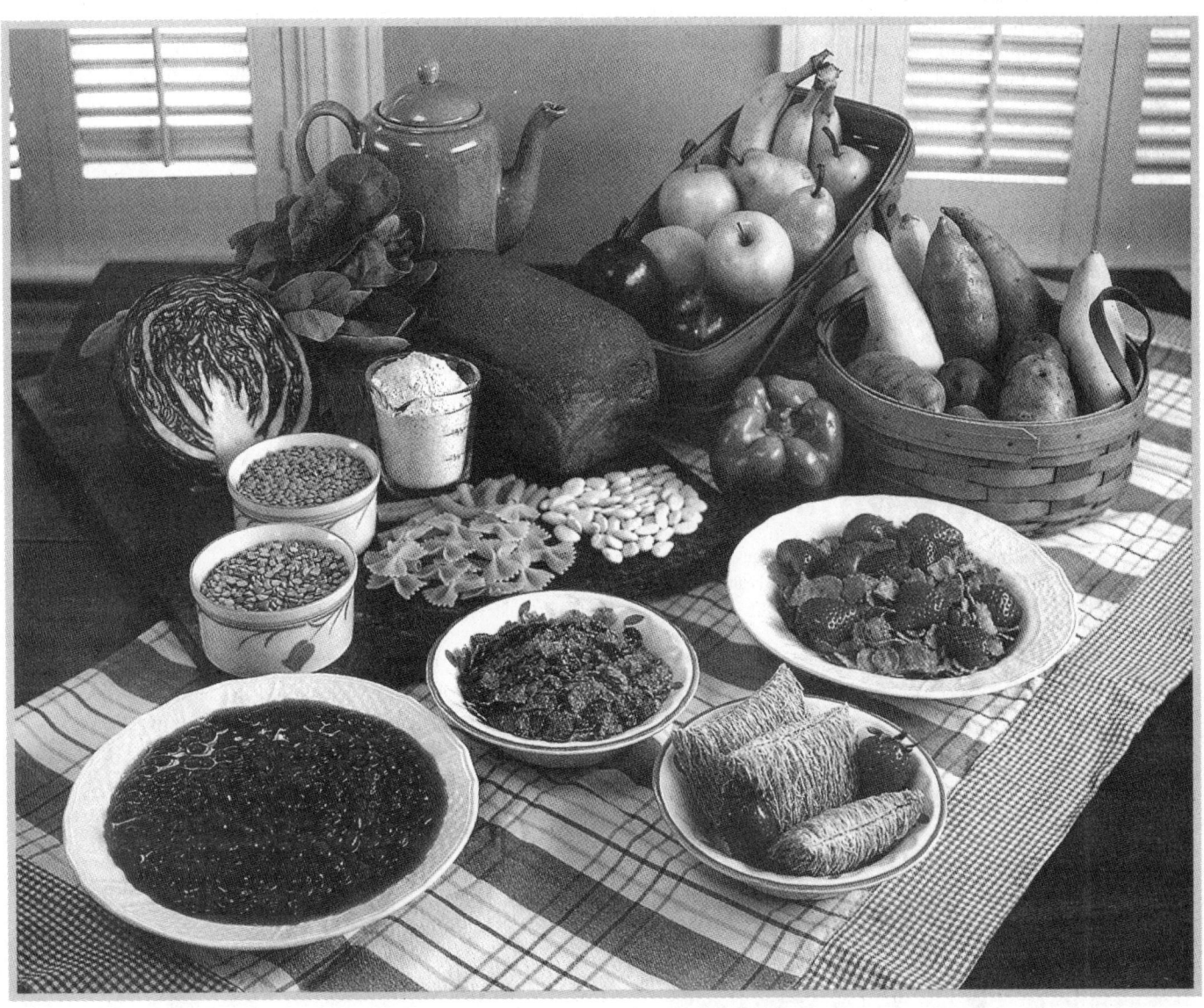

Insoluble fiber, found in the foods above, may hamper the absorption of calorie-dense dietary fat, according to recent studies.

symptoms, which include constipation and/or diarrhea, abdominal pain, flatulence, and mucus or blood in the stool.
• **Diabetes:** As with cholesterol, soluble fiber traps carbohydrates to slow their digestion and absorption. In theory, this may help prevent wide swings in blood sugar level throughout the day. Additionally, a new study from the Harvard School of Public Health, published in the Feb. 12 issue of the *Journal of the American Medical Association*, suggests that a high-sugar, low-fiber diet more than doubles women's risk of Type II (non-insulin-dependent) diabetes. In the study, cereal fiber was associated with a 28 percent decreased risk, with fiber from fruits and vegetables having no effect. In comparison, cola beverages, white bread, white rice, and french fries increased the risk.
• **Heart Disease:** Clinical studies show that a heart-healthy diet (low in saturated fat and cholesterol, and high in

NUTRITIONAL HEALTH

Slow Going

A word of caution: When increasing the fiber content of your diet, it's best to take it slow. Add just a few grams at a time to allow the intestinal tract to adjust; otherwise, abdominal cramps, gas, bloating, and diarrhea or constipation may result. Other ways to help minimize these effects:

- Drink at least 2 liters (8 cups) of fluid daily.
- Don't cook dried beans in the same water you soaked them in.
- Use enzyme products, such as Beano or Say Yes To Beans, that help digest fiber. ∎

—R.P.

fruits, vegetables and grain products that contain soluble fiber) can lower blood cholesterol. In these studies, cholesterol levels dropped between 0.5 percent and 2 percent for every gram of soluble fiber eaten per day.

As it passes through the gastrointestinal tract, soluble fiber binds to dietary cholesterol, helping the body to eliminate it. This reduces blood cholesterol levels, which, in turn, reduces cholesterol deposits on arterial walls that eventually choke off the vessel. There also is some evidence that soluble fiber can slow the liver's manufacture of cholesterol, as well as alter low-density lipoprotein (LDL) particles to make them larger and less dense. Researchers believe that small, dense LDL particles pose a bigger health threat.

Recent findings from two long-term large-scale studies of men suggest that high fiber intake can significantly lower the risk of heart attack. Men who ate the most fiber-rich foods (35 grams a day, on average) suffered one-third fewer heart attacks than those who had the lowest fiber intake (15 grams a day), according to a Finnish study of 21,903 male smokers aged 50 to 69, published in the December 1996 issue of *Circulation*. Earlier in the year, findings from an ongoing U.S. study of 43,757 male health professionals (some of whom were sedentary, overweight or smokers) suggest that those who ate more than 25 grams of fiber per day had a 36 percent lower risk of developing heart disease than those who consumed less than 15 grams daily. In the Finnish study, each 10 grams of fiber added to the diet decreased the risk of dying from heart disease by 17 percent; in the U.S. study, risk was decreased by 29 percent.

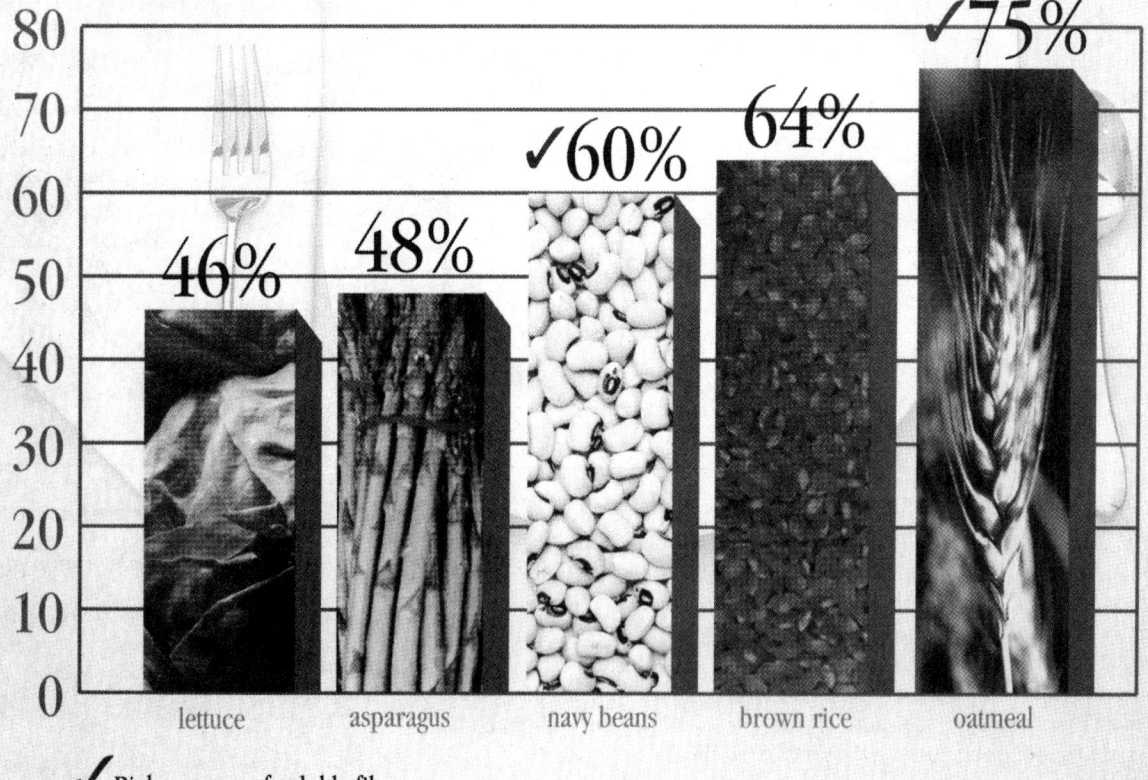

Something to Chew On

Which of these foods—lettuce, asparagus, navy beans, brown rice, oatmeal—are your best bet for cholesterol-fighting soluble fiber? Only oatmeal and navy beans. But when 1,009 Americans answered that question in a 1996 survey, many picked the other three foods as well. The percent that thought a particular food was rich in soluble fiber is below.

- lettuce: 46%
- asparagus: 48%
- navy beans: ✓60%
- brown rice: 64%
- oatmeal: ✓75%

✓ Rich sources of soluble fiber.

Archway Cookies Inc. survey

14. Bulking Up Fiber's Healthful Reputation

These results indicate that high-fiber diets may help blunt the effects of smoking and other risk factors for heart disease.

- **Obesity:** Because insoluble fiber is indigestible and passes through the body virtually intact, it provides few calories. And since the digestive tract can handle only so much bulk at a time, fiber-rich foods are more filling than other foods—so people tend to eat less. Insoluble fiber also may hamper the absorption of calorie-dense dietary fat. So, reaching for an apple instead of a bag of chips is a smart choice for someone trying to lose weight.

But be leery of using fiber supplements for weight loss. In August 1991, FDA banned methylcellulose, along with 110 other ingredients, in over-the-counter diet aids because there was no evidence these ingredients were safe and effective. The agency also recalled one product that contained guar gum after receiving reports of gastric or esophageal obstructions. The manufacturer had claimed the product promoted a feeling of fullness when it expanded in the stomach.

An Apple a Day and More

Recent research suggests that as much as 35 grams of fiber a day is needed to help reduce the risk of chronic disease, including heart disease. A fiber supplement can help make up the shortfall, but should not be a substitute for fiber-rich foods. "Foods that are high in fiber also contain nutrients that may help reduce the risk of chronic disease," Saltsman notes. In addition, eating a variety of such foods provides several types of fiber, whereas some fiber supplements contain only a single type of fiber, such as methylcellulose or psyllium.

To fit more fiber into your day:
- *Read food labels.* The labels of almost all foods will tell you the amount of dietary fiber in each serving, as well as the Percent Daily Value (DV) based on a 2,000-calorie diet. For instance, if a half cup serving of a food provides 10 grams of dietary fiber, one serving provides 40 percent of the recommended DV. The food label can state that a product is "a good source" of fiber if it contributes 10

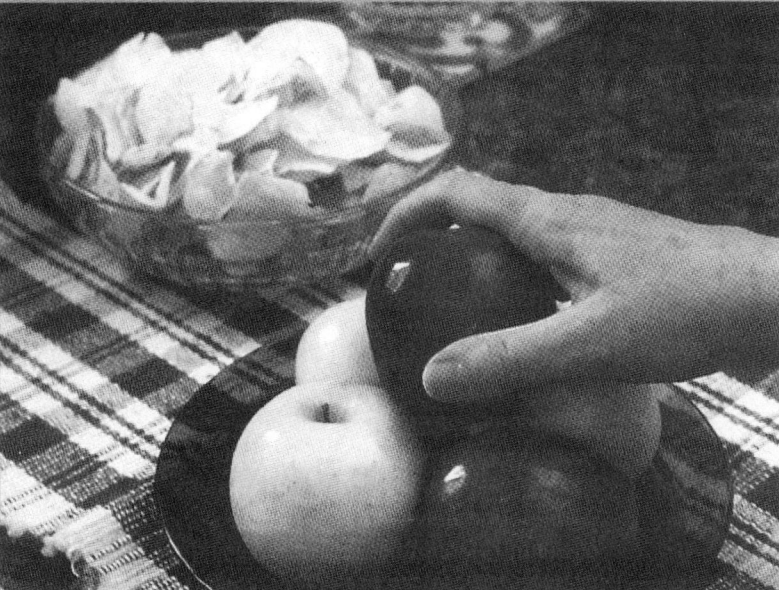

> **Reaching for an apple instead of a bag of chips is a smart choice for someone trying to lose weight.**

percent of the DV—2.5 grams of fiber per serving. The package can claim "high in," "rich in" or "excellent source of" fiber if the product provides 20 percent of the DV—5 grams per serving.
- *Use the U.S. Department of Agriculture's food pyramid as a guide.* If you eat 2 to 4 servings of fruit, 3 to 5 servings of vegetables, and 6 to 11 servings of cereal and grain foods, as recommended by the pyramid, you should have no trouble getting 25 to 30 grams of fiber a day.
- *Start the day with a whole-grain cereal* that contains at least 5 grams of fiber per serving. Top with wheat germ, raisins, bananas, or berries, all of which are good sources of fiber.
- *When appropriate, eat vegetables raw.* Cooking vegetables may reduce fiber content by breaking down some fiber into its carbohydrate components. When you do cook vegetables, microwave or steam only until they are *al dente*—tender, but still firm to the bite.
- *Avoid peeling fruits and vegetables*; eating the skin and membranes ensures that you get every bit of fiber. But rinse with warm water to remove surface dirt and bacteria before eating. Also, keep in mind that whole fruits and vegetables contain more fiber than juice, which lacks the skin and membranes.
- *Eat liberal amounts of foods that contain unprocessed grains in your diet:* whole-wheat products such as bulgur, couscous or kasha and whole-grain breads, cereals and pasta.
- *Add beans* to soups, stews and salads; a couple of times a week, substitute legume-based dishes (such as lentil soup, bean burritos, or rice and beans) for those made with meat.
- *Keep fresh and dried fruit on hand for snacks.*

"So many foods contain fiber that it's really not that hard to get your intake up where it should be," Saltsman says.

Ruth Papazian is a writer in Bronx, N.Y., specializing in health and safety issues.

B D E
The Vitamin Revolution

It turns out a good diet can't do it all. Chances are you're missing out on these three vitamins.

It's official: We've entered a new age. Experts have long seemed unable to talk about vitamin pills without scoffing. All you get from the supplements, they'd say, is expensive pee. Just eat a balanced diet; that's enough. Well, say good-bye to the era of the scientific sneer.

BY HARRIET A. WASHINGTON

LAST APRIL A PANEL ENLISTED BY the venerable National Academy of Sciences announced that a good diet just isn't good enough: Even people who eat lots of fruits and vegetables seldom get all the B vitamins they need. The panel, which is responsible for setting recommended dietary allowances, approximately doubled the RDA of the B vitamin known as folic acid, or folate, to 400 micrograms for adults. The scientists pointed out that Americans get only about 200 mcg a day on average and suggested that for many people supplements are the way to go.

In explaining the new embrace of vitamin pills, researchers tend to emphasize folic acid's role in preventing birth defects. But for many advocates, there's more than one motive at work. Evidence is mounting that the vitamin, along with B-6 and B-12, has the power to protect against heart attacks, and possibly strokes, too.

And the B's aren't the only vitamins making supplements respectable. Often forgotten, vitamin D is calcium's silent partner in building strong bones; adequate levels are crucial to staving off osteoporosis as well as for everyday well-being. Yet there's an unrecognized epidemic of vitamin D deficiency, says Michael Holick, an endocrinologist and vitamin D specialist at Boston University Medical Center. Up to 40 percent of Americans over the age of 50 fall short of the amount they need, he says.

Vitamin E is another nutrient that many researchers wish we would pop. Studies show this antioxidant probably protects against heart disease and might deter Alzheimer's, Parkinson's, and other diseases of age. But the benefits accrue only if you regularly get amounts well above those provided by a sensible diet.

All these tidings might well tempt you to cruise your neighborhood market's supplement aisle, stocking up on the entire alphabet. Rein in your cart. There's no evidence that the average American diet leaves people deficient in the *other* vitamins—A, C, and K.

These nutrients are necessary, no question. Vitamin K helps blood to clot, promotes the healing of wounds, and is critical for strong bones. Furthermore, your very ability to read these words comes courtesy of your stores of vitamin A, essential to making the pigments that enable you to see.

But it's easy to get plenty of A and K from your diet. And that's fortunate because, in the case of A at least, supplements are hazardous. Overdosing can be hard on your liver and if you're pregnant can cause serious birth defects. You might suppose you could avoid danger by instead taking supplements of beta-carotene—a building block of vitamin A that your body uses only as needed. Yet even beta-carotene isn't risk-free. A few years ago scientists were shocked to discover that when smokers took high doses they raised their chances of developing lung cancer.

Perhaps no vitamin illustrates the need for caution better than that celebrity of supplements, vitamin C. Without enough C your muscles and ligaments would lose their stretch, like old rubber bands. You'd be plagued by bleeding gums, fatigue, and wounds that wouldn't heal. Some researchers believe C's benefits extend to warding off heart attacks and strokes, and bolstering the immune system against colds, flu, and even cancer.

No wonder many people take huge doses. Yet last April a study suggested the vitamin may have a Jekyll-and-Hyde character: At 500 milligrams daily—a dose higher than the RDA but lower than the amount frequently taken to beat back colds—it may cause the kind of genetic damage that can lead to cancer. Until all the facts are in, says Chris Rosenbloom, a spokeswoman for the American Dietetic Association, it's wise to rely on your diet for C; if you want to supplement, take no more than 500 mg daily.

So it's a troika of vitamins—the B's, D, and E—that's bringing us into this new era. The view from here: You may scorn junk food and swill milk by the quart, but you *still* ought to think about whether you're falling short on these crucial nutrients. Here's how to know whether you need extra—and how much.

> **B is for buzz. Big buzz. Three of the B's are starting to look like powerful protection for your heart.**

The B Vitamins

WHEN THE GOVERNMENT'S advisory panel raised the RDA for folic acid in April, the scientists identified their primary target as premenopausal women—that is, anyone who might get pregnant. The panel said these women should take 400 mcg of folic acid daily to prevent birth defects such as anencephaly, in which the brain fails to fully develop, and spina bifida, an incomplete closing of the spinal column. The advice was aimed at all premenopausal women rather than pregnant ones because damage to a fetus can occur before a woman knows she has conceived.

But the life these vitamins save may be your own. "It looks like getting B vitamins—from foods or supplements—is nearly as important as stopping smoking, lowering high cholesterol, and controlling blood pressure in preventing a heart attack," says epidemiologist Eric Rimm of Harvard University.

Last February Rimm and his colleagues reported that women who got ample folic acid and B-6 suffered heart attacks only about half as often as women who took in meager amounts. The finding may help explain a longstanding puzzle in heart disease: Half of all heart attack victims have cholesterol levels that are in the desirable range. Increasingly, scientists are looking into a substance called homocysteine as a likely culprit in some of these cases. Homocysteine is thought to scar blood vessel walls, setting the stage for artery-narrowing deposits. Unfortunately, your body busily produces this chemical whenever it digests animal protein.

Now follow along: Experts think that folic acid, B-6, and B-12 help dispose of homocysteine before it can wreak havoc on arteries. The recent study from Harvard—which followed 80,000 women for 14 years—is the first to show a direct link between these vitamins and a reduction in the risk of heart disease.

It remains possible, of course, that something else was protecting the women who had high levels of B vitamins; indeed, it's likely that these vegetable lovers or vitamin takers exercised more and smoked less. "The jury is still out," says endocrinologist JoAnn Manson of Harvard Medical School, "but the evidence supporting folic acid's role is strong, very promising."

Let's assume you're sold on the B's. Do you really need a supplement? After all, the Food and Drug Administration requires enriched grains to be fortified with folic acid. The rule covers rice or flour that's had the germ and bran removed and nutrients added back. Enrichment doesn't make white bread preferable to whole wheat, but it does mean that most every serving of bread or cereal moves you toward your goal.

So you *could* get all you need from a daily bowl of fully fortified cereal, which delivers 400 mcg of folic acid. But could you stand the monotony? You could vow to eat more lentils and spinach and to drink more orange juice, and more power to you. But keep in mind that the folic acid in food is fickle—unstable and also more difficult for your body to use than the synthetic variety used in vitamin pills or sprayed onto cereal. Levels in food vary according to growing conditions and may easily be halved by exposure to heat, air, or light. The title of a recent editorial in the *New England Journal of Medicine* summed the facts up this way: "Eat Right *and* Take a Multivitamin."

As for B-6, it's found in a wide variety of foods including chicken, turkey, bananas, watermelon, and potatoes. Nevertheless, many people don't get enough—15 percent of young women and up to half of women over 50, according to the government panel.

Vitamin B-12 is also thought to play an important part in sweeping your body clean of homocysteine. Moreover, researchers long ago established that it's crucial in the formation of red blood cells as well as in the functioning of the nervous system. A severe deficiency can produce symptoms that range from irritating to horrifying—from tingling or loss of feeling in the hands and feet to irreversible dementia. The vitamin is plentiful in milk, meats, and other animal products. However,

D is for durable bones. This often-overlooked vitamin is as crucial as calcium. But don't count on the sun—or milk—to provide you with enough.

because people tend to produce less stomach acid with age, up to a third of those over 50 have trouble absorbing the nutrient from food.

To B or not to B? To serve you well, these vitamins must be in the proper balance. An overload of folic acid can disguise symptoms of a B-12 deficiency, for example. Besides, excessive doses of some B's can be dangerous in their own right. High doses of niacin—sometimes used to control cholesterol—can harm the liver and shouldn't be taken except under a doctor's supervision.

The bottom line: Take a once-a-day multivitamin. Most contain 400 mcg of folic acid, 2 mg of B-6, and 6 mcg of B-12. And make sure your diet is rich in fruits and vegetables.

Vitamin D

IRONICALLY, AMERICANS' DESIRE to do the right thing for their health may be leading to rampant vitamin D deficiency. "Anyone who doesn't drink much milk and doesn't get out in bright sun very often is a candidate for supplements," says Suzanne Murphy, a nutrition scientist at the University of California at Davis.

The vitamin is vital to the health of your bones, not to mention the quality of your days. Although calcium gets all the attention in osteoporosis prevention campaigns, it's D that shepherds calcium to your bones. If you lack vitamin D, an abundance of calcium won't keep your skeleton strong. What's more, a shortage of D can bring on muscle aches, weakness, and symptoms resembling those of arthritis.

"We see many people with deep bone pain who doctors thought had arthritis but who turn out to be deficient in vitamin D," says endocrinologist Holick. "Their lives improve tremendously when they receive supplements."

It might seem easy to get enough vitamin D, considering that every carton of pasteurized milk is fortified with it. Not only that, your body is a vitamin D factory fueled by sunlight. With 15 minutes of sun exposure thrice weekly, you can make all the D you need.

But studies show that milk doesn't always deliver as promised. "Three-quarters of all milk sold contains less than the label states, and 15 percent of skim milk contains no vitamin D at all," says Holick. And D-rich foods like liver and fatty fish probably don't make a daily appearance on your table. Meanwhile, rising rates of skin cancer have put a chill on many a summer afternoon. Sunscreen with a sun protection factor of more than 8 can reduce vitamin D synthesis by 80 percent. "Sunscreen doesn't create problems for most people because they don't put it on properly," says Holick. "But older adults apply it correctly and religiously." Yet these are just the people who could use a boost in production, not a barrier to it, since the body's efficiency at manufacturing D drops with age.

Even if your sunscreen use is spotty, catching some rays is more complicated than it sounds. From November to February in the northern hemisphere, the ozone layer absorbs a good deal of sunlight before it can hit the earth. In much of the United States during winter months you simply can't get the kind of sunlight it takes for adequate D production.

Some people face a year-round hurdle to getting their daily D. "Melanin acts like sunscreen," says Holick, "so many African Americans have insufficient levels."

The D decision: Depending on where you spend your winters, you may do just fine until the age of 50 with a faceful of sun for 15 minutes three times a week (before you put on your sunscreen). After that, you could likely use a supplement.

But D is not a more-the-merrier kind of vitamin. Overdoses—more than about 2,000 international units daily—can cause headaches and fatigue. If you really go overboard with supplements you might wind up with kidney stones and calcified heart valves. Reckless megadosing can even be fatal.

The bottom line: For young African Americans, or for young people of any race who spend the winter above 42 degrees latitude (think of a line running from Boston to the California-Oregon border), a multivitamin will do the trick; most contain 400 IU of vitamin D. If you're older than 50 and avoiding the sun, add a separate calcium-plus-D supplement, to total 600 to 800 IU. Don't take *two* multivitamins, as you may end up with an overdose of vitamin A.

Vitamin E

IN THE PAST DECADE scientists have made a strong case for vitamin E's powers to safeguard the heart. In one of the most persuasive studies, people with heart disease were given 400 or 800 IU of the vitamin or a dummy pill; those taking either dose of E turned out to be only half as likely to suffer a heart attack as the placebo group. Such research has prompted many investigators to recommend vitamin E to heart patients or people at risk—and to take it themselves.

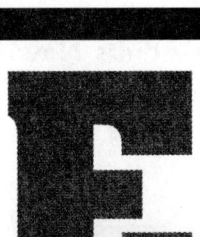

E is for exceptional. Though researchers are skeptical by nature, plenty of them take this vitamin to keep their hearts healthy.

Evidence for other benefits is in the promising-but-preliminary category. Just last year, says Tufts nutrition scientist Jeffrey Blumberg, one study showed that patients in the early stages of Alzheimer's disease who took high doses of the vitamin deteriorated more slowly than similar patients given a placebo. On the other hand, the support for cancer prevention is weak, says epidemiologist Rimm, who's been investigating vitamin E for years. A well-publicized study last March showed fewer deaths from prostate cancer among Finnish men who took supplements. But a number of other sizable studies have failed to register the benefit.

Taken as a whole, though, the research has convinced Blumberg and many other researchers that the RDA should get an upward shove next year from the current setting of 30 IU. More than a minimal boost in the RDA would constitute an implicit endorsement of supplements. The fact is, for a do-gooder vitamin, E keeps company with some oily characters: nuts, margarine, and mayonnaise. Sunflower seeds are a good source, but you'd need to eat a few cups of them to get a decent dose.

Capsule advice on E: A supplement provides cheap, low-risk health insurance, especially for anyone with heart disease or risk factors such as a family history of the condition.

The pills come in natural and synthetic versions. You can tell what's what by checking the label: The prefix *d-* identifies natural, *dl-* synthetic. Natural vitamin E is more potent and absorbed twice as efficiently as the man-made variety. You'll notice that it's also twice as expensive.

Whichever you choose, resist the temptation to load up. Vitamin E is quite safe, but it does inhibit blood clotting, so it should be treated with respect. More than 1,000 IU daily may cause bleeding. If you regularly take aspirin, warfarin, or another blood-thinning medication, ask your doctor what dose of vitamin E is safe for you.

The bottom line: To reduce the risk of cardiovascular disease, researchers generally suggest 100 to 400 IU daily. For people who have heart disease or are at particularly high risk, the recommendation climbs to between 400 and 800 IU. That's also the dose advised for those hoping to keep Alzheimer's at bay. Most multivitamins contain only about 30 IU, so you'll need to purchase a straight E supplement.

Harriet A. Washington is a writer in New York City.

Unit 4

Unit Selections

16. **How Fitness Savvy Are You?** *Consumer Reports on Health*
17. **How Fit Are You?** *Consumer Reports on Health*
18. **Rebel against a Sedentary Life,** Katherine Griffin
19. **The Skinny on Weight Loss,** *Consumer Reports on Health*
20. **The Pressure to Eat,** Kelly Brownell and Bonnie Liebman
21. **Does Food Control You?** Winifred Yu
22. **Binge-Eating That Plagues Adults Now Recognized as a Disorder,** *Environmental Nutrition*

Key Points to Consider

❖ Explain why the concepts of balance and moderation are crucial to any discussion regarding physical fitness or weight control.

❖ How important is regular exercise to optimal health? Why?

❖ Why should exercise be included in weight control programs?

❖ What advice would you give to someone who was considering going on a diet to lose weight?

❖ Are Americans too weight-conscious? Explain. How does American society encourage or contribute to weight control problems? What changes would you suggest?

❖ How do you feel about people who are overweight? Has weight control been a problem for you? If so, what have you done about it?

❖ Do you exercise on a regular basis? If not, why not? What would it take to get you to exercise on a regular basis?

❖ How could you help someone who has an eating disorder?

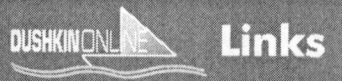 **Links**   www.dushkin.com/online/

15. **American Society of Exercise Physiologists (ASEP)**
    http://www.css.edu/users/tboone2/asep/toc.htm
16. **Health Links**
    http://www.hslib.washington.edu
17. **U.S. Department of Health and Human Services**
    http://www.os.dhhs.gov

These sites are annotated on pages 4 and 5.

Exercise and Weight Control

Recently, a new set of guidelines, dubbed "Exercise Lite," has been issued by the U.S. Centers for Disease Control and Prevention in conjunction with the American College of Sports Medicine. These guidelines call for 30 minutes of exercise, 5 days a week, which can be spread over the course of a day. The primary focus of this approach to exercise is improving health, not athletic performance. Examples of activities that qualify under the new guidelines are walking your dog, playing tag with your kids, scrubbing floors, washing your car, mowing the lawn, weeding your garden, and having sex. From a practical standpoint, this approach to fitness will likely motivate many more people to become active and stay active. "How Fitness Savvy Are You?" examines some of the most common misconceptions that people have regarding exercise and helps the reader sort out fact from fallacy regarding the do's and don'ts of exercise. "Rebel against a Sedentary Life" chronicles the change in philosophy from "No Pain, No Gain" to "Exercise Lite."

Since the benefits of exercise can take weeks or even months before they become apparent, it is very important for an individual to choose an exercise program and stick with it. The essay "How Fit Are You?" provides the reader not only with assessment tools for measuring aerobic fitness, upper and lower body strength, and flexibility and balance but with helpful suggestions on how to improve each component of fitness.

For the first time in our history, the average American is now overweight when judged according to standard height/weight tables. In addition, more than 25 percent of Americans are clinically obese, and the numbers appear to be growing. Why is this happening, given the prevailing attitude that Americans have toward fat? In "The Pressure to Eat," an interview with Kelly Brownell, professor of psychology, epidemiology, and public health at Yale University, Dr. Brownell asserts that a major part of the problem stems from the wide availability of high caloric foods that are low in cost, heavily promoted, and good tasting. Other factors include: a sedentary lifestyle, excessively large serving sizes, and social pressures such as the need to belong.

One of the most interesting aspects of our obsession with fat is that it is not limited to obese individuals. Young women of normal body weight who feel they are fat are of particular concern because some of them become so obsessed with their body weight that they turn to starvation as a way to control it. Still others resort to vomiting and purging their systems with laxatives in an attempt to control weight. Both anorexia and bulimia are serious eating disorders that may have deadly consequences. "Does Food Control You?" by Winifred Yu discusses the issue of body image and suggests that how we look has become a significant component of our self-worth. Yu contends that we have become preoccupied with a quest for the perfect body, and in doing so, we have lost much of the joy and pleasure of life. In addition to these two eating disorders, a third, termed "Binge-Eating Disorder (BED)," has recently begun to get media coverage. The essay "Binge-Eating That Plagues Adults Now Recognized as a Disorder" provides the reader with a brief definition of BED and discusses the nature and scope of this widespread eating disorder.

America's preoccupation with body weight has given rise to a billion-dollar industry. When asked why people go on diets, the predominant answer is for social reasons such as appearance and group acceptance, rather than concerns regarding health. Why do diets fail? One of the major reasons lies in the mind-set of the dieter. Many dieters do not fully understand the biological and behavioral aspects of weight loss, and consequently, they have unrealistic expectations regarding the process. "The Skinny on Weight Loss" addresses several common myths surrounding weight loss.

Being overweight not only causes health problems, it also carries with it a social stigma. Overweight people are often thought of as weak-willed individuals with little or no self-respect. The notion that weight control problems are the result of personality defects is being challenged by new research findings. Evidence is mounting that suggests that physiological and hereditary factors may play as great a role in obesity as do behavioral and environmental factors. Researchers now believe that genetics dictate the base number of fat cells an individual will have, as well as the location and distribution of these cells within the body. The study of fat metabolism has provided additional clues as to why weight control is so difficult. These metabolic studies have found that the body seems to have a "set point," or desired weight, and it will defend this weight through alterations in basal metabolic rate and fat-cell activity. While this process is thought to be an adaptive throwback to primitive times when food supplies were uncertain, today, with our abundant food supply, this mechanism only contributes to the problem of weight control.

It should be apparent by now that weight control is both an attitudinal as well as a lifestyle issue. Fortunately, a new, more rational approach to the problem of weight control is emerging. This approach is based on the premise that you can be perfectly healthy and look good without being pencil-thin. The primary focus of this approach to weight management is the attainment of your body's "natural ideal weight" and not some idealized, fanciful notion of what you would like to weigh.

"Exercise Lite" and the concept of achieving your natural ideal body weight suggest that we need to take a more realistic approach to both fitness and weight control and serve to remind us that a healthy lifestyle is based on the concepts of balance and moderation.

How fitness savvy are you?

Thirteen questions to send you safely into your exercise benefit zone.

It's January—time to put those New Year's resolutions into action. But before you pull on the running shoes or lift those weights, brush up on your fundamental fitness know-how. If you head off in the wrong direction, you could do yourself more harm than good—or at least end up discouraged and back on the sofa.

Last summer, we quizzed some 650 readers on the 13 questions that follow. You'll find the answers and a brief review of each topic beginning on page 4. You'll also have a chance to see how your peers fared. Rest assured that no one aced this exam. In fact, most got fewer than *half* the answers right—and no one got more than 10 right. So don't sweat it. The scoring box at the end will put your performance in perspective.

The quiz

❶ You should drink fluids whenever you start to get thirsty during exercise.
True ___ False ___

❷ The body burns more calories during hot weather.
True ___ False ___

❸ The health benefits of exercise begin to kick in when you raise your heart rate into your "exercise benefit zone."
True ___ False ___

❹ Your maximum heart rate is the level you achieve during strenuous exertion.
True ___ False ___

❺ It's best to stretch your muscles for a few minutes before warming up.
True ___ False ___

❻ Weight training is dangerous for people with high blood pressure.
True ___ False ___

❼ Which can raise your level of "good" HDL cholesterol?
 a. Aerobic exercise
 b. Strength training
 c. Stretching
 d. All of the above

❽ Running and other types of high-impact

16. How Fitness Savvy Are You?

exercise can lead to osteoarthritis.
    True ___ False ___

9 You can prevent muscle soreness by taking a pain reliever after a hard workout.
    True ___ False ___

10 The best first step for sedentary people is to do strength-training exercises for their leg muscles.
    True ___ False ___

11 To build strength, you need to push your muscles to the point of exhaustion.
    True ___ False ___

12 The more frequently you perform strength-training exercise, the more muscle you'll build.
    True ___ False ___

13 You shouldn't exercise when you have a head cold.
    True ___ False ___

Turn to next page for answers.

How fitness savvy are you?

Here are the correct answers to our 13 questions—and a look at how many readers got them right.

If you're keeping score, award yourself one point for each right answer; then check the scoring box at the end.

❶ **You should drink fluids whenever you start to get thirsty during exercise.**

☑ **False.** (29% of the readers we tested answered correctly.)

You should drink fluids *before* you get thirsty. By the time you're thirsty, your body is already becoming dehydrated. Dehydration impairs the ability to regulate body temperature, which can leave you vulnerable to heat-related problems or hypothermia, depending on the temperature of your surroundings. Thirst is a particularly unreliable indicator in older people. To prevent trouble, try to drink two 8-ounce cups about two hours before a hard workout, another cup every 20 minutes during the workout, and an additional cup or two within a half-hour afterward.

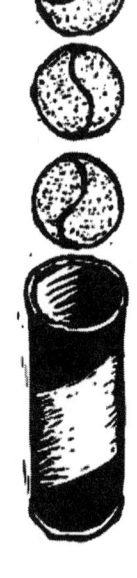

What to drink? Plain old water is fine for everyone except perhaps marathon runners and other endurance athletes. And unlike sports drinks or fruit juice, water is calorie-free.

❷ **The body burns more calories during hot weather.**

☑ **False.** (67% correct)

It may feel as if you're burning more calories during warm-weather exercise, since you're more likely to be sweating. But that's water loss aimed at keeping the body cool; you actually burn more calories during a cold-weather workout, keeping the body *warm*.

❸ **The health benefits of exercise begin to kick in when you raise your heart rate into your "exercise benefit zone."**

☑ **False.** (33% correct)

Raising your heart rate enough to improve your aerobic capacity is clearly beneficial, especially for strengthening your heart and lungs and boosting your athletic performance and overall endurance. But the old "exercise prescription" that specified a target heart rate has fallen by the wayside. Regular exercise that never reaches that aerobic threshold has major health benefits, too. Moderate exercise—such as brisk walking, bicycling, gardening, or even cleaning the house—reduces blood pressure, stress, and anxiety. It helps control weight, especially since you can sustain that degree of activity longer or do it more often. And it can save your life: Death rates from coronary heart disease, cancer, and all causes combined are far lower in moderate exercisers than in nonexercisers; but they're only a little lower in heavy exercisers than in moderate exercisers. The same holds true for the risk of developing type II diabetes.

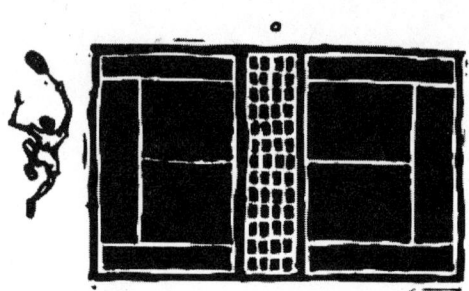

❹ **Your maximum heart rate is the level you achieve during strenuous exertion.**

☑ **False.** (49% correct)

Not many people would "max out" during even an intense workout. Maximum heart rate, after all, is defined as "the highest value attainable during an all-out effort to the point of exhaustion." So for estimating your maximum without having to experience it, there's a rough formula: Subtract your age from 220. (The traditional "exercise benefit zone" mentioned above is typically defined as 60 to 85 percent of that maximum, 90 percent for trained athletes.)

❺ **It's best to stretch your muscles for a few minutes before warming up.**

☑ **False.** (18% correct)

It's the other way around: First you warm up, *then* you stretch. That's because warm muscles are more pliant than cold ones, and thus easier to stretch and less likely to be injured. A good warm-up routine might include several minutes of an easy exercise such as marching in place or light calisthenics. Or gently go through the motions of the exercise you're about to perform. To stretch properly, gradually extend the muscle just to the point of discomfort—not beyond—and hold that position for at least 15 seconds. After your workout, cool down by doing the exercise at a gradually decreasing pace for two or three minutes. Then stretch again.

❻ **Weight training is dangerous for people with high blood pressure.**

☑ **False.** (70% correct)

While patients with hypertension have traditionally been advised to avoid strength-training workouts for fear of further elevating their already high blood pressure, newer evidence has shown that such exercise is safe for hypertensives—provided they do it properly. In fact, some studies suggest that strength-training exercise can actually help *lower* blood pressure. The key to safety is to be sure to exhale during the exertion phase of each exercise and to stick with moderate weights. Straining (holding your breath) and lifting much heavier weights can indeed cause blood pressure to spike. To play it safe, people with hypertension should consult a doctor for guidance before starting any sort of exercise regimen.

❼ **Which can raise your level of "good" HDL cholesterol?**

☑ **Aerobic exercise.** (32% correct)

Aerobic exercise and strength-training exercise can both help improve cholesterol levels—but they contribute in complementary ways: Aerobic exercise raises HDL, while strength training lowers the "bad" LDL. So when it comes to cholesterol, an exercise regimen that includes both forms of exercise really packs a one-two punch.

⑧ Running and other types of high-impact exercise can lead to osteoarthritis.

☑ **False.** (64% correct)

Research shows that the pounding of high-impact exercise won't lead to osteoarthritis, the painful degenerative joint disease—at least not among exercisers with healthy hips and knees who train only moderately. What's moderate? Jogging no more than 5 miles, three or four times a week. Pain or stiffness the next day is a signal that you're overdoing it. To further minimize the risk, alternate high-impact workouts with low-impact routines, such as bicycling or swimming. Wear highly shock-absorbent footwear. And when you have a choice, choose more yielding surfaces for your workout—for example, a cinder track, a dirt road, or even asphalt rather than concrete for running, or a wooden court for basketball.

⑨ You can prevent muscle soreness by taking a pain reliever after a hard workout.

☑ **True.** (33% correct)

A 1991 study found that using an anti-inflammatory pain reliever, such as ibuprofen (*Advil, Nuprin*), *before* a strenuous workout can help prevent soreness afterward. Further research suggested a better strategy: Wait until *after* a workout to decide whether it was strenuous enough to warrant taking the pain reliever regularly for a day or two. That way, you won't mask the pain of a developing injury during your workout, and you won't risk gastrointestinal side effects needlessly. Moreover, taking a prophylactic dose immediately after the workout prevents pain just as effectively as taking it in advance—and it's more effective than waiting for the pain to develop.

Nondrug preventive measures can help, too, if you expect to feel sore: Stretch the muscles more thoroughly than usual (after warming up—see question #5); then warm up and stretch again several times a day until any soreness has come and gone. Once or twice a day, do a few minutes of gentle exercises—ideally, an easy version of the activity that caused the soreness in the first place.

⑩ The best first step for sedentary people is to do strength-training exercises for their leg muscles.

☑ **True.** (48% correct)

The reason for having the legs take the first step is that strong legs facilitate most forms of aerobic-style exercise, such as walking and biking. Thus, greater muscle endurance promotes aerobic endurance.

⑪ To build strength, you need to push your muscles to the point of exhaustion.

☑ **True.** (9% correct)

Apparently, 91 percent of our readers would let themselves off easy—that is, *if* they were performing any strength training at all. The reason that you need to do enough repetitions of each weight-lifting exercise to reach exhaustion—meaning you couldn't lift that weight one more time—is to ensure that you force the muscles past the point where they begin producing the proteins that will build larger muscle fibers. That adds muscle strength and bulk. If you stop too soon, you may not quite reach that threshold. For the good news, however, see the answer to the next question.

⑫ The more frequently you perform strength-training exercise, the more muscle you'll build.

☑ **False.** (48% correct)

First of all, the exhausted muscle fibers (see question #11) gain strength not during strength-training workouts, but during the rest period *between* workouts. For maximum benefit, you need to allow 48 hours for full muscle recovery before your next workout. Moreover, training just twice a week builds about three-quarters as much strength as three weekly sessions do; even one workout per week may be enough to stop muscle loss. During each workout, a single "set" of repetitions for each exercise seems to build as much strength as multiple sets do, at least for the first few months. Whether multiple sets provide any advantage after that is not yet clear; but for the average person, who doesn't need to keep building more and more muscle, a single set of each exercise should still be plenty.

⑬ You shouldn't exercise when you have a head cold.

☑ **False.** (80% correct)

There's no reason to force yourself to keep exercising when you have a cold. But if you really want to exercise, there's no reason *not* to—so long as it's just a head cold, involving symptoms such as headache, runny or stuffy nose, sneezing, or a scratchy throat. Symptoms that are felt below the neck or experienced more generally—for example, fever, achy muscles, coughing deep in the chest, diarrhea, or vomiting—can signal the early stages of influenza, pneumonia, or some other potentially serious viral or bacterial infection that requires rest. But then you probably won't feel much like exercising anyway.

How fit are you?

None of the 650 readers who took the quiz last summer earned more than 10 points; most earned 6 points or less. Here's a guide to your score:

0 - 3 points: Time to exercise your mind. (13% of readers)
4 - 5 points: Not bad, but not highly fit. (34%)
6 - 7 points: Well toned, good capacity. (37%)
8 - 10 points: Better than the average fitness trainer. (16%)
11 - 13 points: No cheating! (0%)

How fit are you?

Here's how to find out—and how to improve your aerobic capacity, strength, flexibility, and balance.

Unless you've been exercising regularly throughout your life, you've probably had some disquieting reminders that you're not as physically fit as you once were. You may have trouble bending over, lugging a suitcase, racing for a bus, or keeping your balance on a sloping trail. Declining fitness can not only erode your athletic prowess but also increase the risk of soreness, stiffness, sprains, falls, and eventual disability. It also increases the risk of coronary heart disease, hypertension, diabetes, obesity, and possibly cancer.

Of course, some loss of physical powers is inevitable as you get older. But are you in good condition for someone your age, or are you badly out of shape, with a body that's older than your years? The simple tests described here—developed by James Rippe, M.D., director of the Center for Clinical and Lifestyle Research in Shrewsbury, Mass.—will tell you where you stand. And the suggested exercises will help you improve any weaknesses.

Note that the scoring is based on comparison with other people of your age group—many of whom may be in poor shape. So even if you get what's considered an "average" score, you might still benefit from more exercise. Whatever your score, you can use the test to chart your progress if you start exercising or increase your exercise schedule.

Unless otherwise noted, get the appropriate muscles ready for each test by working them briefly but briskly; then stretch them.

Aerobic-fitness test

A good way to measure aerobic fitness—the ability to exercise without getting winded—is with a walking test. The version described here has been simplified, so you don't have to measure your pulse. Find a measured track or use the odometer of your car to mark out a one-mile course along a level road. Walk the mile as briskly as possible without signs of exhaustion, such as dizziness or breathlessness. Record your time, in minutes and seconds. Then adjust your time as follows: **Men:** Add 15 seconds for every 10 pounds that your weight exceeds 170, or subtract 15 seconds for every 10 pounds under 170. **Women:** Make the same adjustment for every 10 pounds above or below 125 pounds. Check your score against the chart on next page.

▶ *How to improve.* Older people with an "average" score and virtually anyone with a low score could start by taking an easy 10-minute walk three times a week, then gradually increasing the speed and duration. After three months, they should be doing at least three weekly half-hour walks that either feel moderately hard or push their pulse rate to at least 60 percent of maximum (220 minus your age). People with higher scores can start with longer, faster walks—or even runs—and build up to at least the same level described above. (However, pulse rate should not exceed 85 percent for most people, 90 percent for advanced exercisers.) Of course, you can substitute any potentially aerobic activity, such as biking or swimming, for walking or running.

Strength test

Scores on the following tests, which gauge arm and leg strength, reliably reflect strength throughout the upper and lower body, respectively. Warm up the arm or leg muscles, but don't stretch.

Upper-body test. Sit in a chair with your back straight, holding a 5-pound weight in your stronger hand. (You can use either a dumbbell or a 1-gallon plastic jug filled with 5 pints of water or 5 pounds of sand.) Hold your arm straight down at your side, palm facing forward. Keeping your upper arm stationary, do biceps curls: Bend your arm at the elbow and raise the weight to your shoulder, then lower it. Count how many repetitions you can do in 30 seconds. Then check the chart below.

Lower-body test. Strap a 10-pound ankle weight to your stronger ankle, or measure a total of 10 pounds of sand or stones into two old socks and secure them to that ankle. Sit in a chair on enough cushions to keep your feet off the ground, or sit on a table or countertop. With your back straight and thigh stationary, raise your foot by straightening the knee, then bring it back down. Do as many repetitions as you can in 30 seconds. Then consult the chart below.

▶ *How to improve.* At least two strengthening sessions per week, preferably three, will build muscle, and even one weekly session may prevent muscle loss. A single "set" of repetitions for each exercise seems to build as much strength as multiple sets do.

You could choose the elastic-band exercises described in our December 1995 report. Or you could choose the following: For the upper body, do push-ups, bent-over rows, and abdominal crunches (all described on next page), plus biceps curls (described above in the upper-body test); for the lower body, do hamstring curls plus leg extensions (described above in the lower-body test). For each exercise, adjust the resistance so you can initially do only about 8 repetitions. Once you can do 12, increase the resistance so you can again do only 8.

■ **Push-ups.** Lie face down with your palms on your back or bending your knees, push against the floor with your hands to raise your body, stopping just before your elbows lock. If that's too difficult, do a modified push-up with your weight supported on your knees rather than your toes (see illustration above); or do the exercise in a standing position, leaning forward with your hands against a wall. If the regular push-up is not difficult enough, place something under your feet to elevate them. (Warning: Don't do push-ups if you have a bad back.)

■ **Bent-over rows.** Place a weight (either a dumbbell, or a jug filled with water or sand) on the floor next to a bed, couch, or bench. Put one hand and one knee on the bed (see illustration). Bring the weight up to the starting position, about a foot off the floor. Raise the weight to your armpit, then lower it. After 8 to 12 repetitions, turn around and repeat the procedure with the other arm.

■ **Abdominal crunches.** Lie on your back, with palms face down at your sides. Bring your knees up, keeping your feet flat on the floor. Slowly raise your shoulders until the base of your shoulder blades comes up off the floor, then lower your shoulders. To make the exercise harder, place your hands loosely behind your head (but don't pull), do the curls on an incline, or hold a light weight on your chest.

■ **Hamstring curls.** Stand erect, holding the back of a sturdy chair. Lift one foot behind you as high as possible—past the point of initial resistance—by bending your knee, then lower the foot. Repeat with your other foot. To boost the difficulty, wear ankle weights.

Flexibility test

Tape a yardstick to the floor, then place a foot-long strip of tape perpendicular to the stick at the

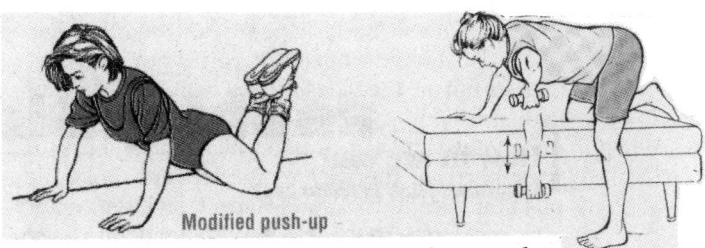
Modified push-up
Bent-over row

15-inch mark. Remove your shoes and sit on the floor with the yardstick between your extended legs, the low end toward you. Keep your heels about a foot apart, on the 15-inch mark. Place one hand over the other, with middle fingers aligned. Lower your head and slide your fingers forward as far as you can (see illustration), without bending your knees or straining. Record the farthest point where you can hold the tips of your middle fingers for two seconds. Do the test three times, then check your best score against the chart.

▶ *How to improve.* If you scored average or below, gradually work up to a minimum of 10 minutes of stretching every other day; if you scored high, it may take more than that minimum to improve—but then again, you may not need to improve. You can get in at least some of that stretching time before and after your workouts (except strength training, which doesn't require preparatory stretching). To log additional time, you could simply stretch longer than usual after you exercise, when your muscles are warmest and most pliable.

Here are four basic stretches:

■ **Hamstring stretch.** Sit with one leg extended. Reach forward along that leg until you feel a gentle stretch in the back of your thigh. Flex from the hips, keeping your back straight.

■ **Single leg pull.** Lie on your back with one knee bent and the other leg flat on the floor. Grip your bent leg with both hands at the back of the thigh, just behind the knee. Gently pull toward your chest until you feel the stretch in your but-

Aerobic-fitness test [1]

Age	High	Above average	Average	Below average	Low
Women					
20-29	<13:12	13:12-14:06	14:07-15:06	15:07-16:30	>16:30
30-39	<13:42	13:42-14:36	14:37-15:36	15:37-17:00	>17:00
40-49	<14:12	14:12-15:06	15:07-16:06	16:07-17:30	>17:30
50-59	<14:42	14:42-15:36	15:37-17:00	17:01-18:06	>18:06
60-69	<15:06	15:06-16:18	16:19-17:30	17:31-19:12	>19:12
70-79	<18:18	18:18-20:00	20:01-21:48	21:49-24:06	>24:06
80-89	<21:18	21:18-23:00	23:01-24:48	24:49-27:06	>27:06
Men					
20-29	<11:54	11:54-13:00	13:01-13:42	13:43-14:30	>14:30
30-39	<12:24	12:24-13:30	13:31-14:12	14:13-15:00	>15:00
40-49	<12:54	12:54-14:00	14:01-14:42	14:43-15:30	>15:30
50-59	<13:24	13:24-14:24	14:25-15:12	15:13-16:30	>16:30
60-69	<14:06	14:06-15:12	15:13-16:18	16:19-17:18	>17:18
70-79	<15:06	15:06-15:48	15:49-18:48	18:49-20:18	>20:18
80-89	<17:06	17:06-17:48	17:49-20:48	20:49-22:18	>22:18

[1] Measurements in minutes and seconds.

Upper-body strength test [1]

Age	Above average	Average	Below average
Women			
20-29	>32	26-32	<26
30-39	>29	23-29	<23
40-49	>27	21-27	<21
50-59	>25	20-25	<20
60-69	>22	19-22	<19
70-79	>21	18-21	<18
80-89	>19	16-19	<16
Men			
20-29	>39	35-39	<35
30-39	>36	32-36	<32
40-49	>34	30-34	<30
50-59	>33	29-33	<29
60-69	>31	26-31	<26
70-79	>28	24-28	<24
80-89	>24	20-24	<20

[1] Number of repetitions.

Lower-body strength test [1]

Age	Above average	Average	Below average
Women			
20-29	>29	26-29	<26
30-39	>28	25-28	<25
40-49	>27	24-27	<24
50-59	>27	23-27	<23
60-69	>25	22-25	<22
70-79	>25	22-25	<22
80-89	>22	19-22	<19
Men			
20-29	>33	29-33	<29
30-39	>32	28-32	<28
40-49	>31	27-31	<27
50-59	>30	27-30	<27
60-69	>29	25-29	<25
70-79	>28	23-28	<23
80-89	>26	21-26	<21

[1] Number of repetitions.

Data for ages 40 to 79 from "Fit over Forty," by James M. Rippe, M.D. (New York: William Morrow, 1996); other data extrapolated by the author. Reprinted with author's permission.

tocks and lower back. Repeat with the other leg.

■ **Twist.** Lie on your back with your arms extended out to the sides, knees bent, and feet together. Swing your hips and knees to the right until your right leg rests on the floor. Then turn your head all the way to the left and hold the position. (See illustration.) Repeat, swinging your hips and knees to the left, and turning your head to the right.

■ **Shoulder-back stretch.** While standing, stretch your arms above your head and lock your fingers together, with palms facing upward. Push your arms slightly back and up until you feel the stretch.

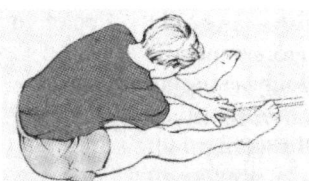

Flexibility test [1]

Age	Above average	Average	Below average
Women			
20-29	>20½	17½-20½	<17½
30-39	>19½	16½-19½	<16½
40-49	>19	14½-19	<14½
50-59	>17½	14½-17½	<14½
60-69	>17	14-17	<14
70-79	>16½	13-16½	<13
80-89	>15	12½-15	<12½
Men			
20-29	>17	13½-17	<13½
30-39	>16½	13-16½	<13
40-49	>16	12½-16	<12½
50-59	>15½	12-15½	<12
60-69	>14	10-14	<10
70-79	>12	9½-12	<9½
80-89	>10	7½-10	<7½

[1] Measurements in inches.

Balance test [1]

Age	Above average	Average	Below average
Women			
20-29	>29.0	22.1-29.0	<22.1
30-39	>22.0	15.1-22.0	<15.1
40-49	>15.5	7.2-15.5	<7.2
50-59	>8.7	3.7-8.7	<3.7
60-69	>4.5	2.5-4.5	<2.5
70-79	>2.6	1.5-2.6	<1.5
80-89	>1.9	1.0-1.9	<1.0
Men			
20-29	>28.0	21.1-28.0	<21.1
30-39	>21.0	14.1-21.0	<14.1
40-49	>14.7	4.1-14.7	<4.1
50-59	>6.7	3.2-6.7	<3.2
60-69	>4.0	2.5-4.0	<2.5
70-79	>3.3	1.8-3.3	<1.8
80-89	>2.5	1.5-2.5	<1.5

[1] Measurements in seconds.

Data reprinted or extrapolated from "Fit over Forty," by James M. Rippe, M.D., with permission.

Hold each stretch for at least 15 to 30 seconds. Repeat the entire sequence as needed to accumulate the minimum 10 minutes of stretching. For more extensive routines, see our March and August 1995 issues.

Balance test

It's preferable to have someone time you for this test, although you could time yourself. If you're age 50 or older, you'll need a stopwatch or a stopwatch feature to measure your time to a tenth of a second. Younger people who don't have such a watch can measure their time in whole seconds, then round off the numbers in the chart to the nearest second (since those numbers are high enough to round off without distorting the results). Frail individuals should have someone stand nearby in case they start to fall.

Raise the foot of your weaker leg and balance on the other foot, keeping your eyes open and your arms hanging limp at your sides. Time how long you can keep your foot raised. Do the test three times, then check the best result against the chart.

> *For more information*
> ■ "Fit over Forty," by James M. Rippe, M.D. William Morrow, 1996. $18.50. Call 800-288-2131.
> ■ Balance exercise program, developed by Yale researchers. Send self-addressed stamped envelope to CRH, 101 Truman Ave., Yonkers, N.Y. 10703-1057.

▶ *How to improve.* Tai chi, a graceful martial art, can sharpen your balance, since many of the maneuvers are done with a foot raised (see our June report). Certain yoga postures can also help.

People with poor balance could also try an effective series of exercises developed by Yale researchers. Here are the first three exercises, to get you started. For each exercise, hold onto a kitchen counter or the back of a sturdy chair with both hands. If necessary, have someone stand nearby.

■ Swing your hips five times in a large clockwise circle, as if you were whirling a hula hoop. Then swing them five times in the opposite direction.

■ Rise up on your toes, hold for five seconds, then come down. Repeat five times.

■ Stand on one foot for five seconds, then do the same on the other foot. Repeat 10 times.

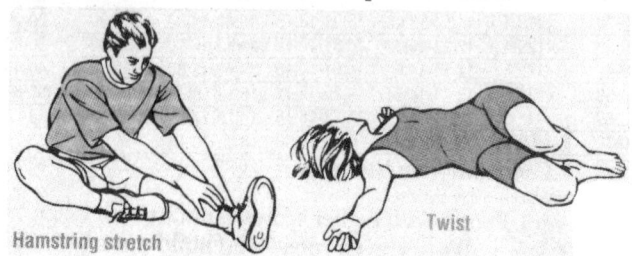

Hamstring stretch | Twist

REBEL AGAINST A SEDENTARY LIFE

Cars. Desk jobs. Escalators. It's hard to be active these days. Yet researchers now know that when it comes to health, the single most important thing you can do is live your life on the go.

By Katherine Griffin

A DECADE AGO MOST of my ideas about exercise came from my housemate John, a former cross-country runner. For exercise to do you any good, he told me, you have to get your heart pounding and keep it that way for at least 20 minutes, or even better, an hour. John's endless energy made him a persuasive advertisement for long runs and killer bike rides. I was sufficiently impressed that I allowed him to haul me out of bed at 6:30 several times a week to go running, a feat I haven't repeated since.

These days John lives nearby, and I still see him bounding off for two-hour runs. But I'm now paying more attention to a neighbor who embodies a strikingly different approach. Her name is Emma, and she's 92 years old. Every morning as I'm drowsily returning to consciousness, the *skritch-skritch* of a rake outside lets me know that Emma has started her workout. She spends a couple of hours each day raking everybody's leaves, up and down our block and around the corners. Her back is bent and her hair a white, wispy puff, but from a distance, watching her stab the rake at the leaves, stuff the leaves into bags, and haul the bags away, you'd swear she wasn't a day over 50.

Emma is modest about her labors. "Don't have anything else I have to do," she says, with a slightly embarrassed shrug. But in my eyes, she's doing more than defying expectations about how someone her age behaves. She's living proof, in my front yard, of the most important health finding of the decade: Just working movement into everyday life can be a veritable fountain of youth.

The irony is, we've discovered this just as we've created a society that compels us *not* to move. Today the average person going about her everyday life burns a whopping 800 fewer calories a day than she would have 20 years ago. That's the equivalent of three hours of daily walking that have simply vanished. Take even a cursory look at how most of us live and it's not hard to see why we move less. Most jobs require nothing more physically taxing than pecking at a computer. Growing numbers of us live in suburbs laid out so it's practically impossible to

HOW "Go for the Burn" BECAME "Easy Does It"

AFTER SOME FALSE STARTS, in 1978 the high priests of fitness declared the road to health was paved with three to five hard workouts a week. The then-20-something boomers dashed out to do right. But just as that dictum became a burden for a generation facing 50, the experts gave everyone a new goal to chase: exercise lite.

1951 Fifteen years after opening the nation's first health club, Jack LaLanne airs "The Jack LaLanne Show." "I'm going to build a new and lovelier you!" he tells his 6 million viewers before putting them through his workout. "We're going to reduce"—pause to touch his rump—"the old back porch!"

1963 Alarmed that baby boom children are weaker than European kids, the new President's Council on Physical Fitness instructs schools to get us exercising. Setting an example, the Kennedys turn family touch football games into a national pastime.

1968 In his best-selling *Aerobics,* Kenneth Cooper of the Cooper Institute argues that four workouts a week prevent heart disease. "I've been called a zealot, yes. But this is an idea that could reshape the lives of millions." Not until 1984 will a study finally tie exercise to longevity.

1977 Once-chubby ex-smoker Jim Fixx brings Cooper's message to the masses with his evangelical *Complete Book of Running.* Everyone perceives an irony when he later dies of a heart attack while running, but he had inherited heart disease.

1982 Jane Fonda's Workout video kicks off the aerobics craze. "Namby-pamby little routines that don't speed up your heartbeat and make you sweat aren't really worth your while."

1987 By touting beauty benefits, the *Buns of Steel* videos trigger another hard-core fitness wave and go on to sell 13 million copies. But when a study finds people who just walk or garden regularly earn exercise's health dividends, experts rethink their advice.

1991 Despite more than a decade of pleas from fitness experts, two in three women get no regular exercise—more than in 1985.

1993 A study at Tufts University finds that lifting weights reverses muscle and bone loss, and may be as important to good health as walking, jogging, swimming, or other aerobic exercise.

1993 Taking the just-get-moving cue, 14 million Americans now go walking at least twice a week, up almost 40 percent in six years. Leading the way is girl-next-door walking enthusiast Kathy Smith.

1996 The surgeon general's report on exercise makes it official: Doing any moderate exercise for 30 minutes a day can help unclog arteries, lower diabetes risk, delay osteoporosis, and lengthen life.

---

go anywhere without getting into a car. There are drive-through restaurants, banks, even liquor stores. In a thousand ways both big and small, our landscape shouts, "All right, nobody move!"

Some 15 percent of us, including my friend John, have compensated for this immobilization by making time for hard workouts. But for the great majority of us who have failed at that, the only answer is to become more active without formal exercise. And that calls for no less than an outright rebellion against the conveniences that cushion our lives.

Emma, for her part, refuses to pay for a gardener—or to let her neighbors hire one. How will the rest of us revolt? I don't know, but we'd better start plotting. Because either we move, or we die.

RESEARCHERS AREN'T JUST playing cheerleader when they say that movement is a genuine magic pill. They've piled up a mountain of proof that activity can stave off the killer diseases that steal vitality and life from millions every year. In 1996 the first surgeon general's report on physical activity exhaustively detailed that evidence. Think of an illness that someone you love has died from—cancer, heart disease—or an ailment that has hobbled someone you're close to—high blood pressure, osteoporosis, diabetes, depression—and chances are that moving around helps prevent it.

Meanwhile, the dangers of a sedentary life have become alarmingly clear. We're used to thinking of cigarettes as the number one health threat, but overused recliners are just as treacherous. Last July Steven Blair, an epidemiologist at the Cooper Institute for Aerobics Research in Dallas, published the first comprehensive study to compare the effects of a lack of exercise with other health dangers. Following 32,000 people for eight years, he found that those whose only risk was inactivity were more likely to die prematurely than those who had high cholesterol, high blood pressure, *and* a smoking habit but who got some exercise each day.

And forget "no pain, no gain" and all those eighties-style exercise mantras. In 1984 University of Pittsburgh epidemiologist Ronald LaPorte found that mail carriers who merely *walked* seven miles a day were as healthy as distance runners. "Workouts" like Emma's are where the vast majority of benefits lie. This means at least 30 minutes per day of activity that's as demanding as a brisk walk. Being about that active, Blair has found, cuts your odds of an untimely death by more than half. The risk for those who follow a hard-core regimen declines further but not by much more. In addition, the experts say, you can pile up activity in short bursts throughout the day.

It sounds simple: Get back to moving

18. Rebel against a Sedentary Life

ARE YOU ACTIVE ENOUGH?

DON'T WORRY IF you can't find the time to get to the gym, experts now say. Accumulating 30 minutes of vigorous movement—taking the stairs, mowing the lawn, pedaling your bike around the block—can offer the same benefits as a full-fledged workout. The trouble is, our lives have become so convenient that even getting bits and pieces of exercise takes a concerted effort. To find out how well you're doing, circle true or false for each of the statements below.

I always take the stairs instead of the escalator.
TRUE or FALSE

I usually walk or ride my bike to do errands.
TRUE or FALSE

I do my own housecleaning and laundry.
TRUE or FALSE

My job involves a lot of walking or lifting.
TRUE or FALSE

I do my own yard work.
TRUE or FALSE

I play active games with children a lot.
TRUE or FALSE

I resist the impulse to find the closest parking space.
TRUE or FALSE

I have stairs in my house.
TRUE or FALSE

I often do exercises while watching TV—at least during commercials.
TRUE or FALSE

My hobbies involve a lot of activity.
TRUE or FALSE

I take a 30-minute walk or go to the gym five times a week.
TRUE or FALSE

.... Total number of trues

> **SIX OR MORE TRUE**
> You're probably managing to work in at least 30 minutes of activity a day.
>
> **FIVE OR FEWER TRUE**
> You need to get moving. Make some small changes to rally yourself.

Walking Away From Convenience

Get out of the car. Whenever possible, go partway to your destination by car, park, then walk the rest. Or even if you simply trade time in the car for time on a bus or train, the walk to and from the station will add valuable active minutes to your day.

Go on three-minute walks. Piling up short periods of activity appears to be as good as exercising all at once, so take "moving" coffee breaks or lunchtime walks.

Swear off E-mail. Communicating by computer is sure to keep you in your chair all day. Walk over and talk to your coworkers face-to-face.

Make chores your workout. Scrub the floor. Weed the garden. Bike to the store. Everyday activities count as exercise as long as they're strenuous enough to leave you slightly winded.

Shun escalators. Elevators may be hard to forswear if your office is on the eighteenth floor. But escalators are usually only a flight or two long—and they're often right next to the stairs.

---

around, a little bit here, a little bit there. But don't fool yourself. The promise of the 20th century was that technology would transform our lives, freeing us from the drudgery of manual labor. For most Americans that promise has been fulfilled, and we aren't begging to chop wood and haul water again. "All through the course of evolution, people had to be active to survive," says Philip James, an obesity researcher at Rowett Research Institute in Aberdeen, Scotland. "Now, for the first time, we have constructed a world in which you have to go out and make a conscious decision to be active."

It was James who calculated that the average person now burns 800 fewer calories each day than she did in 1975. The main culprits? Cars, freeways, offices, and suburbs spreading willy-nilly across the land (the typical American spends 45 minutes each day sitting behind the wheel of a car); televisions glowing in every home (three hours per day); and computers humming in every workplace.

The evils of automobiles and desk jobs are frighteningly familiar to 46-year-old Susan Donahue of Davis, California. Until three years ago her job as a veterinary technician at the local university kept her hopping. "I was always chasing sheep around or carting stuff to the lab," she says. But since becoming the editor of the university's veterinary newsletter, she spends her days behind a terminal, chasing deadlines instead of sheep.

Once movement was gone from her job, she was appalled to realize that she'd turned into the stereotypical sedentary American. "I'd drive to work, drive home, and that was it," she says. Years earlier she had gardened during the week and hiked or skied on weekends. But as she got busier and added a computer to her home, those hobbies slipped out of Donahue's schedule. "When life speeded up," she says, "exercise was the first to go."

Having too much to do, of course, is the epidemic of our era. And Americans pinched for time can find mechanized ways to make any chore far less time-consuming. Can't spare an hour for the lawn? Invest in a sit-down mower and a leaf blower. No time to scrub the car? Drive it through the car wash. Even conveniences that seem innocuous contribute to the decline in activity: Just adding a second phone in your house means you may walk 70 fewer miles a year.

"Everything we do—cleaning, cooking, yard work—burns fewer calories than it used to," says Blair. "It's the accu-

4 ❖ EXERCISE AND WEIGHT CONTROL

mulation of tiny little increments, but they add up to a lot."

Eventually Susan Donahue got fed up. After casting a critical, almost subversive eye on her surroundings, she seized one big opportunity for movement: She gave up the sticker that allowed her to park on campus and started cycling the flat, four-mile round-trip to work. "Instead of mindlessly driving along with all the other driver-drones, I just told myself that I was going to make this happen," she says. "Everything else would have to adapt to it." No more excuses about being too busy, no more oversleeping and flying out the door late.

Three years later she still bikes every day, rain or shine. Sometimes it's a hassle. She has to allow more time to get to work. Her skirt gets stuck in the spokes. Rainy days find her wearing plastic bags over her shoes and looking, she admits, like a fashion outcast. But she won't give up her daily ride. "It's a wonderful thing to work into my day," she says. "Now when I get home I feel energized." So much so that she also takes evening walks with her husband, keeps up with the yard work, and goes on weekend rides with a local bicycle club.

How did Donahue manage to buck the system? Researchers who study why people get moving would ascribe it to some combination of her self-confidence, enjoyment of the activity she chose, and support from others. As a student years before, Donahue had bicycled everywhere, so there was a part of her deep down that knew she could switch from car to bike. And once she was back to cycling, the joy of being outdoors, seeing things she'd otherwise miss, motivated her to stick with it even on cold, windy mornings when the car tempted her. Finally, Donahue's husband was a longtime cycling enthusiast who was thrilled when she started to ride and got her involved with the bike club.

Donahue's path was further smoothed by the fact that she lives in Davis, a town where visionary planners had created a network of bike lanes and greenbelts. Today one in four commuters in Davis cycles to work, compared with 3 percent nationwide.

When Donahue bicycles in other cities, though, she can see why everyone drives. Exhaust fumes and traffic too often make human-powered transport unpleasant and even dangerous. And when she has to hunt around the back of a building before she can find its dirty and poorly lit stairwell, she understands why everyone takes the elevator. Such barriers help explain why people don't make the effort to move and why many experts think that the only sure way out of our bind will be to change our environment.

"Ideas have been floated that range from feasible to ridiculous," says Blair, who mentions levying a tax on recliners, funneling highway money into bike and walking paths, requiring office buildings to have centrally located and attractive stairs, and restricting driving in downtown areas to get people out walking.

This kind of social engineering may sound preposterous, but think back 20 years. Who would have imagined no-smoking restaurants and bars, or forlorn smokers huddled outside office buildings? Now that we know sitting around is as perilous as smoking, shouldn't we, as a society, create opportunities to bustle about, so it's not just the determined few who make movement routine?

In the meantime, those of us who want to thrive at Emma's ripe age will have to change our lives on our own, each finding her own carpet of leaves to attack on sunny—as well as chilly—mornings.

"Don't like to sit around all day," Emma says.

Such a simple idea. Why does it have to be so complicated?

Katherine Griffin has been a staff writer at the magazine since 1989.

> Now that we know sitting around is as perilous as smoking, why don't we create more opportunities to bustle about?

The skinny on weight loss

The truth behind these common myths can help you lose weight when you need to—and stop worrying when you don't.

Slimming Insoles help you lose weight "with every step you take." The *Svelt-Patch* "melts away body fat" even "while you sleep." *Absorbit-ALL Plus* supplements will "zap 3 inches from your thighs." Those and numerous other dubious claims exploit the most enduring of all weight-loss myths: There must be some way—short of taking possibly harmful drugs—to slim down quickly and easily. That myth can lead you to neglect the more demanding steps that really can help you lose weight.

Other weight-loss myths are less obvious but no less harmful. They can lead to needless or fruitless efforts to lose weight. Some may even be damaging to your health.

❶ **Myth: You can tell whether or not you need to lose weight by your appearance or by the size of your clothing.**

Truth: Many Americans, brainwashed by all the emaciated models they see, have a distorted image of a healthy physique. That's particularly true of those with a wide, big-boned frame, who couldn't possibly slim down to the supposedly ideal waiflike proportions. The decision to lose weight should be based primarily on whether your weight poses any health risk, not on whether you look as thin as you think you should.

Start by calculating your body-mass index (BMI); that measures how fat you are—a primary determinant of risk—by correlating weight to height. To figure your BMI, multiply your weight in pounds by 705, divide by your height in inches, then divide by your height again. In general, the risk of disease—notably coronary heart disease, diabetes, and several common cancers—is lowest for BMIs between 21 and 25; then it increases slightly between 25 and 27, substantially between 27 and 30, and dramatically for scores over 30. (A BMI below 21 is also linked with increased risk—but only because skinniness sometimes results from underlying health problems, not because it's intrinsically unhealthy.)

But you need to check more than just your BMI. For one thing, your BMI does not distinguish between muscle and fat, the real culprit. Further, body fat poses a substantially greater risk in people who have or are susceptible to such illnesses as coronary heart disease, stroke, and diabetes than it does in other people. And regardless of your current BMI, the risk of disease generally starts to rise if you've gained more than about 10 pounds as an adult.

Where the weight sits on your body also affects your health. Fat on the belly is linked with increased blood-cholesterol levels, hypertension, diabetes, and possibly breast cancer, regardless of your overall weight. So even if you have a desirable BMI, a chubby belly increases your risk of disease more than plump hips or thighs do. Women are at increased risk if the ratio of their waist to hip measurements exceeds 0.8, men if the ratio exceeds 1.0. To calculate your ratio, measure your waist at its narrowest point and your hips at their widest; then divide the waist measurement by the hip measurement.

❷ **Myth: Most overweight people could slim down if they just used a little self-control.**

Truth: Losing weight is hard. For one thing, your genes have determined the range of possible weights you could reasonably expect to sustain; even if you forced yourself below that range, your body would almost inevitably swing back. In addition, weight loss, particularly rapid loss from diet alone, slows the body's metabolic rate—its basic rate of burning calories. So a person who slims down to 150 pounds, for example, generally must consume fewer calories to maintain that weight than another 150-pound person who has never been overweight.

The good news is that losing just a little weight can substantially reduce your risk of disease. And improving your diet and exercise habits will improve your health even if you don't lose any weight at all.

❸ **Myth: Strength training won't help you lose weight, since it adds pounds of muscle and burns few calories.**

Truth: A typical strength-training session—with machines, free weights, or flexible bands—uses up calories at least as fast as moderately paced walking does. More important, muscle tissue burns calories faster than fat tissue, even when you're resting. So building muscle can increase the number of calories you burn throughout the day; that can help you not only lose weight but keep it off. And muscle is denser than fat, so even if you merely lost fat and added muscle, without losing any weight overall, you'd still become trimmer—and healthier.

❹ **Myth: Vigorous exercise promotes weight loss better than moderate exercise.**

Truth: A vigorous workout does burn more calories than a milder workout of the same duration. But a long, moderately intense workout burns more calories than a brief, strenuous one. And most people can

The fen-phen fiasco

Last September, the U.S. Food and Drug Administration persuaded the maker of two weight-loss drugs—dexfenfluramine (*Redux*) and fenfluramine (*Pondimin*)—to pull them off the market. The FDA acted after learning that up to 30 percent of users developed leaky heart valves. Fenfluramine and, to a lesser extent, dexfenfluramine, had recently become popular as part of "fen-phen," a prescription "cocktail" for weight loss that paired either drug with the appetite-curbing stimulant phentermine (*Ionamin*). Here's what to do if you've taken one of the withdrawn drugs—and what you should know about the alternatives.

The dangerous drugs

For unknown reasons, both drugs seem to damage the heart valves in the same way they curb appetite—by boosting production of the brain chemical serotonin. None of the carefully controlled studies originally submitted to the FDA had even hinted at that problem. But then none of the studies had used the drugs the way many doctors prescribed them in real life: for long periods of time, in combination with other drugs, and in people who were not truly obese.

All former users of fenfluramine or dexfenfluramine should be checked for heart-valve leakage. In particular, those with possible indications of leaky valves—chest pain, fainting, palpitations, or a recently diagnosed heart murmur—should undergo an ultrasound imaging test of the heart called an echocardiogram.

A number of invasive medical or dental procedures—including deep cleaning of the teeth—can cause bacterial endocarditis, a potentially deadly heart infection, in people who have valve disease. So even former users who have no symptoms of the disease should ask their doctor whether they need an echocardiogram if they're about to undergo an invasive procedure. Antibiotics would have to be given before treatment if the test revealed significant leakage.

New drugs and herbs

Despite the recent debacle, the FDA has approved a new weight-loss drug, sibutramine (*Meridia*), and will probably soon approve another, orlistat (*Xenical*). Both drugs are about as effective as the withdrawn drugs, helping a substantial minority of obese people reduce their weight by an average of 10 percent.

Unlike the withdrawn drugs, sibutramine does not increase secretion of serotonin. But all three drugs make serotonin work more effectively. (Sibutramine is also a stimulant, which further reduces appetite.) Despite the related mechanism, sibutramine does not seem to harm the heart valves. But it can cause other problems, notably increased blood pressure. While that rise is usually small, all sibutramine users must have their blood pressure monitored carefully; people with poorly controlled hypertension should avoid it entirely.

Orlistat fights obesity by inactivating certain intestinal enzymes needed to absorb dietary fat. That can produce bloating, gas, and loose stools if you consume lots of fat. It may also block absorption of fat-soluble vitamins, including vitamins A, D, and E, so users should take a multivitamin supplement. (Early concerns about a possible breast-cancer risk are apparently unfounded.)

The safety of the new drugs won't be clearly established until they've been used extensively. So consider them only if you're truly obese—with a BMI over 30 or a BMI over 27 plus multiple risk factors for obesity (see story)—and have really tried and failed to lose weight without drugs.

Herbal fens

In the wake of the FDA ban, supplement makers have been flooding health-food stores with concoctions such as *Herbal Phen-Fen*, *PhenTrim*, and *Phen-Cal*. Those names clearly imply that the products offer the weight-loss power of fen-phen without the risk. But there's no good evidence that any of them can help people lose weight. Further, most of them contain ephedra, or ma huang, which has been linked with numerous problems, including nervousness, insomnia, headache, high blood pressure, irregular heart rate, even heart attack and stroke. And some contain chromium, which isolated reports have linked with anemia, kidney failure, and mental impairment.

---

exercise at a moderate pace for much longer than they can exercise strenuously.

For the average person, building up to sessions lasting at least 45 to 60 minutes, four to five times a week, is generally the most effective exercise regimen for weight loss. Two or preferably three times a week, you should devote some of those minutes to strength training. You could devote the rest to exercises like brisk walking, hiking, bicycling, cross-country skiing, or energetic dancing: They're vigorous enough to burn calories at a reasonable clip, yet sufficiently moderate, interesting, and easy on the joints that the average person could do them for a fairly long time.

◆ **Myth: The best weight-loss diet is a strict, very low calorie regimen.**

Truth: Extreme diets rarely work in the long run. The sharp drop in your metabolic rate after rapid weight loss makes you likely to put the pounds back on. In addition, extreme diets increase the risk of gallstones. And some low-calorie diets—especially those that limit you to only a few foods, such as the popular grapefruit or cabbage-soup diets—might harm your health by depriving you of needed nutrients.

Instead of crash-dieting, try to make changes you can live with. The most healthful approach is to replace high-calorie fatty or sugary foods with more nutritious, lower-calorie foods like whole grains, beans, fruits, and vegetables. If you're already eating a healthful diet—or want to try a more aggressive approach—you could also reduce the size of your portions, particularly of any higher-calorie foods.

◆ **Myth: A low-fat diet will definitely help you lose weight.**

Truth: While the typical American diet has become less fatty, the typical American has become fatter, in part because the average intake of calories has actually gone up (see illustration). When people adopt a low-fat diet, they often compensate by eating

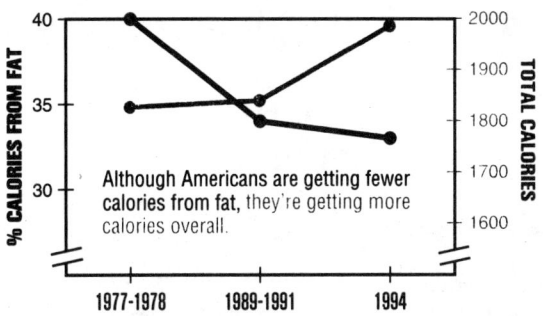

Less fat, but fatter

Although Americans are getting fewer calories from fat, they're getting more calories overall.

more than they did before. And many of the new foods manufactured to be low in fat have nearly as many calories as the regular versions, since manufacturers adjust for the loss of palate-pleasing fat by adding extra carbohydrates or protein. So if you want to lose weight, you need to watch the calories, not just the fat.

◆ **Myth: Cream, butter, lard, and other animal fats are more fattening than vegetable oils like canola and olive.**

Truth: Animal fats—as well as certain tropical oils, such as coconut and palm oil—are indeed worse for you than vegetable oils. But that's not because they're more fattening; rather, it's because they're high in saturated fat, which raises blood-cholesterol levels and the risk of coronary disease as well as possibly raising the risk of certain cancers. All fats, regardless of the source, provide the same number of calories, and thus pose the same potential for weight gain.

◆ **Myth: Carbohydrates make you gain weight, while protein helps you lose it.**

Truth: Several popular diet books have resurrected the antiquated notion that substituting protein for carbohydrates can melt away fat. But both of those dietary components contain four calories per gram, and the body socks away unused calories from both sources equally efficiently. Further, there's little evidence for the claim that protein helps curb the appetite.

Some diet gurus claim that carbohydrates raise blood levels of the hormone insulin, which in turn increases appetite and also helps convert carbohydrates to body fat. But carbohydrates may boost insulin only in people with insulin resistance, a metabolic disorder that prevents efficient use of the hormone. And there's no evidence that carbohydrates lead to weight gain even in those people. On the contrary, high-carbohydrate foods such as rice, pasta, and bread—preferably whole-grain versions—should be the mainstay of a healthful diet, though you need to go easy on the adornments, like butter and sauce. High-carbo foods are low in calories and fat, high in certain minerals and B vitamins and, if whole grain, high in fiber.

Summing up

Judge the need to lose weight by your BMI, your body type, and the size of your waist and hips—not by your appearance. If you do need to lose:

■ Do lengthy workouts at the fastest pace that you can comfortably sustain—generally a moderate one. Spend some of that time strength training.

■ Instead of going on a crash diet, replace high-calorie foods with lower-calorie, healthier fare, such as produce and whole grains. If necessary, you can cut the portion sizes as well.

■ Watch your calorie intake even if you're already watching your fat intake.

■ Don't avoid carbohydrates; in fact, eat plenty of them—but go easy on the toppings.

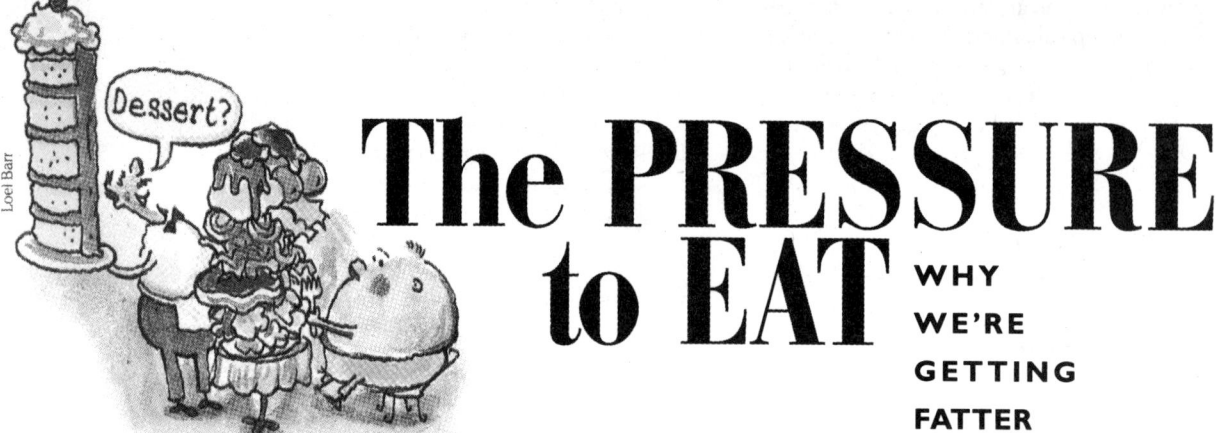

The PRESSURE to EAT
WHY WE'RE GETTING FATTER

Q: Why is there an obesity epidemic in the U.S.?

A: There are several logical places to look for the answer. Our culture and the medical profession may be looking in the wrong places.

Culture has blamed obesity on the individual. We assume that people are overweight because of personal failings, that they're lazy, weak, and gluttonous. An imperfect body reflects an imperfect person.

Q: Don't people need to watch what they eat?

A: Yes, but the pressure on people to take responsibility for what they eat is staggering already, and I wonder whether more pressure will be counterproductive and make people even more obsessed with what they eat.

A good example is the Shape Up America! program, which is spearheaded by former Surgeon General C. Everett Koop. Its basic message is that the American public should weigh less and exercise more. Is there anyone in America who doesn't know that?

Q: What's wrong with the medical profession's approach to obesity?

A: People are in hot pursuit of the obesity gene, and perhaps something will come from genetic discoveries that will help some people lose weight. But, I ask you, do genes explain the epidemic and will they provide the solution? I don't believe so.

Developing drugs to solve the obesity problem might help some people, but the effort might be likened to developing drugs to repair the damage caused by smoking, and not attending to its cause.

And searching for the gene for obesity may be like searching for the gene to discover who will get lung cancer once they smoke. Yes, it would be interesting, but the cause of the lung cancer is smoking, not biology.

Q: What's causing obesity rates to soar must be something that has changed recently.

A: Right. The prevalence of obesity has increased dramatically since 1980. And obesity is on the rise in country after country, as each becomes more like America.

Can we explain the increase because we have less willpower than we did ten years ago? Are we so different? Can we explain it with biology? Has the gene pool changed in ten years? Evolution takes millions of years. We ignore the obvious.

Q: The constant pressure to eat?

A: Yes. I believe that Americans are exposed to a toxic food environment. The word 'toxic' is not too strong. There are dangerous agents in the environment that are widely available and that cause people to be sick.

Americans have unprecedented access to a poor diet—to high-calorie foods that are widely available, low in cost, heavily promoted, and good tasting. These ingredients produce a predictable, understandable, and inevitable consequence—an epidemic of diet-related diseases.

Q: Is the food industry to blame?

A: The food industry certainly contributes, but it's hard to know whether the industry is responding to demand from consumers or is shaping food preferences. Either

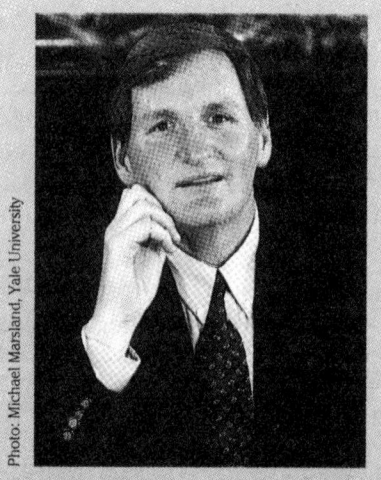

Kelly Brownell is a professor of psychology, epidemiology, and public health at Yale University in New Haven, Connecticut. He is one of the nation's leading obesity experts and is a member of *Nutrition Action Healthletter*'s Scientific Advisory Board. Brownell spoke to *Nutrition Action*'s Bonnie Liebman by telephone.

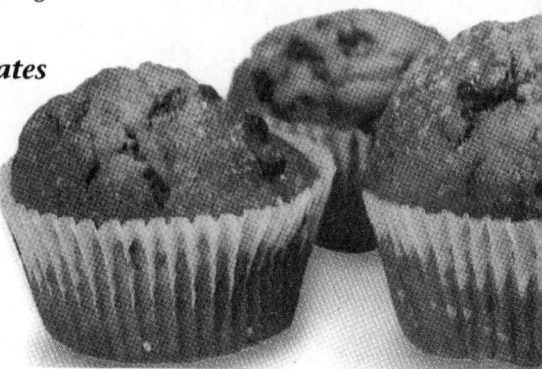

Au Bon Pain Blueberry Muffin (1)
430 calories & 18 grams of fat

20. Pressure to Eat

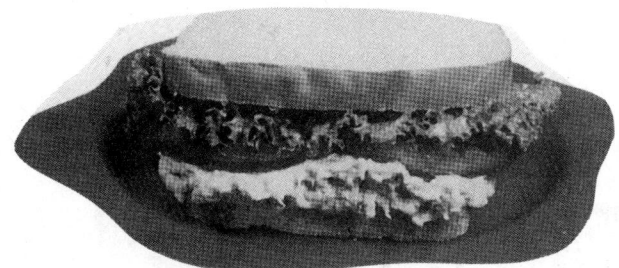

Deli Tuna Salad Sandwich with Mayo
833 calories & 56 grams of fat

way, the environment is terrible.

The *New York Times* recently ran an article on McDonald's. It said that three new McDonald's come on line every day, that a corporate goal is to have no American more than four minutes from one of its restaurants, and that seven percent of Americans eat at McDonald's on any given day. And that's only one chain.

This is capitalism at its best to be sure, but what effect is it having on us? McDonald's signs now say 'billions and billions served.' When it becomes 'trillions and trillions,' will we be better off?

Q: *Why is the fast food industry so successful?*

A: It has made many marketing breakthroughs. One was serving breakfast. Others were the drive-in window and package meals—what McDonald's calls super-value meals. And now we have very large sizes—what they call supersizes.

The industry's influence is so pernicious and pervasive that many, perhaps most, American children recognize the word 'supersize' as a verb. It's just part of our culture.

Q: *It's not just fast food. Our studies show that a typical meal at an ordinary restaurant has 1,000 calories, and that's without the dessert or appetizer.*

A: One of the first things people from other countries notice when they visit the U.S. are the large portions served in restaurants. In most of the world, there's no such thing as a doggie bag.

Q: *And food is available everywhere, all the time.*

A: Yes. It seems like every service station has been remodeled to put a food market inside. You can drive down the road in many communities and pass five or six service stations, fast food restaurants, and convenience stores in less than a mile.

One Exxon station near my home has not only a food market with the usual chips and snack foods, but also a Dunkin' Donuts franchise inside it. And a Texaco station off the interstate had a food market, Dunkin' Donuts, and Subway.

Fast food is infiltrating our culture. There are fast food restaurants inside some schools. Malls have food courts. Fast foods are showing up on airline flights and in airports. It's basically everywhere.

Q: *And schools that don't house fast food chains serve hamburgers, pizza, tacos, or other fast foods anyway.*

A: Right. You can argue that we're biologically programmed to eat such food because it's high in fat and sugar. Laboratory rats will eat that kind of food if you give them access to it, and they can become quite obese.

Animals—and people—evolved in an environment where food was scarce and calorie expenditures were high. Under those conditions, being programmed to eat high-calorie food is adaptive. Those ancient genes wouldn't be a problem if the environment weren't so damaging.

Q: *The ancient genes programmed our ancestors to eat high-calorie foods to sustain people in times of scarcity?*

A: Exactly. But there's no scarcity today, and we expend far fewer calories. The environment has only changed over the past hundred years, and it takes thousands or millions of years for evolution to catch up and change our ancient genes. The environment has changed too quickly.

Q: *What about sedentary lifestyles?*

A: This is terribly important. The toxic environment is a combination of food and lack of physical activity. The remote control, video games, the automobile, television, and to some extent the computer are all part of the toxic environment because they discourage people from being physically active.

Q: *Aren't there barriers to physical activity?*

A: Some people live in neighborhoods where they can't go outside because walking or running is too dangerous, and they don't have money to join health clubs. Plus, given that we're becoming fatter as a society, it becomes less appealing to exercise.

And energy-saving devices are part of who we are. We can't get rid of the remote control or the computer. Those devices will continue to creep into our daily lives so there'll be even less need to be physically active. That means that people are going to have to get physical activity on their own time and in their own way.

4 ❖ EXERCISE AND WEIGHT CONTROL

Pizza Hut Pepperoni Lover's Pan Pizza *(2 slices)*
700 calories & 34 grams of fat

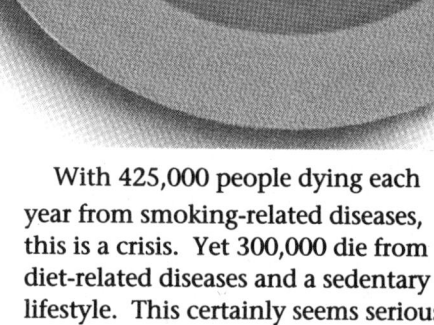

Q: *Do other countries have less-toxic environments?*

A: Yes. And they have less obesity, too. There's an alarming increase in obesity, like we see in the U.S., but they start at a lower level. As the environment changes, those countries will have more diet problems, as we do.

Q: *What about the social pressure to eat? Has junk food become synonymous with fun?*

A: As in most cultures, food has tremendous social meaning. People can feel like they aren't part of the group if they don't eat like everybody else does.

Food also has personal meaning. It can be a person's best friend, and it allows some people to numb out from a difficult world. Some people look forward during the day to being alone with their food in the evening. It represents comfort, soothing, and nurturance that may not come from other people.

Q: *Is that a result of the toxic environment?*

A: Some people would be drawn to food regardless of the environment, but just as the alcohol industry glorifies drinking and makes people feel cool and part of a group if they drink, the food industry makes eating seem pretty special.

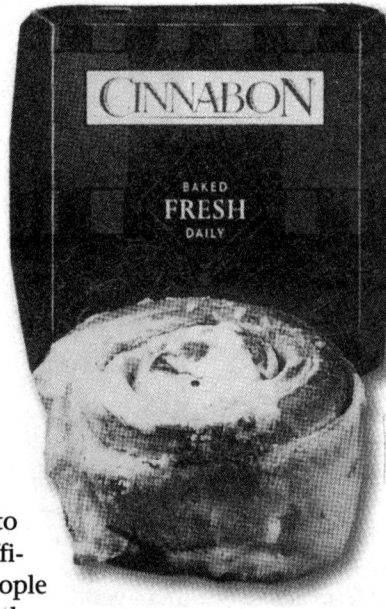

Cinnabon
670 calories & 34 grams of fat

Q: *What's the answer?*

A: I recommend that we develop a militant attitude about the toxic food environment, like we have about tobacco. And that leads to certain actions to change the American diet to be more healthy.

The specific proposals I've made are: subsidize the cost of healthy foods, so they cost less; increase the cost of bad foods, so they cost more; regulate food advertising aimed at children; and develop more opportunities for people to be more physically active.

Q: *How do people react to your bad-food-tax proposal?*

A: The knee-jerk response has been: 'Where does it end? Are you going to tell us how to lead our lives and intrude on personal decisions?'

But if you went back 20 years and said 'I propose we recover money from the tobacco companies to repay states for expenses caused by smoking' or 'we should ban smoking in public places' or 'take Joe Camel off the billboards,' people would have thought you were crazy. Government intrusion, they would have charged.

But all that changed as we recognized the overwhelming toll produced by smoking. It became so serious that society overlooked the intrusion on individual rights for the greater social good.

With 425,000 people dying each year from smoking-related diseases, this is a crisis. Yet 300,000 die from diet-related diseases and a sedentary lifestyle. This certainly seems serious to me.

Q: *So even though french fries aren't as addictive or harmful as cigarettes, in both cases there's an industry manipulating us, from a young age, to do something unhealthy?*

A: Exactly right. I have asked myself whether Joe Camel is different than Ronald McDonald. One could claim that they both encourage children to adopt habits that could be bad for their health.

Q: *Aren't our growing waistlines a sign of the food industry's success?*

A: There are probably many factors that explain the growing national waistline. But it's difficult to be optimistic about the future when we see record levels of obesity in our children and phenomenal sales of snack foods, fast foods, and soft drinks.

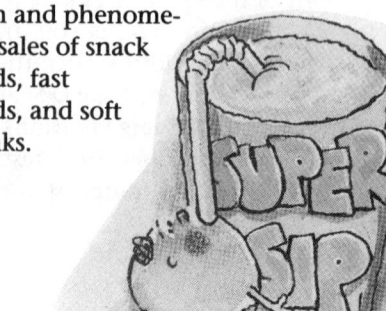

Supersize Foods, Supersize People

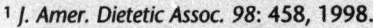

"The food industry is selling food in larger portions," says Marion Nestle, chair of the Department of Nutrition and Food Studies at New York University.

"There's been a steady progression of restaurants and manufacturers dropping small sizes. Starbucks doesn't have 'short' drinks on its menu any more, only 'tall,' 'grande,' and the even-larger 'venti.'"

Nestle and colleague Lisa Young asked 100 college students taking a nutrition course to bring in a bagel, baked potato, muffin, or cookie that they considered "medium."[1] Then they compared those foods to serving sizes that the U.S. Department of Agriculture—which advises the public on how much of what to eat—calls "medium." The results:

- A typical medium baked potato was seven ounces, instead of the USDA's four ounces.
- A typical medium bagel was four ounces, double the USDA's two ounces.
- A typical medium muffin was six ounces, triple the USDA's two ounces.

"It's a great sales technique," says Nestle. "People buy larger sizes because they perceive them as good value. If they're going to spend all this money on food, especially in a restaurant, they figure they might as well get a lot to eat."

And more food doesn't cost much more. At many United Artists movie theaters, a small drink (22 oz.) costs $2.50, a medium (32 oz.) costs $2.75, and a large (44 oz.) costs $3.00.

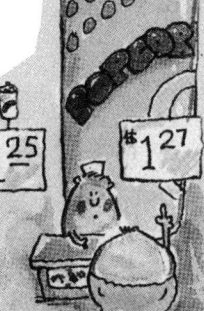

Why is it profitable to sell giant servings? "Only about 20 cents of every food dollar goes to the producer of the food," explains Nestle. "The rest is for packaging, transportation, advertising, and marketing." And those costs don't change much as the serving size soars.

Movie and a Measuring Cup

OK, so foods come in bigger sizes. Does that make us eat more? Yes, says Brian Wansink, director of the Food and Brand Research Lab at the University of Illinois at Champaign-Urbana.

Wansink sent 79 parents home with a video and either one- or two-pound bags of M&Ms plus either a "medium" or "jumbo" movie-theater-sized tub of popcorn for each family member.

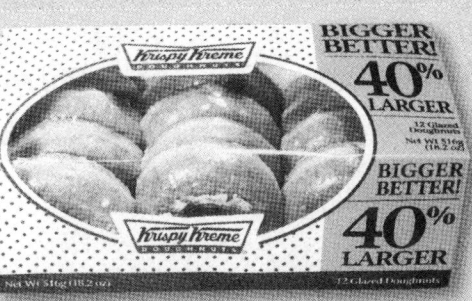

"On average, people ate 112 M&Ms from the one-pound bag and 156 from the two-pound bag," says Wansink. Likewise, the average person ate roughly half a tub of popcorn, whether it was medium or jumbo (which held twice as much).

"People can often eat about 50 percent more of hedonistic foods like candy, chips, and popcorn when they come in bigger packages," says Wansink. "With other foods, the increase is usually about 25 percent."

Why? "I think we're hard-wired to believe that bigger equals cheaper. So people feel that it costs nothing to use more."

More evidence: People poured themselves about 20 percent more bottled water when it came in a two-liter container instead of a one-liter container.[2] But when the containers were labeled "tap water," they poured the same amount from each.

"People see tap water as free, so there's no size quantity discount," says Wansink. "And for most products, you don't save money by buying a larger size."

Drop Anchor

Signs in supermarkets can also encourage people to buy more food.[3] In Wansink's studies, people buy more of an item—often twice as much—if the sign uses:

- *Multiple-unit pricing*, like "2 for $1.50" instead of "75 cents each."
- *Quantity limits*, like "limit 4 per customer" ("limit 12 per customer" sells even more).
- *Suggested quantities*, like "Snickers bars—buy 18 for your freezer."

"Just putting a specific number on a sign will stimulate shoppers to buy more than the one or two they ordinarily would," says Wansink. "When consumers shop, they anchor on a suggested number to buy and then adjust that up or down, depending on the circumstances."

Most people anchor on one or two, and usually buy one to three of the item. "But when the sign suggests a different, higher number," he explains, "many consumers unconsciously adopt this as their new anchor and adjust down a few units from that."

How to avoid eating more?

- Include in your shopping list the *amount* of each item to buy.
- At restaurants, don't hesitate to ask for a doggie bag. You'll have tomorrow's lunch already made.
- Offer to share an entree, appetizer, or dessert. You'll save money and calories. —Bonnie Liebman

---

[1] *J. Amer. Dietetic Assoc.* 98: 458, 1998.
[2] *Journal of Marketing* 60: 1, 1996.
[3] *Journal of Marketing Research* 35: 71, 1998.

Article 21

Walk It Off

Does Food Control You?

There's a difference between worrying about your weight and being obsessed

By Winifred Yu

In a culture that puts a premium on appearances, body weight has become a measure of worth: Thin is good, fat is bad. So it's not surprising that most of us experience what experts call "normative discontent" with our bodies: We lament our jiggling thighs and upper arms, fret over fat grams and calories, and desperately rearrange our hectic schedules to fit in exercise.

But for some people, weight—and the food and exercise that affect it—is an all-consuming obsession. Maybe it's dwelling on every calorie they ingest. Or focusing too much on fat grams. Or calculating the amount of exercise they'll need after every dessert. In any case, an obsession with weight can dominate a person's life.

"It's not the person who says, 'I've eaten too much today and will have only a bite of pie for dessert,'" says Dori Winchell, a psychologist in Encinitas, Calif., who specializes in eating disorders. "It's when food controls you rather than you controlling the food."

Distinguishing an obsession

Clinically, an obsession with weight is a characteristic of all three major eating disorders: anorexia nervosa, bulimia and binge eating. On its own, however, it is categorized as an "eating disorder otherwise unspecified." The sufferer does not have a major disorder. In fact, she may even be at a normal, healthy weight. People who are obsessed simply spend the majority of their days contemplating their weight and anything that might affect it. Especially food.

"If a person is at a normal weight and has had a pretty stable weight pattern for five to 10 years, but she still continues to worry about her weight, count calories, avoid fats, or weigh her food at every meal, there's probably an obsession going on," says Susan Head, a clinical psychologist at Duke University Diet and Fitness Center in Durham, N.C.

So how do you know if you're obsessed with weight? Here are some telltale signs:

- *Your diet interferes with other aspects of your life.* Maybe you avoid social situations for fear of overeating.

People who are obsessed spend the majority of their time thinking about their weight and anything that might affect it—especially food.

Or maybe you don't frequent certain restaurants because you'll be tempted by a favorite dessert. The problem is that your food intake dictates how you end up living the rest of your life.

- *You restrict what you eat.* Do you confine yourself to certain foods that you designate as "safe"? Ban entire categories of food from your diet? Impose a daily calorie limit that you hold as gospel? Unless you have a health condition that requires you to limit your intake of, say, fat or cholesterol, such restrictions are unnecessary and often unhealthful.

"You can't always eat just cottage cheese and carrot sticks," says Debra Hauser, M.S.W., Ph.D., who offers eating-disorder treatment at the Yale Center for Eating and Weight Disor-

21. Does Food Control You?

> ## Overcoming an Obsession
>
> **Take risks with your diet.** If you restrict fat intake to 10%, try adopting a more moderate goal of 15% of calories for a week, says Susan Head of Duke University Diet and Fitness Center. "When you see that your weight hasn't changed, it will prove to you that you can veer."
>
> **Challenge your restrictions.** "If you find yourself omitting certain foods for no other reason than you've decided they're bad, try introducing them back into your diet," says Head. Make a list of forbidden foods, then allow yourself to eat a "mildly" restricted food. Keep your calories the same, and weigh yourself only at the start and end of the week.
>
> **Set a weight range.** Instead of holding yourself to 130 pounds, allow yourself to weigh 130 to 135. Setting a range alleviates some of the tension that goes with occasional and normal weight fluctuations.
>
> **Examine your life.** Consider keeping a journal to assess your emotions. According to Debra Hauser., M.S.W. Ph.D., most obsessions are born of such problems as loneliness, depression, and vocational dissatisfaction. Confronting the real issue may help you overcome your preoccupation with weight. —*W.Y.*

ders in Connecticut. "Nor can you eat everything you want all the time."

- *You're rigid in your thinking.* Some people don't feel good about themselves unless their weight is at a magic number. To maintain that number, each day they eat only a certain number of calories or exercise for a set amount of time. Or maybe they set strict rules, such as not allowing themselves to eat after a certain hour. This inflexible mind-set leads to unnecessary feelings of guilt when a rule is violated.
- *You spend most of your day thinking about food.* A person with normal eating habits may think about food 10% to 15% of the day, according to Frances Berg, M.S., author of *Afraid to Eat: Children and Teens in Weight Crisis* (Healthy Weight Network, 1997). But if you think about it more than 30% of the time, you may be a dysfunctional eater, and obsessed with your weight.

Getting help

Changing the obsessed mind-set typically requires professional help. But most people won't seek help unless their obsession is impinging on other aspects of their lives, Hauser says. The fact that so many women are like this doesn't help matters, because the pattern is often viewed as "normal" and not something that requires attention. "People have to be pretty unhappy to come to therapy," she says.

If you suspect you're spending too much time dwelling on your weight, there are steps you can take to alleviate the obsession (see "Overcoming an Obsession").

The goal is to return to more balanced thinking and eating. "You want to go beyond food," Winchell says. "Healthy is moderation. It means sometimes eating too much, sometimes not eating enough. It's you making the choice based on your needs, not the food making the choice based on weight issues."

Winifred Yu is a freelance writer who lives in Voorheesville, N. Y.

Binge-Eating That Plagues Adults Now Recognized As A Disorder

We've all binged from time to time. Whether it was downing an entire quart of ice cream because of feeling blue or caving in to the temptation of trays of hors d'oeuvres and pitchers of eggnog during the holidays.

But those are occasional binges. Most of us find it hard not to overeat during festive occasions or when strong emotions get the better of us. It's only a problem if it becomes an out-of-control, more-than-occasional thing. Then it's what medical experts have dubbed "binge-eating disorder," a serious medical condition, says Karen Eselson Belding, Psy.D., clinical director at The Renfrew Center in Philadelphia, which specializes in eating disorders.

"Binge-eating disorder is when an individual repeatedly consumes extremely large quantities of food—several thousand calories at a time—in an effort to cope with whatever is bothering them emotionally, like depression, grief or boredom," explains Belding.

This pattern of eating far beyond fullness is estimated to affect 2% to 5% of Americans. That's much more common than either anorexia nervosa (starvation) or bulimia nervosa (bingeing and purging)—more well-known eating disorders. (Less than 1% of the population is anorexic, while bulimia affects 1% to 3%.)

Newly Recognized Status. Only recently has the American Psychiatric Association proposed binge-eating as a psychiatric illness with specific criteria. They include:

- Consuming extremely large amounts of food, totaling several thousand calories, in a short period of time (for example: 2 to 3 hamburgers plus 2 to 3 orders of fries, followed by a gallon of ice cream).
- Consuming food rapidly.
- Recurring episodes of binge-eating—at least twice a week over six months.
- Bingeing alone.
- Feeling a lack of control or inability to stop during a binge.
- Post-binge feelings of self-hatred, guilt, depression or disgust.
- No purging, fasting, excessive exercise or other compensation for calories ingested.

As is true of most people with eating disorders, binge-eaters let food control their lives. Many sleep for eight hours or more after a binge, because they are physically sick from all the food ingested. As a result, they find their work, family and social lives suffer. Yet because binge eaters are good at hiding their behavior, close family members and friends often don't know they binge.

Not Anorexia or Bulimia. This same secrecy and obsession with food characterizes anorexia nervosa and bulimia. Yet body weight distinguishes the three conditions. Those with anorexia are noticeably gaunt because they simply starve themselves; there's no bingeing involved. Those with bulimia tend to be within a desirable weight range, because they compensate for their binges by fasting, purging (e.g. vomiting or taking laxatives) or engaging in strenuous exercise.

In contrast, those who binge-eat are typically significantly overweight or obese, because they do not engage in compensatory behaviors to off-set the calories they eat, says Seda Ebrahimi, Ph.D., director of the Eating Disorders Treatment Program at McLean Hospital in Belmont, Massachusetts.

Nevertheless, explains Ebrahimi, because they aren't starving themselves or subjecting their gastrointestinal tracts to constant vomiting or diarrhea, the medical consequences of binge-eating are generally much less than for either bulimia or anorexia. That's not true, however, if the person has diabetes, hypertension or another chronic weight-triggered condition. In such cases, serious consequences *can* occur from repeated binges, like poor control of diabetes.

The Classic Binge-Eater. Another difference separates this disorder from other eating disorders—who it strikes. Anorexia and bulimia sufferers are 90% to 95% female (and typically adolescents or young adults). Binge-eating disorder, on the other hand, doesn't usually begin until early adulthood, and those who suffer often don't seek help until middle-age. Moreover, more than one-third are men; less than two-thirds are women.

Do You Have a Problem?

If you agree with most of these statements, you may have a binge-eating problem and should seek help.

- Do you frequently find yourself eating unusually large amounts of food in a short period of time?
- Are there times when you cannot stop eating, even if you want to?
- Do you ever feel extremely guilty or depressed after bingeing?
- Do you feel more determined to diet or to eat healthfully after a binge?

Source: Journal of the American Dietetic Association, Vol. 96, No. 1, with permission.

Classic binge-eaters see themselves as failures. They've tried numerous diets, losing and regaining the same weight many times over. Surveys show that nearly one-third of enrollees in weight-loss programs meet the criteria for binge-eating disorder. Strikingly, almost three-quarters of those in Overeaters Anonymous (OA) meet the criteria, probably because OA approaches overeating as an addiction, similar to alcoholism or gambling.

Experts are not sure what causes binge-eating disorder, but believe it has a psychological basis, with binge eaters perceiving situations as more stressful than others do. Up to half of people with the condition have a history of depression. Moreover, many sufferers say binges are triggered by anger, sadness, boredom, anxiety or some other negative emotion.

Hope and Help. Treatment options for binge-eating disorder include cognitive behavior therapy, psychoanalysis and antidepressant medications, such as fluoxetine (*Prozac*).

During cognitive therapy, a therapist teaches patients to understand the connection between feelings and episodes of bingeing. "We work with clients to help them eat in response to physical hunger rather than emotion," says Adrienne Ressler, M.S., C.S.W., a body image specialist at The Renfrew Center. To do this, clients are asked to identify their feelings when they feel the urge to binge, by asking themselves: Am I sad? Happy? Fearful? Whatever their feelings, they need to learn to identify these triggers and nurture them in ways other than eating, explains Ressler. For example, counselors teach a technique called "pausing"—switching to another activity, such as telephoning someone, going for a walk or taking a shower.

Typically, counselors do not give binge-eaters a strict diet to follow. Instead, they give general guidelines for meal planning, to help regulate food intake. At the Renfrew Center, for example, all foods are "legalized," so clients do not label foods as "good" or "bad," which can cause feelings of deprivation that might trigger bingeing, says Ressler. Because eating disorders create a feeling of isolation, group therapy is recommended to help binge eaters open up to and learn from others who suffer from the same condition.

If you suspect someone has binge-eating disorder, help the person seek treatment from a qualified program specifically designed to treat eating disorders. (See below.)

—*Julie Walsh, M.S., R.D.*

Where to Turn for Help

The following organizations and university-based hospitals specialize in eating disorders. For a clinic in your area, call one of the associations below.

- American Anorexia/Bulimia Association (212) 575-6200
- Eating Disorders Research Program, University of Minnesota (612) 627-4494
- National Eating Disorders Organization (918) 481-4044
- Nutrition Research Clinic, Baylor College of Medicine (713) 798-5757
- Overeaters Anonymous (505) 891-2664
- Renfrew Centers (800) RENFREW
- Stanford University School of Medicine, Behavioral Medicine (415) 723-5868
- Yale Center for Eating and Weight Disorders (203) 432-4610

Unit 5

Unit Selections

23. **The Postmodern Guide to Cold Relief,** Bill Shapiro
24. **Alcohol and Health: Straight Talk on the Medical Headlines,** Charles H. Hennekens
25. **The War over Weed,** Tom Morganthau
26. **Will You Pay for Your Past as a Smoker?** Harvard Health Letter

Key Points to Consider

❖ Do you think America has a drug problem? Defend your answer.

❖ How might a person decide when drug use has become drug abuse?

❖ What responsibility does the U.S. government have in the area of preventing drug abuse? What responsibility do communities have in the area of drug abuse?

❖ Should insurance companies pay medical costs incurred as a result of drug abuse? Why or why not?

❖ Given society's ambivalence toward alcohol, how can we best curb the problem of alcohol abuse?

❖ What factors should a person consider before making the decision to use alcohol to safeguard health?

❖ Should marijuana be made available for medical purposes? Why or why not? What potential problems could arise as a result of this action?

❖ What restrictions, if any, should be placed on the use of tobacco products?

❖ Recently the mass media has been charged with contributing to the growing drug problem by portraying drugs in an appealing manner. Do you feel this charge is justified? Why or why not?

❖ Some states are considering passing laws that would make it a crime to abuse drugs during pregnancy. How do you feel about this?

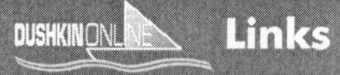 **Links**   www.dushkin.com/online/

18. **National Institute on Drug Abuse (NIDA)**
    http://165.112.78.61
19. **University of California at San Francisco/Drug Dependence Research Center (DDRC)**
    http://itsa.ucsf.edu/~ddrc/about.html
20. **University of Chicago**
    http://uhs.bsd.uchicago.edu/~bhsiung/tips/tips.html

These sites are annotated on pages 4 and 5.

Drugs and Health

As a culture, Americans have come to rely on drugs not only as a treatment for disease but also as an aid for living normal, productive lives. This view of drugs has fostered both a casual attitude regarding their use and a tremendous drug abuse problem. The term "drug abuse" conjures up visions of derelicts, dark alleys, and wasted lives. In reality, this description is accurate for only a small minority of drug users. That is not to say that drugs are not responsible for destroying many lives, but rather that drug abuse has become so widespread that there is no way to describe the typical drug abuser, except to say that he or she could be anyone.

What accounts for the casual attitude toward drug usage? There is no simple explanation for why America has become a drug-taking culture, but there is certainly evidence to suggest some of the factors that have contributed to this development. From the time that we are children, we are constantly bombarded by advertisements about how certain drugs can make us feel and look better. While most of these ads deal with proprietary drugs, the belief is created that drugs are a legitimate and effective way to help us cope with everyday problems. Growing up, most of us probably had a medicine cabinet full of over-the-counter (OTC) drugs, freely dispensed to family members to treat a variety of ailments. This familiarity with OTC drugs, coupled with rising health care costs, has prompted many people to diagnose and medicate themselves with OTC medications without sufficient knowledge of their possible side effects. While most of these preparations have little potential for abuse, that does not mean that they are innocuous. OTC drugs are relatively safe if taken at the recommended dosage by healthy people. The risk of dangerous side effects rises sharply when people exceed the recommended dosage. Another potential danger associated with the use of OTC drugs is the drug interactions that can occur when they are taken in conjunction with prescription medications. The gravest danger associated with the use of OTC drugs is that an individual may be using them to control symptoms of an underlying disease and thus preventing the early diagnosis and treatment of the disease. Bill Shapiro, in "The Postmodern Guide to Cold Relief," explores the major categories of cold medications currently being marketed for the relief of cold symptoms and provides useful information for making an informed decision regarding their use.

Alcohol, nicotine, and caffeine are the most widely used and abused drugs in America, but they do not get nearly as much media coverage as do the more exotic and illicit drugs, such as cocaine, crack, PCP, and marijuana. Does this mean that these drugs are not as dangerous? When it comes to tobacco and alcohol, the answer is a resounding "no." Clearly alcohol and tobacco are far and away the leading causes of death and disability related to drug usage. How can we as a society expect to significantly curtail drug usage in general if we sanction the use of two drugs with such a deadly track record?

Marijuana, perhaps more than any other drug, has stirred considerable debate regarding the criteria being used to legalize or decriminalize a given drug. To date there is not a single case of an individual dying as a result of a marijuana overdose. And despite all the allegations regarding the damaging impact that smoking this substance will have on the lungs, there is yet to be a single case of lung cancer or chronic obstructive lung disease among long-term marijuana users who have never smoked tobacco products. The stage is ripe for a serious and rational debate on legalizing the medical use of marijuana. In "The War over Weed," Tom Morganthau addresses the issue of "medical marijuana" and provides the reader with the argument on both sides of the issue.

Of the drug problems facing this nation, alcohol use is clearly one of the most complex. While we deplore alcohol for the countless deaths and disabilities it causes each year, we openly sanction moderate use of alcohol in a variety of social situations. This ambivalence even permeates the scientific community. While it is clear that heavy alcohol use results in significant damage to a variety of organ systems, the same cannot be said of moderate use. Several recent studies have reported that moderate alcohol use increases a woman's risk of breast cancer, and at the same time, several studies have suggested that moderate alcohol use may help prevent coronary artery disease. At issue here is the meaning of the term moderation. What constitutes moderate alcohol use? Is it the same amount for all people and at all ages? "Alcohol and Health: Straight Talk on the Medical Headlines" addresses the pros and cons of using alcohol from a physician's perspective.

Few people today continue to harbor any misconceptions about the health hazards associated with prolonged use of tobacco. Most realize that this drug is associated with emphysema, lung cancer, strokes, and heart disease, but they may not be aware that smoking can cause retinal damage, impotence, cold fingers, and low-back pains. Given the amount of bad press that tobacco has had over the last few years, why is it that so many Americans continue to smoke? Some argue that they continue to smoke because they have done it for so long that quitting wouldn't make any difference with regard to their health. "Will You Pay for Your Past as a Smoker?" examines the benefits associated with stopping smoking and concludes that, while they are substantial regardless of how long you have smoked, the actual rate of recovery varies with each organ system and the degree of damage sustained.

As a culture, we have grown up believing that there is, or should be, a drug to treat any malady or discomfort that befalls us. Would we have a drug problem if there were no demand for drugs? We have seen the enemy and it is us!

The Postmodern Guide to Cold Relief

So many pills, such a simple ailment

BY BILL SHAPIRO

There are sneezes, and there are sneezes. And then there was Hurricane Ethel. The sheer thunder of Ethel took everyone in the pharmacy by surprise, including the pink-nosed woman in the Yankees cap who unapologetically claimed it as her own. Pacing aisle six, she studied the cold remedies—all 72 feet of them. Back and forth. Back and forth. She chose one; looked it over, replaced it. Back and forth again. She was confused. And sick. And sick of being confused. So she marched up to the pharmacist with an armful of boxes and, this being New York, addressed him with a resounding "Yo!" As in, "Yo, how the hell am I supposed to figure out which one of these to take?"

How indeed? With some 2,800 products on the market, a stroll down cold remedy lane leaves the consumer with almost as many questions. The situation is so overwhelming that while shoppers spend 53 seconds at the shelf choosing the average item, they take a full two and a half minutes to decide on a cold medication, according to Meyer's Research Center, a market-research firm in New York City.

One reason for this product glut is that colds are a very popular ailment: The average adult catches two to four of them a year. But since only a few ingredients are considered effective, sometimes all a pharmaceutical company can do to catch the consumer's eye is change a flavor or tweak a delivery system. Pill or capsule, elixir or gel cap, grape or orange: Such distinctions create the illusion of variety, but when it comes to treating your cold, they usually don't amount to a hill of beans.

Of course, purists argue that it's best to avoid this whole circus altogether—that when you dry up a runny nose or suppress a cough, you're monkeying around with the body's own system for getting rid of the cold. But experts say that by the time your symptoms kick in, your body's well on its way to shedding the virus and healing itself. Medication won't speed this process, but it won't slow it down either. So if you'd rather not sneeze, wheeze, or sniffle your way through the day, here's frontline advice to help you choose a medication that's right for your cold.

Steer clear of multisymptom remedies.

THE RAMBO STRATEGY is certainly tempting: Assault all symptoms at once, and kick the daylights out of that wimpy little sniffle. But experts describe several pitfalls to this approach.

For one thing, symptoms usually hit sequentially over a few days—first sore throat and achiness, then congestion, then runny nose, then sneezing and coughing. If you immediately dose up with an all-in-one pill, you'll be taking more medication than you need and subjecting yourself to some not-so-pleasant side effects.

Say you've got woeful congestion and a nasty headache but not much of a cough. If you go for the killer combo drug, you'll end up with way more cough medicine than you need, plus an antihistamine that may put you to sleep. On the other hand, if you're sneezing and coughing to beat the band, a cure-all concoction will load you up with unnecessary decongestant, which can make you as jumpy as a cat.

Worse still, all drugs carry some risk, particularly for people with certain medical conditions, and the more ingredients a medicine has, the greater the chance of a negative reaction. In a recent study at the University of North Carolina's school of pharmacology, professor Celeste Lindley concluded that around 23 million American medicine cabinets contain a potentially dangerous mix of cold remedies and prescription drugs. Decongestants, for instance, which raise your blood pressure, can wreak havoc if you take them on top of diet pills, hypertension medicine, or antidepressants. Some over-the-counter medications can also cause problems for people taking drugs for glaucoma.

So what's the best strategy for dealing with a cold? Pinpoint your most irritating symptoms, and go for the simplest medications that attack them directly. Usually one or more of the following will do just fine: a decongestant to clear up your nose, a pain reliever (ibuprofen, aspirin, or acetaminophen) for your aching head and body, a cough suppressant for your hack, and lozenges or a spray to soothe your sore throat.

Nose sprays are a better bet than oral decongestants.

AS SOON AS A COLD VIRUS sets up shop, the body releases a tsunami of chemicals, and the blood vessels in the infected area—ye olde schnozz—start to swell. Since your nose has greater blood flow per cubic centimeter of tissue than even your brain or liver, the swelling hits it particularly hard.

Oral decongestants work by constricting blood vessels throughout the body, including ones that supply blood to the nose. The catch is that they also agitate the central nervous system, so you might feel double-espresso-like side effects: nervousness, restlessness, insomnia. That's why many medication experts, such as Leslie Hendeles, a professor of pharmacy at the University of Florida in Gainesville, prefer nasal sprays to pills.

"Why stimulate the whole body with the poor man's Dexedrine when you can target the nose?" he asks. Sprays with oxymetazoline (which lasts eight to 12 hours) or phenylephrine (four hours) work faster than pills and and are less likely to produce side effects, but—and this is a big but—using them for more than three days may lead to "rebound" congestion. That's when you feel even more stuffed up than you did from the cold, and the drug no longer works.

If you're still congested on day four and decide to go the oral route, look for pseudoephedrine; it's the easiest single-ingredient formula to find, and it won't spike your blood pressure as much as phenylpropanolamine, the second most popular decongestant and, incidentally, the main ingredient in some diet pills.

There's no magic bullet when it comes to a sore throat.

SOME MULTISYMPTOM cold remedies advertise that they relieve sore throats, but that's only because the decongestant they contain stops postnasal drip, which can irritate the throat. Many sore throats, however, have nothing to do with postnasal drip; they're either an infection of the throat tissue or an irritation from coughing—and therefore require a more direct approach.

Throat sprays or lozenges containing a topical anesthetic work by temporarily deadening nerve endings in the throat. Gargling with warm salt water will also allay soreness, as will sucking on a plain-jane hard candy, which stimulates saliva flow and keeps the tissue moist.

MANY MEDICINE CABINETS CONTAIN A POTENTIALLY DANGEROUS MIX OF COLD REMEDIES AND PRESCRIPTION DRUGS.

Figure out what kind of cough you've got before dosing up.

IF YOUR DRY, hacking cough is keeping your family awake at night or earning you glares during yoga class, formulas with codeine (available without a prescription only in some states) or dextromethorphan are the most effective suppressants—also known as antitussives. They actually turn off the brain's cough center. But you don't want to suppress a so-called productive cough, which brings up phlegm; this is the body's way of cleaning your system.

For those wet, thick coughs, doctors used to recommend an expectorant called guaifenesin ("think g for gunk" was the mnemonic reminder) to thin and loosen mucus in the lungs. But the evidence supporting guaifenesin's effectiveness has come under attack from researchers and pharmacists. Michael Smith, a pediatrician who specializes in respiratory viruses and who has conducted the most comprehensive review of cold medicines to date, could find only one study on guaifenesin that met his criteria for scientific validity. The study showed no significant thinning or loosening of mucus.

"Guaifenesin," says Hendeles, who testified before Congress about the ingredient's ineffectiveness, "simply doesn't work for a cough."

The best way to treat a productive cough, doctors say, is to drink plenty of liquids (at least six eight-ounce glasses a day) to thin the mucus. And again, stay away from those multisymptom remedies: Some contain an expectorant *and* a suppressant, which work at cross-purposes and can cancel each other out.

Ignore the hype on the front of the box.

HOW MUCH STRONGER is an "extra-strength" pill? How much faster is a "fast-acting" cold tablet? What is a "pediatric formula"?

The truth, says the University of North Carolina's Lindley, is that "you just don't know because there is no standard requirement about what those words have to mean."

A "maximum-strength" medication, for instance, usually provides a larger dose than similar products by the same manufacturer. But in a multisymptom formula, it's often unclear which ingredient is beefed up. The decongestant? The painkiller? The expectorant? All three? Or consider the term "sinus formula." The only difference between Sudafed's sinus formula and its single-ingredient nasal decongestant is a dose of plain, old acetaminophen.

The only way to understand what you are really getting, says Lindley, "is to turn the box over and compare the ingredients and the dosages to those in other products."

Timed-release formulas really do work.

YOU'RE SUPPOSED TO POP to a second decongestant at noon, but the boss buzzes by. And the phone rings. And the copy machine breaks. Before you know it, it's 1:15 and you're as stuffed as a Thanksgiving turkey.

The solution? Take one timed-release pill (sometimes called sustained-release or extended-release) in the morning, and you'll get the correct doses of medicine at the right times throughout the day. Here's how it works: The pill's outer coating starts to dissolve in your stomach almost immediately, releasing a full dose. Four hours later an inner coating dissolves, releasing another full dose. And so on, usually for up to 12 hours.

DRUGS DON'T KILL THE VIRUS, BUT THEY DO TREAT A COLD'S SYMPTOMS.

Capsules have an even more impressive delivery system. Their outer coating also dissolves right away, so all the tiny pills inside are released at the same time. But different groups of pills are programmed to dissolve at certain intervals throughout the day, dosing you regularly.

Taking medicine right away won't cut your cold short.

"A COLD WILL LAST a week if you treat it and seven days if you don't," says Hendeles. That's because cold medications, even at their maximum doses, don't kill the virus, cure the infection, or even change its course; they merely relieve the symptoms.

One good bet for skirting this rule may be to go natural. Several studies suggest that taking one 500-milligram tablet of vitamin C four times a day can lessen both the symptoms and the duration of a cold. In one study zinc lozenges were shown to halve the length of the typical cold. Also, the herb echinacea may prevent and shorten some varieties of this miserable ailment.

You don't need to take an antihistamine.

EVEN THOUGH you'll find antihistamines in numerous cold products, the vast majority of pharmacists and researchers believe that they provide cold sufferers with next to no relief. Why?

Colds are reactions to viruses, and antihistamines go to work on the body's response to allergens. Antihistamines intercept histamines, the sneeze-inducing chemicals released in an allergic reaction. And histamines don't even play a supporting role in a cold.

"There's simply no pharmacologic basis for using antihistamines to treat the common cold," says Karen Tietze, an associate professor of clinical pharmacy who wrote the chapter on cold medicines in the pharmacists' Bible, the American Pharmaceutical Association's *Handbook of Nonprescription Drugs*.

Some scientists do, however, give antihistamines a nod. In a recent study Jack Gwaltney, chief of virology at the University of Virginia's medical school and a man on the cutting edge of cold research, found that cold sufferers who took an antihistamine called clemastine fumarate sneezed 50 percent less often and produced about 35 percent less mucus than those who took a placebo.

But even if further studies bear this one out, there's no getting around an antihistamine's whopping side effects: dryness of the eyes, nose, and mouth; impaired motor skills; and major drowsiness. In fact, antihistamines are one of the main ingredients in P.M. formulas.

Of course, an antihistamine's sedative effect might well be its main selling point, says Victor Padron, an associate professor of pharmacy at Creighton University in Omaha, Nebraska. "Taking an antihistamine forces me to slow down and rest," he says. "And that in itself is curative."

Avoid this whole song and dance with an ounce of prevention.

FORTUNATELY, two amazingly low-tech measures can help you avoid getting a cold in the first place: Wash your hands frequently, and don't share your air with a sick person.

These strategies work because you catch a rhinovirus, the type responsible for most colds, by inhaling it or picking it up from a hard, nonporous object. Around an office the virus may lurk on doorknobs, coffeepots, telephones, and keyboards; at home any surface that gets touched a lot is suspect. Keeping your hands away from your eyes and nose means no transmission, and washing your hands with soap and warm water wipes out any bugs. If you share a cubicle with someone who is coughing or sneezing, open a window or sit near a vent—anything to keep from inhaling too much of what she's exhaling.

Even if you follow all of these precautions, you'll probably still catch a cold or two this year. And even if you adhere to the minimalist approach at the drug counter, you will endure a couple of wretched days when your nose feels soggy, your throat feels froggy, and your brain completely shuts down. Which is nature's way of steering you toward the best cure of all: an extended dose of Oprah and the soaps.

Bill Shapiro is a writer in New York City.

STRAIGHT TALK ON THE MEDICAL HEADLINES

Alcohol and Health

THE STORY

Fountain of youth: A drink a day can help you live longer — *Boston Herald*, Dec. 11, 1997

Studies confirm relationship of alcohol to breast cancer — *New York Times*, Feb. 18, 1998

Which of these is the truth: Is alcohol a life-extending elixir or a soothing poison? It's actually a combination of these, depending on how much you drink, your general health, and personal risk factors for a host of health problems, including heart and liver disease, many cancers, and alcoholism.

In the United States, public health campaigns have traditionally urged people to avoid alcohol or cut back on their drinking. And rightly so — heavy drinking is the second leading cause of preventable death in the US, right behind cigarette smoking. Alcohol is implicated in up to half of all fatal traffic accidents. Heavy drinking clearly contributes to liver disease, a variety of cancers, a weakening of the heart muscle, high blood pressure, strokes, and depression, and can take a terrible toll on families and relationships. Even moderate drinking interferes with a host of medications or magnifies their negative side effects.

A new countermovement, though, is touting the apparent benefits of a drink a day on the heart and circulatory system. These recommendations are spurred by studies from around the world showing that alcohol offers some protection against heart disease, the leading cause of death in the US and other developed countries.

The latest, and largest, of these was published in the December 11, 1997 *New England Journal of Medicine*. Researchers from the American Cancer Society, the World Health Organization, and Oxford University looked at causes of death and death rates in half a million men and women, all of whom had answered a questionnaire in 1982 about their drinking, smoking, and other habits. Over the following 10 years, moderate drinkers — those who had a drink a day — were 20 percent less likely to die than people who didn't drink at all, thanks to substantial reductions in death from heart disease.

The overall picture masks some important trends. Even though moderate drinking was associated with an overall lower death rate from heart disease, alcohol's protective effect was relatively small among those at low risk for heart disease and more powerful among those at high risk for it. As expected, deaths from alcoholism; cirrhosis of the liver; cancers of the liver, mouth, throat, larynx, or esophagus; and injuries or accidents were highest among the heaviest drinkers. And when the researchers looked at causes of death for women, they found a greater risk of dying from breast cancer among women who reported having at least one drink a day compared with nondrinkers.

Other researchers found a similar connection between drinking and breast cancer in an analysis of six long-term studies that included more than 300,000 women, published in the February 18 *Journal of the American Medical Association*. Among women who averaged one or fewer drinks a day, the breast cancer risk was 9 percent higher than it was among nondrinkers. (This doesn't mean that 9 percent of women who have a drink a day will develop breast cancer. Rather, it's the difference between 11 of every 10,000 women developing breast cancer — the current US risk — and 12 of every 10,000 developing the disease.) Among those who reported having two to five drinks a day, breast cancer rates rose by 41 percent.

A study of more than 5,000 Italian women, published in the March 4 *Journal of the National Cancer Institute*, also found a connection between increasing amounts of alcohol and breast cancer. The researchers calculated that more than 20 grams of alcohol (slightly more than one drink) a day and little physical activity accounted for about 20 percent of breast cancers; and

From Health News, March 31, 1998, pp. 1-2. © 1998 by the Massachusetts Medical Society. All rights reserved. Reprinted by permission.

more than 40 percent among premenopausal women.

Parallel lines of research are showing that we can't view alcohol as all bad or all good. Finding your own balance of benefits and risks may be challenging, but it's well worth the effort.

— *The Editors*

THE PHYSICIAN'S PERSPECTIVE

Charles H. Hennekens, MD
Associate Editor

Given the way medical science works, and the way the media interact with scientists, you will probably see more conflicting headlines about alcohol and health in the months to come. Most studies, and the news reports that follow them, examine a single connection — alcohol and heart disease, alcohol and breast cancer, alcohol and mortality. While such narrowly focused studies clearly advance what we know about the impact of alcohol on the body, they don't reflect the broader reality. The alcohol you consume in a glass of wine, beer, or spirits alters mood and metabolism, and influences a variety of organs, including your brain, stomach, intestines, liver, and many glands. The complexity of alcohol's effects make it difficult to untangle its benefits from its risks.

Small amounts of alcohol offer some people subtle physical benefits. A drink before a meal can improve one's appetite and aid digestion, and may also keep bowel movements regular. Furthermore, many people look forward to having a drink at the end of a long, stressful day or enjoy the occasional drink with friends — emotional or psychic benefits that may improve health and well-being.

The scientific jury is still out on the degree to which light to moderate amounts of alcohol may benefit the heart, despite what the headlines may claim. A number of large, carefully constructed studies support the hypothesis that drinking small to moderate amounts of alcohol helps prevent the development of coronary heart disease. We think that alcohol itself is playing this role by raising levels of protective HDL cholesterol or by preventing the formation of small clots that can block blood vessels in the heart. It may, however, be something about people who drink in moderation that is the real cause. For example, according to a large national survey on American eating habits, moderate drinkers are more likely than nondrinkers or heavy drinkers to exercise, watch their diets, and get adequate sleep, each of which may have an independent and beneficial impact on heart disease.

Moderate drinking carries risks as well as benefits. It may interrupt sleep, or degrade the quality of sleep. It is notorious for impairing judgment. And even modest amounts of alcohol can interact with medications in harmful ways. Some antidepressants, sedatives, painkillers, and anticonvulsants can amplify the effects of alcohol, causing inebriation at lower intakes. Alcohol can also amplify the harmful side effects of some medications. Finally, research has consistently shown that moderate drinking increases the likelihood of dying from liver disease, strokes caused by bleeding inside the brain, breast cancer, and suicide and accidental deaths.

One thing is clear: Assumptions that the average person should begin to have a drink a day are premature, or even misguided. None of us is the mythical average person. Each of us has a unique personal and family history, as well as habits that predispose us to or protect us from diseases. So alcohol offers each of us different risks and benefits.

Alcohol offers abundant risk and no net benefit for pregnant women, recovering alcoholics, people with a family history of alcohol abuse, anyone with liver disease or a weakening of the heart muscle (cardiomyopathy), and anyone taking medications that may interact with alcohol.

Assuming that you don't fall into any of those categories, the

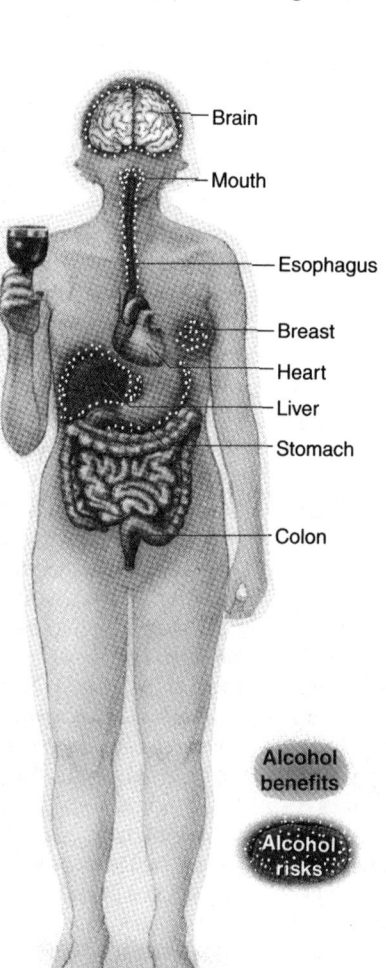

balance between risk and benefit is harder to calculate. Let me give several examples. A 23-year-old man reaps no net benefit from a drink or two a day, because he is at very low risk for developing heart disease and is at high risk for accidental, often alcohol-related, injury or death. Furthermore, there's no getting an early start since any possible "heart benefits" of alcohol aren't stored up for the future. A 55-year-old man who has high cholesterol levels and whose mother died of a heart attack may benefit from a drink a day, assuming he doesn't fall into any of the categories mentioned above. For a 55-year-old woman with high cholesterol and a family history of breast cancer, the risk-benefit calculation is more complicated. Heart disease kills five to six times more women each year than breast cancer, 236,000 compared with 44,000. And the increase in breast cancer associated with a drink a day or less is small. So on the face of it, the occasional drink may offer a net benefit. But a woman who is more afraid of developing breast cancer than heart disease may want to choose to avoid alcohol.

The health benefits of an alcoholic drink a day are substantially smaller than those offered by exercise and eating right. So a healthy lifestyle offers you the best chance of avoiding disease and living longer. You can best determine whether or not the occasional drink should be part of that healthy lifestyle by talking with your physician and taking an inventory of your health and health risks.

If you decide that it should, the key word must be moderation. Given the complexity of alcohol's physiological, metabolic, and psychological effects, the difference between a little bit of alcohol and a lot may be the difference between preventing disease and premature death, and causing it.

NATIONAL AFFAIRS

It can be a seductive argument: why not let sick people ease their pain by smoking pot? But drug warriors say 'medical marijuana' could lead to legalization—and the country does not seem ready for that. BY TOM MORGANTHAU

The War Over Weed

CONSIDERED SOLELY AS AN EXAMPLE OF practical politics, the campaign for Proposition 215 was brilliant. It was fought and won in California, a bellwether state whose law on ballot initiatives makes it uniquely open to grass-roots political movements. It attacked a policy, the U.S. drug war, about which many opinion leaders have large doubts. It mobilized a politically potent interest group—doctors—to defend their right to practice their profession as they see fit, and it appealed to voters' compassion for people with cancer, AIDS and other deadly diseases. It used the federal government as a scapegoat and made cops and prosecutors look like dolts. On Election Day, Prop 215 scored a clean kill, 56 percent to 44. Now the fun begins.

Simply put, Prop 215 and Proposition 200, a similar measure passed in Arizona last fall, pose a frontal challenge to the American prohibition against drugs—which is exactly what some, though not all, backers of these initiatives wanted to do. By convincing voters there are humane reasons to relax current laws against marijuana use, a Hungarian-born billionaire named George Soros and his helpers created a muddle that may take years to sort out. Like many political controversies, this one is headed for the courts. After the initiative passed, Gen. Barry McCaffrey, the drug czar, publicly warned doctors not to break federal law by prescribing marijuana. That prompted a group of California physicians to file suit claiming that their rights to advise their patients were being infringed. The policy is, who controls America's drug laws—the federal government or the voters of California and Arizona? The political issue is whether we Americans, fighting what seems to be an endless war, want to move toward greater tolerance of marijuana and other drugs. That is not overstatement: the Arizona law permits the use of heroin, LSD and methamphetamines if a user gets prescriptions from two doctors.

Marijuana is the soft spot in the national opposition to drugs. Millions have tried it at some point in their lives and found that it was pleasurable and not particularly addictive. To that reservoir of latent tolerance, the backers of Prop 215 shrewdly added the irresistible notion of helping people in pain—people like 77-year-old Hazel Rodgers of San Francisco, who regularly smokes pot to relieve the symptoms of glaucoma and her anxiety about having been diagnosed with breast cancer. Drug warriors like McCaffrey are thus forced into the no-win position of trying to deny the weed to thousands of patients who say it makes them feel better. Never mind the fact that current medical research suggests pot doesn't do anything for glaucoma, or that other prescription drugs alleviate pain and anxiety. And never mind the fact that the fine print in the California law makes it a sham. Though sold to the voters as a way of helping people with terrible illnesses, the law specifically permits pot use for almost any complaint—even migraine headaches. It sidesteps federal law by specifying that pot use is legal if a doctor merely "recommends" it orally. That may mean doctors will not lose their licenses because they didn't *prescribe* the drug. It also means there will be no paper trail for narcs to follow.

Considering the fact that poll after poll reveals no sign that U.S. voters want to legalize pot or any other drug, this outcome is arguably perverse. It greatly disturbs groups like the Partnership for a Drug-Free America, which points out that marijuana use among teenagers is rising steadily and that the California law contains no age restrictions. The theory here is that marijuana is a "gateway" to harder drugs. That isn't Reefer Madness alarmism: reliable research shows that virtually all heroin and cocaine addicts started out with pot.

What worries drug warriors now is the possibility that would-be users will find friendly doctors to give them oral approval and then buy the weed on the black market or at so-called cannabis buyers' clubs, which serve as middlemen between illicit growers and their middle-class clientele. That will surely create large problems for cops trying to suppress the underground pot trade, and it could produce a new class of criminal defendants who could claim their doctors said pot was a good thing to do. Ultimately, it may lead to a test case in which some prosecutor will press charges against an old lady like Hazel Rodgers. "The sense of frustration here is just huge," says a U.S. Justice Department official. "The dilemma is that in trying to look tough [to deter pot use], we wind up looking draconian."

What we have here, thanks to the voters of California and Arizona, is a nightmare of drug warriors everywhere—and a small but potentially significant breach in the national resolve against drugs. Earnest appeals by McCaffrey and many others failed to stop these slippery proposals at the ballot box, and it is time for clear leadership from the top—from Bill Clinton, the man who didn't inhale. Should we legalize pot, or not? That question is clearly implied in the controversy over medicinal marijuana. It is an issue that all Americans, ready or not, must confront honestly and resolve.

With MATT BAI *and* PATRICIA KING *in San Francisco and* DANIEL KLAIDMAN *in Washington*

Can Marijuana Be Medicine?

The claims are unproven, but many patients say the drug helps them. By GEOFFREY COWLEY

SUSAN NELSON SPENT most of 1978 watching her husband, Don, retch almost constantly. His body fought so hard to expel the chemicals used to treat his testicular cancer that, after 18 months, his battered esophagus ripped, causing tissue damage that has plagued him ever since. A decade later, it was Susan's turn. She developed lymphoma in 1989, and she, too, underwent chemotherapy. But in four months of treatment, she vomited only once. Instead of heading for the bathroom when she felt a surge of nausea, she took matters into her own hands: she fired up a joint.

Susan Nelson is no dopehead. She grew up in a military family, and never even experimented with pot as a '60s teenager. But she wasn't about to relive her husband's experience. The anti-nausea drug her doctor prescribed did wonders for her digestion, but it also lowered her inhibitions, causing inexplicable urges to throw plates and roll burning logs on the living-room floor. Smoking marijuana may have broken the law (she bought it from fellow patients), but it didn't break her dishes. "When I smoked it," she recalls, "you could still trust me."

Americans may frown on recreational pot smoking, but as recent votes in California and Arizona make clear, a lot of people favor leaving folks like the Nelsons alone. The states' initiatives won't have much practical effect (they free doctors to recommend marijuana without creating legal supplies of the drug). Still, the measures have revived an important and long-neglected question: does pot ever make good medicine? Federal drug-enforcement officials say the drug is both useless and dangerous. They're challenging the new initiatives in court and vow to punish doctors who prescribe pot to their patients. But proponents claim marijuana can help control glaucoma, forestall AIDS-related wasting, ease the nausea brought on by cancer chemotherapy and counter the symptoms of epilepsy and multiple sclerosis. The claims are largely unproven, but they warrant some serious attention.

Marijuana's basic mode of action is well known. Several years ago, researchers discovered that the body makes a chemical closely resembling THC, the main active ingredient in cannabis, and that the brain has receptors designed specifically to receive it. The receptors are concentrated in the brain regions responsible for motor activity, concentration and short-term memory. As anyone who ever inhaled will attest, marijuana can disrupt all those functions.

The question is whether it can do anything else. For nearly three decades the government has listed marijuana as a "schedule I" drug, a designation reserved for substances with no apparent medical value and a high potential for abuse. Barry McCaffrey, director of the Office of National Drug Control Policy, stoutly defends that ruling, saying there is "no convincing scientific evidence" that marijuana offers benefits that a person can't get from approved prescription drugs.

Where glaucoma is concerned, McCaffrey has a point. It's well known that smoking marijuana can reduce pressure within the eye, a hallmark of the disease. But the drug may also reduce the blood supply to the optic nerve—the last thing a glaucoma sufferer needs—and it doesn't seem to prevent blindness. Even if marijuana could save eyes, smoking it enough would take extraordinary effort. "In order to substantially reduce eye pressure," says Dr. Harry Quigley of Johns Hopkins University's Wilmer Eye Institute, "you'd have to be stoned all the time." When researchers tried dissolving THC in eye drops, they succeeded only in irritating people's eyes, but other compounds proved more useful. As a result, glaucoma patients can now choose from a number of potent topical treatments. The latest, a once-a-day eye drop called Xalatan, is virtually free of major side effects.

Marijuana may not cure glaucoma, but it has other claims to respectability. People have used it for centuries to stimulate appetite, and an unknown number now use it to combat the wasting associated with AIDS. No one knows how much good it's doing—the drug-control agencies have recently thwarted studies intended to answer that question—but some experts suspect the benefits are modest. The wasting syndrome doesn't stem solely from a lack of appetite, says Dr. Donald Kotler, an immunologist at New York's St. Luke's–Roosevelt Hospital. The patient may have an intestinal infection that blocks the absorption of nutrients, or a neck tumor that interferes with swallowing.

Skeptics also note that the FDA has already approved several effective remedies for wasting. To stimulate appetite, patients can take Marinol, a synthetic version of THC that comes in pill form, or Megace, a derivative of the hormone progesterone. In premarketing studies, AIDS patients who took Megace for 12 weeks gained an average of 11 pounds, while those getting a placebo lost 21. Since AIDS takes a particular toll on muscle tissue, the FDA has also approved several muscle-building steroids (testosterone and its kin) as AIDS treatments. Patients with good insurance can also get synthetic human-growth hormone, a bone-and-muscle builder that costs $1,000 a month.

Yet as many patients have discovered, plain old pot may still have a valuable role. Keith Vines, a 46-year-old San Francisco prosecutor, considers himself a stalwart in the war on drugs. As an assistant district attorney, he has spent years putting street dealers in jail. As an AIDS patient, he has seen his body threaten to disintegrate. "Three years ago my ribs were protruding," he says. "I was terrified to get on the scale." He wanted to enroll in a study of human-growth hormone, but participants had to eat three meals a day, and eh could hardly force down one. He tried several drugs—including Ma-

25. War Over Weed

The Medical Bottom Line

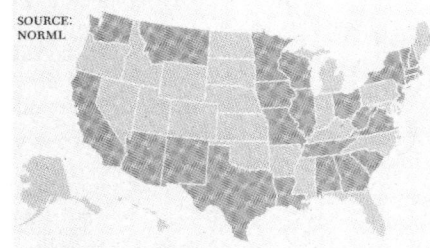

States with medical-marijuana laws

SOURCE: NORML

Though largely illegal since 1937, marijuana may prove an effective alternative to more commonly prescribed drugs for some diseases. California, Arizona and Massachusetts are leading the fight to make marijuana more readily available. They aren't alone: 26 states and the District of Columbia have passed various laws and resolutions establishing therapeutic-research programs, allowing doctors to prescribe marijuana, or asking the federal government to lift the ban on medical use.

CONDITION	MARIJUANA TREATMENT	CONVENTIONAL TREATMENT
Cancer chemotherapy Often causes extreme nausea and vomiting	● Active ingredient THC reduces vomiting and nausea, alleviates pretreatment anxiety	● Marinol (synthetic THC): Commonly used but can cause intoxication. Pill form only, hard to swallow if you're vomiting. ● Serotonin antagonists such as Zofran (ondansetron): Can be taken intravenously but more expensive than Marinol
AIDS-related wasting Low appetite, loss of lean (muscle) mass	● Improves appetite	● Marinol: Boosts appetite, but smokable marijuana allows better dose control ● Megase (megestrol acetate): Stimulates appetite and may reduce nausea. Currently being compared to Marinol for cancer patients.
Pain and muscle spasms Associated with epilepsy and multiple sclerosis	● Reduces muscle spasms; may ease incontinence of bladder and bowel and relieve depression	● Dantrium (dantrolene sodium): Capsules or injection can relax nerves and muscles to calm spasms. Can cause liver damage. ● Lioresal (bactofen): Tablet alleviates spasticity but also causes sedation. Sudden withdrawal can cause hallucinations and seizures.
Glaucoma A progressive form of blindness due to increased pressure inside the eyeball	● When smoked, it reduces pressure within the eye. But it may also reduce blood flow to the optic nerve, exacerbating the loss of vision.	● Xalatan (latanoprost): Once-a-day eye drop. Low rate of side effects. Changes eye color in some users. ● Beta-blocker eye drops: Can cause lethargy and trigger asthma attacks ● Miotic eye drops: Allow eye to drain faster but constrict the pupil, dimming vision ● Carbonic anhydrase inhibitors: Decrease production of fluid in the eye, but can cause numbness and weight loss

rinol, which often left him too blasted to function—but nothing worked until he joined a local buyers' club and started smoking pot. Once he took that leap, he qualified for the human-growth-hormone study, put on 45 pounds and managed to salvage his job. "Without marijuana," he says earnestly, "I would be dead."

Like AIDS-related wasting, the nausea from cancer chemotherapy is readily treated by prescription drugs. But those drugs are expensive, they don't always work and they're not always harmless. Their warning labels are littered with phrases like "hives," "impotence," "difficulty breathing," "tremors and rigidity" and "leukopenia" (a drop in white blood cells). Marijuana isn't risk-free—its smoke contains a number of carcinogens—but it's less toxic than many prescription drugs. There is no recorded instance of a death from overdose. And because people consume it one puff at a time, feeling the effects as they go, they can easily tailor their intake to their needs.

That's a big advantage for people with chronic pain or with spastic disorders such as multiple sclerosis. Whereas prescription drugs may zonk them out for the whole day, marijuana lets them respond directly to their symptoms. No one has conducted trials to gauge marijuana's genuine therapeutic effect on pain and spasms. But that doesn't much concern 39-year-old Andrew Hasenfeld, who was diagnosed with multiple sclerosis in 1980. He tried the prescription drug bactofen, but it never relieved the spasms, the stiffness, the sensation of "being all locked up." He resorted to marijuana six months ago, at the urging of fellow sufferers in Amherst, Mass., and the result was dramatic. "There's no comparison with any drug I could buy in a pharmacy," he says.

Few people would argue that Andrew Hasenfeld, Keith Vines or Susan Nelson belongs behind bars. ("I'm already in a wheelchair,") says Hasenfeld. "Isn't that enough?") And though recreational pot smokers can get involved with harder drugs, it's hard to see

how easing one's nausea, wasting or muscle spasms could cause what the drug office describes as "a downward spiral of self-destruction." Still, federal regulatory policy can't rest entirely on individual testimonials. As McCaffrey argues in a forthcoming "myths and truth" position paper, "drug policy must be based on science, not ideology." Approving marijuana as a prescription drug would require organizing clinical trials, identifying appropriate uses and finding ways to regulate its cultivation and sale. Those aren't insurmountable obstacles; morphine has been used medically for years. But federal policy has long discouraged clinical research with marijuana. The drug-control office is now pledging that "any serious marijuana research request will be considered." Perhaps that will begin to clear the smoke.

With MARY HAGER *in Washington,* ADAM ROGERS *in New York,* CLAUDIA KALB *in Boston and* PATRICIA KING *in San Francisco*

Old Habits

Will You Pay for Your Past as a Smoker?

People often grimace when they see themselves in old photos wearing outdated clothes or twisting to once-popular dance music. But when they see a cigarette dangling from their lips or between their fingers, embarrassment may turn to dread.

Until the 1960s, cigarette smoking was considered fun and glamorous—and without consequence. In 1964, the U.S. Surgeon General declared smoking a health hazard, ten years after scientists first discovered that tobacco caused cancer in mice. Ultimately, it took decades for the whole truth about smoking to be revealed. Congress banned TV and radio ads for cigarettes in 1971, but it wasn't until 1982 that the Surgeon General announced that smoking was the major cause of cancer death in the United States.

Over the past 45 years, researchers have unearthed mountains of evidence to support what everyone now knows: smoking is bad for your health. Indeed, it is considered the biggest preventable cause of mortality in this country. Cigarettes cause 30% of heart disease deaths, 30% of cancer deaths, and a whopping 80% to 90% of all lung cancers. They also increase people's risk of developing mouth, throat, esophageal, bladder, and possibly pancreatic cancer.

Most Americans have gotten the message loud and clear. About 46 million of them have kicked the habit, and half of all U.S. adults who ever smoked have quit. From 1965 to 1994, the proportion of current smokers dropped from 42% to 26%.

Many of those former smokers have come full circle: they watch what they eat, get regular exercise, and may even preach to others about the virtues of vegetarianism or the dangers of sedentary living. Although they have a healthy lifestyle now, many wonder if their years of smoking took an irreversible toll on their bodies.

The good news is that heart disease risk is cut in half within a year of quitting and lung cancer risk is halved within 10 years. The not-so-good news is that former smokers are still much more likely than nonsmokers to develop these diseases for at least 15 years after they've stopped smoking.

Fortunately, these statistics apply to populations and not necessarily to individuals. People can reduce their chances of getting chronic diseases by doing the things may of them are already doing— eating plenty of fruits and vegetables, which may prevent some cancers, and staying physically active, which reduces heart attack and stroke risk. But, most important, former smokers should stay away from second-hand smoke. Indeed, this may be the single biggest preventive measure they can take.

Researchers have long known that second-hand smoke raises lung cancer risk, but a May 1997 report from the ongoing Nurses' Health Study is the largest and most comprehensive to date showing that passive smoke also promotes heart disease. Harvard researchers followed 32,046 nonsmoking women age 36–61 for 10 years

> **Avoiding second-hand smoke is important for everyone's health, but it is particularly critical for ex-smokers.**

26. Will You Pay for Your Past as a Smoker?

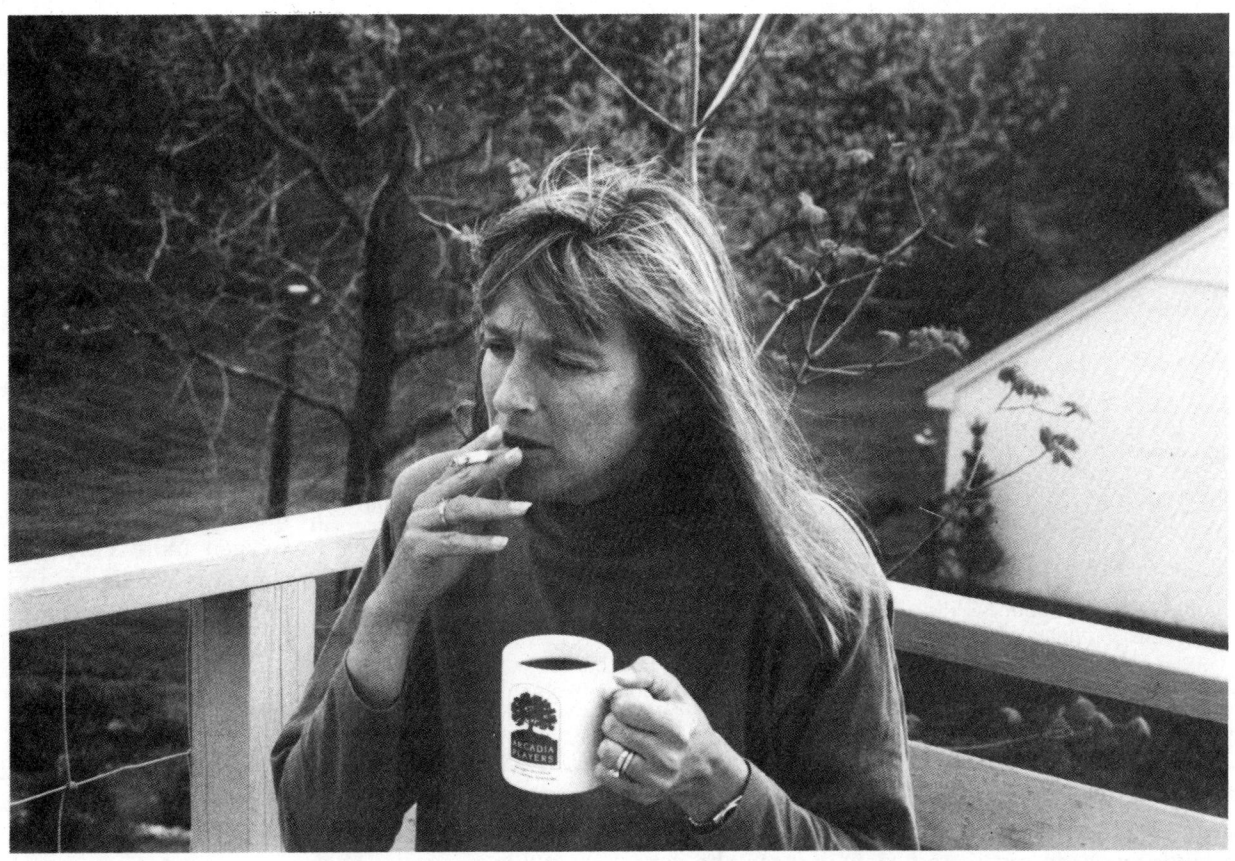

Photo by Pamela Carley

Quitting smoking at any time can literally save your life. The damage caused by smoking isn't reversed overnight, but avoiding second-hand smoke, getting regular exercise, and eating lots of fruits and vegetables may help repair the process.

and found that those who were regularly exposed to other people's smoke at home or at work were 91% more likely to have a heart attack than those who weren't.

The study, which made headlines across the country, startled both doctors and the public and strengthened the cases of plaintiffs who had sued companies that forced employees to work for years under smoky conditions. Although previous studies had hinted at a link between second-hand smoke and heart attack, no one realized the association was so strong. The researchers estimated that second-hand smoke is responsible for between 30,000 and 60,000 heart disease deaths each year—far more than the 3,000 lives it claims from lung cancer.

The chemicals in cigarette smoke increase cardiovascular risk by reducing the body's oxygen supply, raising blood pressure, lowering levels of "good" high-density lipoprotein (HDL) cholesterol, and making blood platelets more likely to stick together and form clots that can trigger a heart attack.

Avoiding second-hand smoke is important for everyone's health, but it is particularly critical for those who used to smoke, because these people continue to have greater risk for heart disease and lung cancer more than a decade after they quit. To reduce your exposure to someone else's smoke:

- ask others not to smoke in your home; if someone must smoke inside, limit them to rooms where windows can be opened,
- only patronize restaurants where smokers are segregated from nonsmokers, and sit as far as possible from the smoking section, and
- encourage friends and loved ones who smoke to quit and politely tell people you are bothered by their smoke.

What's the damage?

Various parts of the body recover from smoking at different rates; some damage is reversed almost immediately. For example, the level of carbon monoxide, a toxic gas in cigarette smoke (and car exhaust) formed by the incomplete combustion of carbon, declines to normal within 8 hours of snuffing out one's last cigarette; carbon monoxide deprives the body of oxygen by binding to *hemoglobin*, the oxygen-carrying molecule in red blood cells.

You've come a long way, baby

Disease	If you smoke	After you quit
Heart disease	Risk raised 70% compared to that of nonsmokers.	Within 1 year, risk drops by 50% compared to that of continuing smokers. After 15 years, risk is close to that of nonsmokers.
Stroke	Risk raised 2- to 3-fold compared to that of nonsmokers.	Risk drops steadily. After 5 to 15 years, risk is close to that of nonsmokers.
Lung cancer	Risk is 7–20 times higher than that of nonsmokers.	Within 10 years, risk drops by 50% compared to that of continuing smokers. After 15 years, risk is 4 times that of nonsmokers.
Chronic obstructive pulmonary disease (COPD)	Risk of death is 9 times that of nonsmokers.	After 20 years, risk of death remains elevated 2- to 8-fold compared to that of nonsmokers.

Source: U.S. Surgeon General's report on smoking cessation, 1990, and other government sources.

However, other damage, such as that done to the lungs, takes longer to repair, and some of it may be permanent. For example, smoking causes more than 80% of all cases of emphysema, an irreversible lung disorder that affects 2 million Americans. Emphysema and chronic bronchitis (inflammation of the airways) are the two respiratory ailments doctors refer to as chronic obstructive pulmonary disease (COPD), a condition in which the passages that allow air to flow in and out of the lungs become inflamed, narrowed, or damaged, making every breath a struggle.

People usually develop emphysema in their 50s or 60s after having smoked for many years. Early symptoms include coughing, shortness of breath, and labored breathing. Individuals with mild emphysema may get winded easily but can still carry out their daily activities; those with more severe disease may have trouble performing even the simplest tasks, such as making a bed or walking up a flight of stairs.

In advanced cases, people may not be able to get through the day without using an oxygen tank to help them breathe. Although there is no way to reverse the damage that has been done by COPD, there are several treatments that can make the disease easier to live with. Some people take part in pulmonary rehabilitation programs, for example, where they learn special exercises to build up their endurance and strengthen the muscles used to draw air into the lungs.

A normal lung is composed of clusters of tiny air sacs called *alveoli*, which expand and contract as a person breathes; each sac abuts a web of vessels where carbon dioxide in the blood is exchanged for newly breathed oxygen. In people with emphysema, the fragile walls of the alveoli have been broken down by enzymes called *elastases*; as a result, the air sacs merge and lose their elasticity, and the breathing muscles are unable to push air out of the enlarged sacs.

Former smokers have already taken the most important step toward preventing emphysema: quitting smoking. Getting regular exercise is also important; when muscles are well conditioned, they use oxygen more efficiently, putting less strain on the heart and lungs. Some studies have suggested that a diet rich in vitamin C (found in citrus fruits, potatoes, red and green peppers, collard greens, and broccoli) and other antioxidants improves the lung function of both smokers and nonsmokers.

While everyone knows that smokers are at greatest risk for lung cancer, people may not be aware that many former smokers are also at particular risk. Indeed, more than 50% of all newly diagnosed lung cancer cases in the United States are among ex-smokers. That's because lung cancer develops slowly, after many years of smoking or exposure to environmental carcinogens such as radon or asbestos. Some people may have quit too late—after their lungs have already undergone cellular changes that will later develop into cancer.

Although the number of U.S. smokers dropped substantially over the past three decades, lung cancer rates continued to rise until the 1990s, when the disease's incidence and mortality began to decline for the first time.

Smoke screen?

Many former smokers wonder if they should get an annual chest x-ray to screen for early signs of lung cancer. The official answer is no: neither the American Cancer Society nor the U.S. Preventive Services Task Force advises screening except for people with symptoms that point to lung cancer, such as chronic chest pain and a deep, wheezing cough. That's because early lung tumors are difficult to detect on x-rays; by the time they grow large enough to be seen, the tumors have usually metastasized (spread) to other parts of the body.

Studies have shown that x-ray screening doesn't reduce lung cancer death rates across the board, but periodic chest x-rays for other conditions occasionally detect some early tumors that can be surgically removed. When lung tumors are excised when they are still small and localized, the disease's 5-year survival rate jumps dramatically—from 14% to 48%.

People may find it hard to believe that in an affluent society such as the United States, no one has developed a better screening method for a disease that causes more deaths per years than any other form of cancer. Part of the reason is that decades of antismoking messages have had an unintended consequence: lung cancer patients are too often viewed as deserving their fate, even though there is ample evidence that nicotine is one of the most addictive substances available and many people started smoking long before anyone knew of the harm it could cause. The disease simply doesn't engender the same sympathy in the public mind, nor the same attention from scientists, as breast and prostate cancer.

The last word

Long-time smokers sometimes rationalize that there is no use quitting now—they are addicted and the damage has been done. But this isn't necessarily the case; quitting at any time can literally save your life. Although the damage isn't all reversed overnight, avoiding second-hand smoke, getting regular exercise, and eating lots of fruits and vegetables may help the repair process. Indeed, the future for ex-smokers is a promising one: the benefits of quitting only get better with time.

Unit 6

Unit Selections

27. **Rethinking Birth Control,** Julia Califano
28. **Condoms: Barriers to Bad News,** Tamar Nordenberg
29. **America: Awash in STDs,** Gracie S. Hsu
30. **Your Sexual Landscape,** Beth Howard

Key Points to Consider

❖ Do you think that birth control has contributed to increased promiscuity and the rapid spread of sexually transmitted diseases? Why or why not?

❖ How could sex education be improved so that it would be more effective in reducing teenage pregnancies, abortions, and the spread of AIDS and other STDs?

❖ Do you feel at risk of contracting AIDS or other STDs? If not, why not? If you do, what are you doing to reduce your risk?

❖ How do the "conservative" and "liberal" positions on sex education differ? Which do you support? Why?

❖ What could be done to help women feel more comfortable with their own anatomy?

❖ What are some of the key factors to consider when choosing a contraceptive method? Explain.

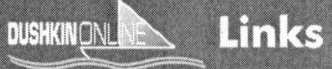 **Links** www.dushkin.com/online/

21. **Men's Health**
    http://www.menshealth.com/new/guide/index.html
22. **Planned Parenthood**
    http://www.plannedparenthood.org
23. **Sex and Gender**
    http://www.bioanth.cam.ac.uk/pip4amod3.html
24. **University of Maryland/Women's Studies**
    http://www.inform.umd.edu/EdRes/Topic/WomensStudies/

These sites are annotated on pages 4 and 5.

Human Sexuality

According to Dennis Barbour, president of the Association of Reproductive Health Professionals, the contraceptive choices that Americans have are safe and effective, but a method that is good for one woman may not work for another. Some of the factors that must be considered in making a contraceptive choice include the health of the individual, frequency of sexual activity, number of partners, future plans for having children, effectiveness rates, side effects, convenience, and cost.

Birth control itself has been a source of controversy and confusion. In the 1970s one of the most popular contraceptive devices was the IUD (intrauterine device). This form of birth control was very effective and convenient to use. This all changed rather abruptly in the 1980s as it fell victim to legal and medical issues. The IUD named the Dalkon Shield was linked to pelvic inflammatory disease, infertility, and sometimes death. The litigation that ensued prompted several other manufacturers to remove their IUDs from the market. Over the past few years, new contraceptives are once again starting to appear in the marketplace. Depo-Provera, Norplant, and the female condom were the first wave of new contraceptive devices to enter the U.S. market in more than a decade. In addition to these, several others are currently under development, including contraceptive vaccines, a male birth control pill, male condoms that promise greater comfort, a two-capsule version of the Norplant device, creams and gels with anti-HIV and spermicidal properties, and barrier methods that release spermicides. The article "Rethinking Birth Control" examines the contraceptive choices currently available and compares them on the basis of their cost, failure rate, ability to prevent sexually transmitted diseases, and potential drawbacks.

While the concept of "safe sex" is nothing new, the degree of open and public discussion regarding sexual behaviors is. With the emergence of AIDS as a disease of epidemic proportions and the rapid spreading of other sexually transmitted diseases (STDs), the surgeon general of the United States initiated an aggressive educational campaign based on the assumption that knowledge would change behavior. If STD rates among teens are any indication as to the effectiveness of this approach, then we must conclude that our educational efforts are failing. Conservatives believe that, while education may play a role in curbing the spread of STDs, the root of the problem is promiscuity, and promiscuity rises when a society is undergoing a moral decline. The solution, according to conservatives, is a joint effort between parents and educators in which students are taught the importance of values such as respect, responsibility, and integrity. Liberals, on the other hand, think that preventing promiscuity is unrealistic, and instead the focus should be on establishing open and frank discussions between the sexes. Their premise is that we are all sexual beings, and the best way to combat STDs is to establish open frank discussions between sexual partners so that condoms will be used correctly when they engage in intercourse. "America: Awash in STDs" examines the scope of the STD problem, and presents both the conservative and liberal positions on solving the problem.

While education undoubtedly has had a positive impact on slowing the spread of STDs, perhaps it was unrealistic to think that education alone was the solution, given the magnitude and the nature of the problem. Most experts agree that for education to succeed in changing personal behaviors the following conditions must be met: (1) The recipients of the information must first perceive themselves as vulnerable and, thus, be motivated to explore replacement behaviors, and (2) the replacement behaviors must satisfy the needs that were the basis of the problem behaviors. To date most education programs have failed to meet these criteria. Given all the information that we now have on the dangers associated with AIDS and STDs, why is it that people do not perceive themselves at risk? It is not so much the denial of risks as it is the notion that when it comes to choosing sex partners most people think that they use good judgment. Unfortunately, most decisions regarding sexual behavior are based on subjective criteria that bear little or no relationship to actual risk. Even when individuals do view themselves as vulnerable to AIDS and STDs, there are currently only two viable options for reducing risk of contracting these diseases. The first is the use of a condom and the second is sexual abstinence, neither of which is an ideal solution to the problem. "Condoms: Barriers to Bad News," by Tamar Nordenberg, explains what you need to know about storing and using condoms to maximize their effectiveness.

A discussion of sexual health would not be complete without addressing the issue of vaginal health. Just the mention of the word "vagina" makes many people uneasy, and many women find it unbearable to examine this part of their anatomy. This is unfortunate because this anatomical region of the body has an ecological balance as delicate as that of a tropical rain forest. The net result of this lack of attention is the source of much discomfort and many potential problems. Ironically, most vaginal problems, with the exception of STDs, are the result of using products aimed at helping women feel fresh, such as douches, vaginal deodorants, and scented panty liners. "Your Sexual Landscape" discusses the importance of vulvar self-examination and what to look for. The author also discusses the most common infections that women are likely to experience and the symptoms to look for. Perhaps it is time to remove the shroud of mystique from the vagina so that this anatomical structure can be cared for with the attention to detail that it warrants.

Rethinking Birth Control

If you still believe the IUD is dangerous and the Pill is for women under 35, you may be stuck in a contraception rut. Here's a roundup of the most effective methods for midlife women.

JULIA CALIFANO

Through two years of dating, 10 years of marriage and two kids, Chris, a college professor in Syracuse, NY, relied almost exclusively on a diaphragm for birth control. Indeed, this 40-year-old would still be putting up with the hassle and mess if, at her last checkup, her doctor hadn't suggested she try an intrauterine device (IUD). Persuaded by his argument that it was highly effective, long-lasting and, for most women, nearly free of side effects, she switched. She hasn't regretted her decision. "It's such a pleasure not to have to plan ahead or get out of bed in the heat of passion," she says. "We don't even think about birth control anymore."

By the time a woman turns 35, she's moved an average of eight times, switched jobs seven times and had two children, yet there's only a 50–50 chance that she has ever thought about changing her method of birth control, according to a survey by Ortho Pharmaceutical. But the truth is she should. "A woman's contraceptive needs change as her life changes," says Anita Nelson, M.D., medical director of the Woman's Health Care Clinic at Harbor UCLA Medical Center in Los Angeles. "A barrier method may be great when you're 21 and concerned about AIDS and other sexually transmitted diseases [STD's], but it's probably not ideal when you're 35 and married with kids."

Perhaps more surprising is the staggering rate of unplanned pregnancies among women in their 40s: According to the Alan Guttmacher Institute in New York City, eight out of 10 pregnancies in this age group are unintended—the same rate as for women under age 20.

How can you tell if your current choice is still your best choice? Reassess your birth control periodically, taking your lifestyle, health, sex life and desire for children into consideration. Here's a guide to the options, plus expert advice on what to use when.

The IUD: Unfounded fear

What it is: The current IUD of choice is ParaGard, a piece of plastic with copper inside it that's put into the uterus to stop sperm from reaching eggs for up to 10 years. Another IUD called Progestasert contains hormones; it works for one year.

Benefits: Long-term, reversible, worry-free protection, and an insertion process that's only slightly more involved than a Pap smear. Progestasert also reduces menstrual cramps and the flow of monthly bleeding.

Drawbacks: The copper IUD can cause heavier than usual periods, won't protect you from STD's and shouldn't be used if you're not in a mutually monogamous relationship. Users with multiple partners are at increased risk for pelvic inflammatory disease (PID), an infection that can cause infertility.

What you may not know: Though most people still associate this device with the dreaded Dalkon Shield (an IUD that caused infection and infertility in thousands of women, along with a few deaths, in the '70s), ParaGard is considered one of the best and safest birth control options. In fact, it's the most popular form of reversible contraception outside the U.S., with 85 million users worldwide.

When to consider it: If you're in a mutually monogamous, long-term relationship and have had at least one child (for childless women there's a small risk that the device will be expelled). "An ideal time to switch to the IUD is when you've completed your family but don't want to take the irreversible step of sterilization," says nurse practitioner Kara Anderson, a medical consultant to the Planned Parenthood Federation of America in New York City.

The Pill: Now for Older Women

What it is: This oral contraceptive is a combination of two hormones, progestin and estrogen, that suppresses ovulation.

Benefits: Easy, reliable and offers a wealth of health benefits. After five

A Field Guide to Cost and Effectiveness

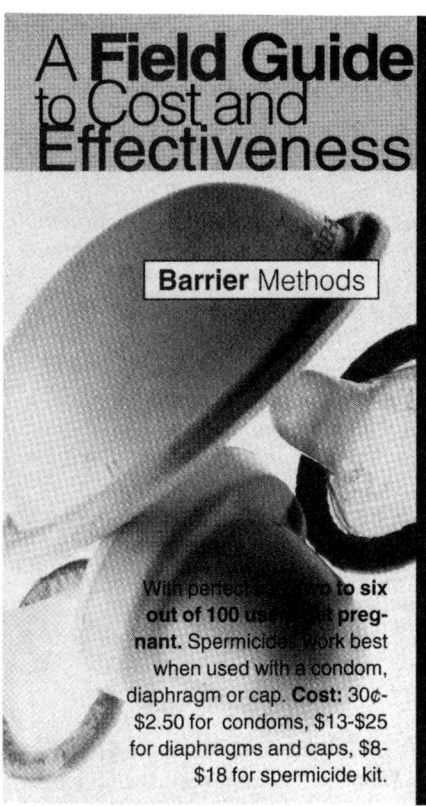

Barrier Methods

With perfect use, two to six out of 100 users get pregnant. Spermicides work best when used with a condom, diaphragm or cap. **Cost:** 30¢-$2.50 for condoms, $13-$25 for diaphragms and caps, $8-$18 for spermicide kit.

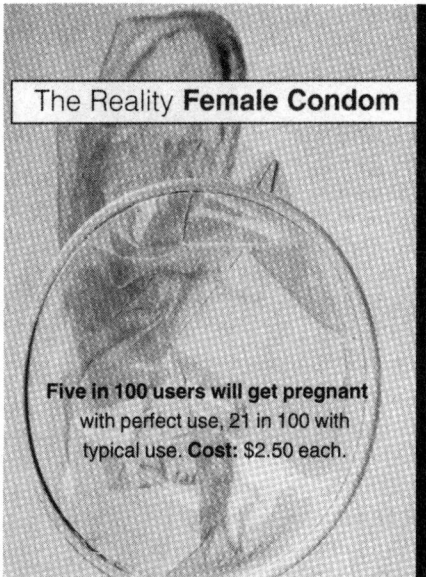

The Reality **Female Condom**

Five in 100 users will get pregnant with perfect use, 21 in 100 with typical use. **Cost:** $2.50 each.

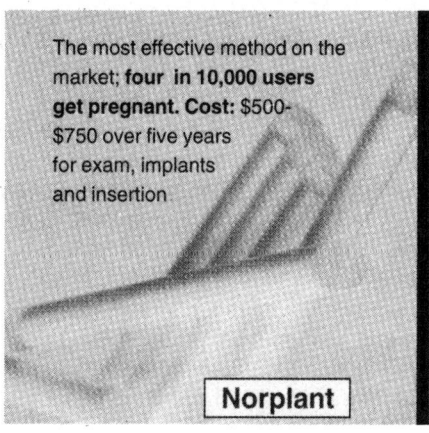

The most effective method on the market; **four in 10,000 users get pregnant. Cost:** $500-$750 over five years for exam, implants and insertion.

Norplant

---

years the Pill halves your risk of endometrial and ovarian cancers, an effect that, for endometrial cancer, may last as long as 15 years after you stop using it. [Experts aren't sure how long the protective effects last for ovarian cancer.] It also reduces the risk of benign breast lumps, ovarian cysts, iron-deficiency anemia and PID.

Drawbacks: Side effects include breast tenderness, nausea, weight gain and headaches (though these usually clear up after two to three months). The Pill must be taken every day, and it doesn't protect against STD's. In addition, studies show it increases the risk of heart attack and blood clots in women over 35 who smoke. Some studies have also shown that the Pill increases breast cancer risk, though a recent analysis of 150,000 users found this risk to be negligible. In most cases, say experts, the health benefits far outweigh the risks.

What you may not know: A study at San Francisco State University found that women who use triphasic pills such as Orthonovum 7/7/7 (in which hormone levels vary throughout the course of the month) experience heightened sex drive compared with women on other types of pills.

When to consider it: If you're in a committed relationship and want a highly effective form of contraception. Contrary to what many believe, the Pill can be ideal for fortysomething non-smoking women. It eases the transition to menopause, says David Grimes, M.D., vice chairman of the department of obstetrics and gynecology at the University of California at San Francisco. "The Pill helps regulate periods, prevent hot flashes and protect against bone loss," he explains.

Norplant: A Five-Year Plan

What it is: Six flexible, matchstick-sized capsules inserted by a doctor just beneath the skin of the upper arm. They release progestin to suppress ovulation for five years.

Benefits: It's effective and convenient—you can't mess up. Norplant is also easily reversible; after removal, any remaining drugs leave the body in about three days. In addition, experts believe Norplant may be as good as the Pill at reducing the risk of endometrial and ovarian cancer.

Drawbacks: Norplant won't protect you from STD's, and it can cause ir-

---

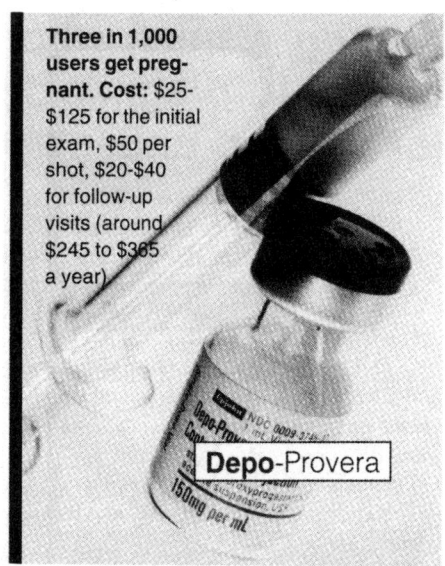

Three in 1,000 users get pregnant. Cost: $25-$125 for the initial exam, $50 per shot, $20-$40 for follow-up visits (around $245 to $365 a year).

Depo-Provera

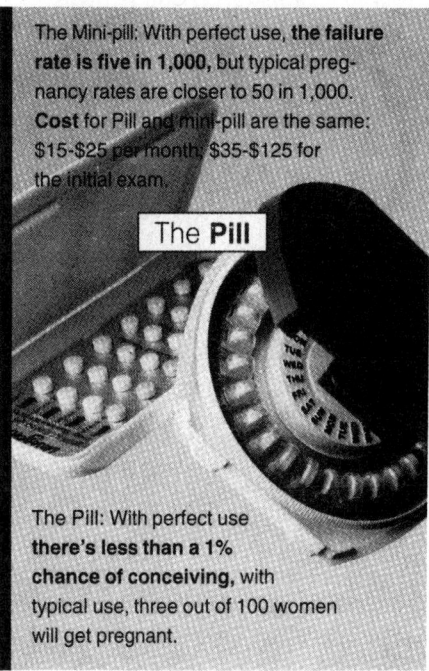

The Mini-pill: With perfect use, **the failure rate is five in 1,000,** but typical pregnancy rates are closer to 50 in 1,000. **Cost** for Pill and mini-pill are the same: $15-$25 per month; $35-$125 for the initial exam.

The Pill

The Pill: With perfect use **there's less than a 1% chance of conceiving,** with typical use, three out of 100 women will get pregnant.

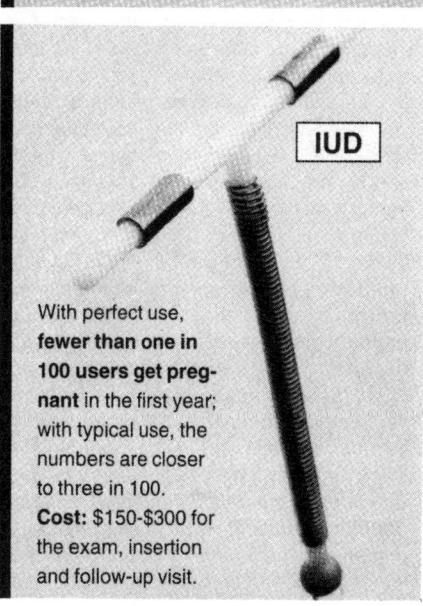

IUD

With perfect use, **fewer than one in 100 users get pregnant** in the first year; with typical use, the numbers are closer to three in 100. **Cost:** $150-$300 for the exam, insertion and follow-up visit.

HUMAN SEXUALITY

Among women who are in their 40s, a staggering eight out of 10 pregnancies are unintended—the same rate as for women under age 20.

regular bleeding during the first year. There have also been a number of lawsuits filed by Norplant users, primarily because of problems such as pain or scarring upon removal. Despite the bad press, experts say such problems shouldn't arise if you use an experienced doctor. (For referrals, call your local Planned Parenthood clinic.)

What you may not know: Norplant is very expensive if used for fewer than three years.

When to consider it: If you're breastfeeding (unlike estrogen in the Pill, progestin doesn't reduce milk flow) and plan to wait several years before having another child or if you've completed your family. You also may want to try it if you absolutely don't want to worry about an accidental pregnancy.

Depo-Provera: Convenience Without Long-Term Commitment

What it is: This injection of synthetic progestin suppresses ovulation for 11 to 13 weeks.

Benefits: Depo-Provera provides many of the health perks of the Pill, and you don't have to take it every day. After about a year, periods may stop completely, which many women consider a welcome side effect.

Drawbacks: Doctor's visits are required four times a year to get the shots, and the effects are not immediately reversible (fertility may not return for an average of 10 months after the last dose). Side effects may include headaches, weight gain, depression and heavier, more frequent periods. Depo-Provera also provides no protection against STD's.

What you may not know: Though many American women think of this method, approved here in 1992, as new, Depo-Provera has been used by more than 30 million women in 100 other countries over the past 30 years.

When to consider it: If you're nursing or trying to space out the arrival of new children, or you can't remember to take the Pill every day.

The Reality Female Condom: Women in the Driver's Seat

What it is: The Reality Condom is a floppy polyurethane tube with an inner ring at the closed end that fits over the cervix, like a diaphragm, and an outer ring at the open end that hangs outside the vagina.

Benefits: Protection against AIDS and other STD's; more spontaneity than with male condoms, since it can be inserted in advance.

Drawbacks: It has about as much sex appeal as a sandwich bag.

What you may not know: The device is reputed to squeak during use (adding a little extra lubricant can alleviate this distraction).

When to consider it: If you're not in a stable relationship or you have a partner who refuses to wear a condom.

Tubal ligation: No More Hassles

What it is: This surgical procedure blocks the fallopian tubes so that sperm and egg never meet.

Benefits: No-worry, contraceptive-free sex for the rest of your life. And, after the cost of the surgery ($1,000-$2,500), you'll never spend another dime on birth control.

Drawbacks: This procedure isn't foolproof: Though only five in 1,000 users become pregnant in the first year, surprisingly, over 10 years the failure rate is one in 50 (2%). And, as with any surgery, the procedure carries risks. Finally, depending on how it's done it can't easily be undone.

What you may not know: Sterilization is the most popular method of birth control in the U.S., chosen by a whopping 42% of contraceptive users.

When to consider it: If you're *sure* you don't want any more children.

The Mini-Pill: Fewer Annoying Side Effects

What it is: This pill contains no estrogen and a very small dose of progestin—hence the name.

Benefits: Since it contains no estrogen, the mini-pill has fewer side effects than the Pill and is not associated with any increased risk of blood clots or breast cancer. It also causes lighter than normal periods, making it a good choice for women who are anemic or who tend to bleed heavily.

Contraception 911

Condoms break, diaphragms slip and even the most responsible woman sometimes misses a Pill. The good news is that postcoital contraceptive options are expanding. An FDA advisory panel recently agreed unanimously that the Pill can safely be used as a morning-after contraceptive. The procedure—taking two doses of two or four pills each, depending on the brand, within 72 hours of unprotected sex—reduces the risk of pregnancy by 75%, though nausea and vomiting are common side effects. Several different Pill brands can be used; check with your doctor for specifics. Note: Don't try this on your own.

An emergency IUD insertion can also be done within five to seven days of unprotected sex and is more than 99% effective. Contact your doctor or Planned Parenthood, or call the new 24-hour Emergency Contraception Hotline (800-584-9911) for a list of doctors who provide emergency contraception in your area. You'll also find a list of local providers on the Internet at http://opr.princeton.edu/ec/.

Alternatives to surgical abortion are on the way. The long-awaited French abortion drug mifepristone, better known as RU 486, is expected to be available in this country later this year. The drug blocks progesterone and causes the uterus to discard its lining along with the implanted egg. It can be used up to nine weeks into pregnancy and may also be used as emergency birth control up to three days after unprotected sex, with fewer side effects than oral contraceptives.

On the horizon: Two FDA-approved drugs already on the market, methotrexate (a chemotherapy drug) and misoprostol (used to prevent stomach bleeding), induce abortion when combined. Since research is still limited on this method, few doctors use it, but that may soon change. Planned Parenthood has received FDA clearance for a large-scale clinical trial to test the technique's safety and effectiveness.

Women who use triphasic birth control pills report experiencing a heightened sex drive.

And it doesn't require a waiting period to get pregnant after you stop taking it.

Drawbacks: It can cause irregular bleeding, offers no protection against STD's and has a significantly higher failure rate than combined oral contraceptives, particularly if you have trouble remembering to take a pill every day.

What you may not know: This method has almost no margin for error. Missing even one day can result in a pregnancy.

When to consider it: If you're nursing (which naturally reduces—but doesn't rule out—fertility); it also seems to slightly increase the quantity and quality of breast milk.

Barrier Methods: STD Protection

What they are: This group includes condoms; diaphragms and cervical caps used with spermicidal jellies or foam; inserts and film. All prevent sperm from reaching eggs.

Benefits: They're safe, cheap and available without a prescription; barrier methods also guard against STD's. Latex condoms provide the best protection against the AIDS virus.

Drawbacks: They interfere with spontaneity and can be messy, and your partner may complain of lessened sensation during sex with condoms. Also, caps can be tricky to insert and diaphragms may increase the risk of urinary tract infections in women.

What you may not know: Lubricated condoms and spermicides help counteract vaginal dryness, a common perimenopausal and postpartum problem.

When to consider them: If you're breast-feeding, planning to get pregnant relatively soon or having sex infrequently. Condoms are the best choice if you want iron-clad protection against AIDS and other STD's. Barrier methods are also handy backups when you forget to take a Pill.

Julia Califano is a writer in Hoboken, NJ

Six Reasons to Switch

If you've been using the same contraceptive since college, it's probably time to take a fresh look at your birth control options. Here are some compelling reasons to reconsider your method:

1. You've settled down with one partner. Provided neither one of you has a sexually transmissible disease, you can switch from condoms to a method you both like better and will use consistently.

2. Your health has changed. If you develop heart disease, high blood pressure or diabetes, you should re-evaluate your current method with your doctor.

3. You're breast-feeding. Consider a nonhormonal contraceptive, such as condoms, a diaphragm or a copper intrauterine device (IUD), or a progestin-only method, such as the minipill, Norplant or Depo-Provera.

4. You've completed your family. Sterilization is only one long-term option. Also consider Norplant, Depo-Provera, the IUD and the Pill.

5. You're contemplating pregnancy. If you're on the Pill, doctors recommend stopping two to three months before conceiving to re-establish your natural cycle. If you use Depo-Provera, it can take up to a year after your last shot to conceive.

6. You dislike your current method. If you hate inserting your diaphragm or can't remember to take the Pill every day, don't grin and bear it—switch.

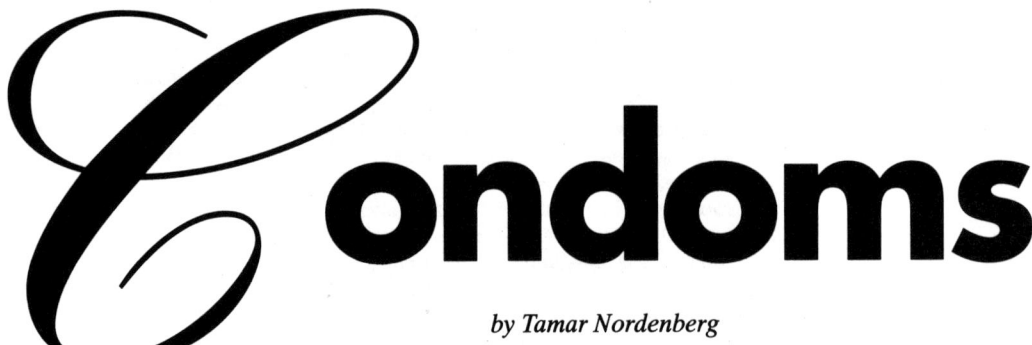

Condoms
by Tamar Nordenberg

Barriers To Bad News

What do condoms have in common with toothpaste and toilet paper?

Not enough, according to Adam Glickman, owner of the Condomania stores in New York and Los Angeles. Glickman, who has sold condoms by the millions to individuals and organizations such as the Peace Corps and Planned Parenthood, says condoms should be viewed as ordinary, like toothpaste and toilet paper. "People have gotten past asking, 'Isn't brushing my teeth every morning a hassle?' Given the world we live in, wearing condoms is something you just have to do, like brushing your teeth. The stakes are too high."

Luis Lopez knows first-hand what's at stake. About 10 years ago, Lopez, now 31 and a health educator with the People With AIDS Coalition of New York, became infected with HIV virus, which causes AIDS, during a casual sexual encounter.

"I thought people with AIDS had purple spots or looked really skinny," Lopez says. "I thought by being discriminating about who I slept with, I could keep myself safe. We know now that makes no sense."

We know now that abstaining from sex is the only foolproof protection from the sexual passage of HIV and other sexually transmitted diseases (STDs). We know, too, that for those who choose to have sex with someone who has *any chance* of being infected, using a latex condom during every sexual encounter can significantly reduce the risk of HIV and other sexually transmitted diseases, while protecting against pregnancy.

For those who can't or won't use latex condoms, the Food and Drug Administration has cleared two alternative barrier methods of birth control, a male condom made of polyurethane and a condom that is worn by the woman. Both help protect against pregnancy and may provide some level of protection from STDs.

Life-Saving Barrier

A male condom, sometimes called a "rubber" or "prophylactic," is a sheath that fits snugly over a man's erect penis, with a closed end to catch the sperm and stop them from entering the woman's vagina. No prescription is needed to buy a condom.

Data show that if a condom is used correctly with every act of sexual intercourse for one year, about three out of every 100 women are expected to get pregnant.

Besides sperm, latex condoms act as a barrier to a wide variety of viruses, bacteria, and other infectious particles. By preventing contact with many sores and minimizing the exchange of infectious fluids, condoms can help prevent the transmission of sexually transmitted diseases, including HIV, gonorrhea, chlamydia, syphilis, herpes infection, and genital ulcers.

Millions of Americans are infected with these diseases each year, and hundreds of thousands of them become seriously ill or die as a result. According to the Centers for Disease Control and Prevention, in the United States, someone is infected with HIV every 13 minutes. CDC estimates that 65 percent of these AIDS cases can be attributed to sexual contact.

The best protection from such diseases is to not have sex or to have a mutually monogamous relationship with someone who is known to be uninfected. However, for those who are sexually active, studies have shown that proper and consistent use of latex condoms is the best defense.

A 1994 European study published in the *New England Journal of Medicine* looked at HIV transmission rates of heterosexual couples with one HIV-infected partner. The study compared the transmission rates for couples who used condoms consistently to those who didn't. Of the 123 couples who consistently used condoms, none of the HIV-free partners became infected during the study, whereas 12 of the 122 partners who didn't consistently use condoms became infected.

"The scientific evidence is compelling," says Herbert Peterson, M.D., chief of CDC's women's health and fertility branch. "We're not guessing about this."

The spermicide nonoxynol-9, used in some condoms, has been shown to be effective as a contraceptive, and may reduce the risk of transmitting certain STDs. But the spermicide has not been proven to prevent sexual transmission of HIV.

Similarly, lambskin (or natural membrane) condoms, while effective for contraception, should not be used for disease protection because the naturally occurring pores in lambskin are large enough to allow some viruses to pass through.

Hole Check

Since 1976, FDA has regulated condoms to ensure their safety and effectiveness. Currently, manufacturers of American-made and imported condoms electronically test each condom for holes and other defects. Also, before distributing the condoms to retailers, manufacturers perform additional testing on random condoms from each batch, usually involving a "water leak" test to find holes and an "air burst" test to check condom strength.

FDA oversees the testing procedures by periodically inspecting the manufacturing facilities, and the agency tests some condoms in its own laboratories to confirm their quality.

Condoms are sold in various colors, shapes or packaging to suit different personal preferences. But, whether they glow in the dark or taste like strawberries, products that sufficiently resemble a condom must comply with FDA's requirements, even if they are labeled as "novelties." The only condom-like products that need not comply are those that can't be used like condoms. For example, some novelty products have the

Handle with Care

To get the maximum protection against pregnancy and sexually transmitted diseases, remember the following things when using condoms:

• Store condoms in a cool, dry place out of direct sunlight. Don't make the common mistake of storing them in a glove compartment, wallet or purse.
• Don't use a condom if the package is damaged or the rubber material is sticky, brittle, discolored, or otherwise deteriorated. Don't use a condom after the expiration date or more than five years after the manufacturing date.

• *Never reuse a condom.* Use a new condom with each sexual act that involves contact with the penis.
• Handle a condom carefully to avoid damaging it with fingernails, teeth, or other sharp objects.
• Put on the condom after the penis is erect and before intimate contact. Place the condom on the head of the penis and unroll it all the way to the base. Leave an empty space at the end of the condom to collect semen. Remove any air remaining in the tip by gently pressing the air out toward the base of the penis.

• Ensure adequate lubrication during intercourse. When needed with latex condoms, use only water-based lubricants such as K-Y jelly or glycerin. Don't use oil-based lubricants such as baby oil, petroleum jelly, massage oil, body lotion, or cooking oil because they can weaken the latex. Oil-based lubricants may be used with polyurethane, however, without damaging the material.
• After ejaculation, hold onto the rim of the condom and carefully withdraw the penis while it is still erect.

—*T.N.*

HUMAN SEXUALITY

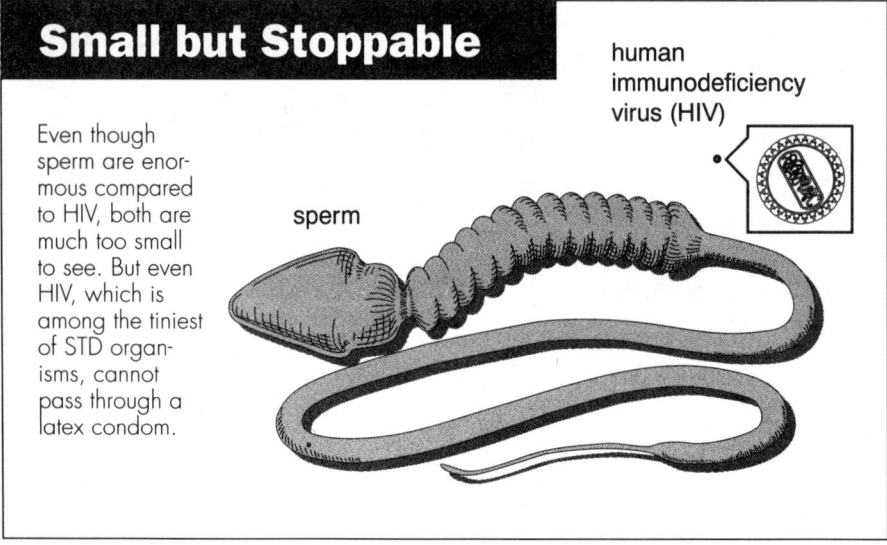

Small but Stoppable

Even though sperm are enormous compared to HIV, both are much too small to see. But even HIV, which is among the tiniest of STD organisms, cannot pass through a latex condom.

---

closed end removed or are sealed so they can't be unrolled.

Correct and Consistent

Although condoms are generally expected to break less than 2 percent of the time—with more than half of the breakages occurring before ejaculation—real-life pregnancy rates over a year of condom use may be as high as 15 percent.

Inconsistent or incorrect use of condoms explains the discrepancy, according to Lillian Yin, director of the division in FDA that regulates condoms and other reproductive devices. One national survey of heterosexual adults with multiple sex partners found that only 17 percent used a condom every time they had sex.

"People say they use condoms," Yin says, "but do they use them each and every time and use them correctly? That's another ballgame. We hear it all the time—'We tried to use it, but ....'"

But what? Partner trust was the most-cited reason for not wearing condoms in a recent study sponsored by the National Institutes of Health. But be careful, CDC cautions, because even a trustworthy partner could unknowingly have a sexually transmitted disease.

Many participants in the NIH study said they didn't always wear a condom because sex feels better without them. Lopez responds, "If you don't use them, you run the risk of something that feels much worse."

Sometimes a couple can't use a latex condom because one partner is allergic to latex. For these people, FDA has approved condoms made from polyurethane.

If a man objects to wearing a condom for some other reason, Planned Parenthood suggests possible replies. For example, to the partner who says, "I guess you don't really love me," the organization suggests responding, "I do, but I'm not risking my future to prove it." If the man still chooses not to wear a condom, the Reality female condom cleared by FDA in 1993 offers an alternative. (See "For the Female.")

Using condoms consistently is a start, but using them correctly is another key to protecting oneself. User error, not poor condom quality, leads to most breakages. But a few simple rules can minimize breaks and leaks. (See "Handle with Care.")

Even when used correctly, condoms aren't perfect, CDC acknowledges, comparing them to other important safety-enhancing behaviors like wearing seatbelts and bicycle helmets. Imperfect as they are, condoms can significantly reduce the rates of unintended pregnancies and sexually transmitted diseases.

"Correct and consistent condom use," says CDC's Peterson, "could break the back of the AIDS epidemic."

Tamar Nordenberg is a staff writer for FDA Consumer.

More Safer Sex Information

CDC National AIDS Hotline
1-800-342-AIDS
(1-800-342-2437)
http://www.cdcnac.org/

CDC National STDs Hotline
1-800-227-8922

Planned Parenthood Federation of America
1-800-230-7526
http://www.ppfa.org/ppfa/

For the Female

The pouch-shaped Reality female condom enables women to protect *themselves* against pregnancy and AIDS and other sexually transmitted diseases.

The female condom is made from polyurethane and, like the male condom, is a nonprescription barrier method of birth control. The device has a closed end that is inserted deep inside the vagina to catch the sperm and an open end that remains outside the body. A female condom should not be used with a male condom because the devices will not stay in place.

Over the course of a year, between 5 percent and 21 percent of women who use the female condom are expected to get pregnant, depending on whether the condom is used correctly with every act of vaginal intercourse. The female condom also provides some level of protection against STDs.

As with other condoms, follow label directions carefully to ensure that the material is not deteriorated or torn.

—T.N.

America: Awash in STDs

by Gracie S. Hsu

A "hidden epidemic" is stalking America, according to the Institute of Medicine, a branch of the National Academy of Sciences. More than 25 infectious diseases transmitted by unprecedented rates of promiscuous extramarital sexual activity are infecting at least 12 million Americans annually.

At current rates of infection, at least one in four Americans will contract a sexually transmitted disease (STD) at some point in life.

The United States bears the dubious distinction of leading the industrialized world in overall rates of STDs.

Two-thirds of the 12 million new cases a year are among men and women under age 25. Indeed, about 3 million teenagers—one in four sexually experienced adolescents—acquire an STD each year.

STDs should concern Americans because they can cause such serious consequences as cervical cancer, infertility, infection of offspring, and death. Most people are unaware that

- an estimated 100,000 to 150,000 women become infertile each year as a result of an STD;
- half of the 88,000 ectopic pregnancies that occur each year are due to a preexisting STD infection;
- 4,500 American women die each year from cervical cancer, which is almost always caused by an STD called the human papilloma virus (HPV).

'STEALTH' DISEASE

"I don't think people understand how common some of these serious consequences are, particularly infertility," says Patricia Donovan, senior associate at the Alan Guttmacher Institute (AGI), a nonprofit research corporation specializing in reproductive health.

"Seventy-five percent of women with chlamydia don't have any symptoms. They don't know until 5 years later, when they have serious pelvic pain, or 10 years later, when they can't get pregnant, that they had this STD that would have been easily curable."

STDs such as chlamydia, gonorrhea, syphilis, and trichomoniasis are nonviral and therefore curable if detected early enough. Other STDs, however, are viral and have no cure. These include HPV, genital herpes, sexually transmitted hepatitis B, and the human immunodeficiency virus, or HIV, which is responsible for 90,000 cases of AIDS annually, a figure that was dramatically expanded in 1993 over previous years due to an official redefinition of AIDS.

As many as 56 million individuals—more than one in five Americans—may be infected with an incurable viral STD other than AIDS.

STDs are "a tremendous problem," says W. David Hager, president of the Infectious Diseases Society for Obstetrics and Gynecology.

"Last fall, a *New England Journal of Medicine* article found that slightly over 21 percent of Americans over age 12 are herpes simplex virus positive," Hager says. "That equals 45 million people.

"Furthermore, huge numbers of coeds on college campuses have HPV. Ninety-five percent of all cervical cancer and dysplasia [abnormal growth of organs or cells] are caused by HPV. And this may only be the tip of the iceberg."

The Institute of Medicine (IOM) estimates that the annual direct and indirect costs of selected major STDs, in addition to the human suffering associated with them, are approximately $10 billion. If sexually transmitted HIV infections are included, the total rises to $17 billion.

Medically, experts agree that the main risk factor for contracting an STD is promiscuity.

PROMISCUITY'S PERIL

"Having more than one lifetime sexual partner connotes risk," says Shepherd Smith, president of the Institute for Youth Development

---

This article originally appeared in *The World & I*, June 1998, pp. 56-61. Reprinted by permission of *The World & I*, a publication of The Washington Times Corporation. © 1998.

The Hidden Epidemic

→ The United States leads the industralized world in overall rates of STDs.

→ STDs can cause cervical cancer, infertility, infection of offspring, and death.

→ As many as 56 million Americans (more than one in five citizens) may be infected with an incurable viral STD other than AIDS, such as genital herpes or hepatitis B.

→ Annual costs of selected major STDs are about $10 billion. Including sexually transmitted HIV, the total rises to $17 billion.

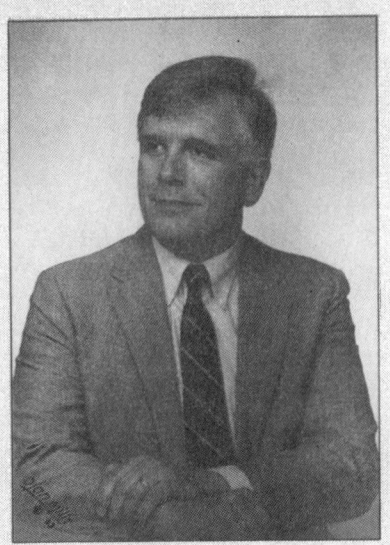

COURTESY OF THE INSTITUTE FOR YOUTH DEVELOPMENT

■ *Promiscuity skeptic:* Shepherd Smith, president of the Institute for Youth Development, says, "The more [sexual] partners, the more risk [for contracting STDs]. It's that simple."

(IYD). "The more partners, the more risk. It's that simple."

Compared with men and women who have had only 1 partner, those who report 2–3 partners are 5 times as likely to have had an STD; those with 4–6 lifetime partners are 10 times as likely; and the odds are 31 times greater for those who report 16 or more partners.

But Americans today are far more promiscuous than in the past. One big reason is that people are initiating sexual intercourse at younger ages, which usually leads to a higher number of partners during their lifetime.

According to a national poll of more than 11,000 high-school-aged youths, 54 percent said they were sexually active, compared with 29 percent in 1970. The proportion of 15-year-olds who have had sex has risen from 4.6 percent in 1970 to 26 percent. And almost one-fifth of the sexually active teens say they have had four or more partners.

In urban areas, the percentage of sexually experienced women aged 15–19 who reported four or more sex partners increased from 14 percent in 1971 to 31 percent in 1988.

"Sexual behavior is putting a sizable portion of high school students at risk," says Richard Lowry, an adolescent-health expert at the federal Centers for Disease Control and Prevention (CDC).

Having several partners is especially dangerous for teenage girls, he says, because studies show that they often have an immature cervix, which may be more easily infected.

While experts agree that promiscuity is a major risk factor, liberals and conservatives generally hold very different values regarding promiscuity. Conservatives usually believe that promiscuity in and of itself is unhealthy and should be prevented by advocating abstinence until marriage and faithfulness within marriage.

Liberals usually argue that promiscuity already exists, that it results from legitimate personal choices, and that it is not necessarily something that can or should be prevented. Rather, people should be educated about their risks so that they can protect themselves with condoms if they choose to have more than one sexual partner.

CONSERVATIVES: PREVENT PROMISCUITY

To conservatives, America's STD epidemic is really a problem of promiscuity, a symptom of society's moral decline, which began with the 1960s sexual revolution.

Joe McIlhaney, president of the Medical Institute for Sexual Health in Austin, Texas, says that "the reason there are more [sexually transmitted] diseases now than 30 years ago is because the ethics and values of society have changed."

There has been, he says, "a weakening of values, not just those having to do with sex, but also of other values like respect, responsibility, integrity." He says parents are not teaching their children these values strongly anymore.

Hager concurs. "Family breakdown and the loss of a great deal of family identity," he says, have contributed to a problem he's seeing become more common among young women: "A majority of young women that we see with STDs come from a situation where they are seeking the love and intimacy that they have missed in their homes."

To reverse the moral decline, conservatives advocate reinstating the traditional values of abstinence until marriage and faithfulness within marriage.

First, "parents should give unambiguous messages regarding appropriate sexual conduct," says the IYD's Smith.

Research shows that parents have the biggest impact of anyone on kids' behavior. And, according to the National Longitudinal Study on

The STD Tidal Wave

STD	Consequences of Infection	Estimated New Cases Annually	Estimated Costs (1990)
Pelvic Inflammatory Disease (PID)	Infertility, ectopic pregnancy	1 million	$4.2 billion
Chlamydia	PID, infertility, ectopic pregnancy; neonatal eye infections; infant pneumonia and chronic respiratory problems	4 million	$781 million
Gonorrhea	PID, infertility, ectopic pregnancy; in newborns causes blindness, septic arthritis, meningitis	1.1 million	$288 million
Genital Herpes*	Babies exposed at birth may die or suffer neurologic damage	200,000–500,000 (31 million currently infected)	$145 million
Trichomoniasis	Vaginal discharge	3 million	Unknown
Urethritis		1.2 million	Unknown
Human Papilloma Virus (HPV)*	Cervical cancer	500,000–1 million (24–40 million currently infected)	Unknown
Epididymitis	Fever, chills, groin pain	500,000	Unknown
Hepatitis B*	Liver cancer	100,000–200,000 (1.5 million currently infected)	Unknown
Syphilis	Stillborn children; in infants, congenital syphilis	120,000	Unknown
HIV*	Death, greater susceptibility to other diseases	40,000 (1 million currently infected)	Unknown

*NONCURABLE STDs
SOURCE: ALAN GUTTMACHER INSTITUTE

Adolescent Health, the largest-ever survey of American adolescents, kids were more likely to abstain from sex if their parents encouraged them to wait until marriage and discouraged birth control.

Kids also need to know that "sex within marriage is truly worth waiting for," Smith continues. "The NORC [National Opinion Research Center] study in Chicago found that the most sexually satisfied Americans are those who are in monogamous married relationships."

Second, "educators and medical professionals need to come around and help the parents to avoid disease and have a consistent message," says McIlhaney. He suggests that schools teach a character-based sex education program, because "values are the foundation on which good character is built."

"Young people will behave at the level of greatest expectation," says Hager. "If your expectation of young people is that they will engage in sexual activity, you aren't teaching them appropriate restraints.

"If your expectation of young people is that they can abstain, your educational program and expectations will give them enough hope that they will be able to abstain."

LIBERALS: PREVENT UNPROTECTED SEX

Unlike conservatives, liberals think that preventing promiscuity is unrealistic and not even necessarily desirable.

Instead, they envision a culture where people are open and comfortable with their sexuality so each person would be able to negotiate with his sexual partner about what he wants or doesn't want from sex. Preventing promiscuity, therefore, is not the goal; preventing unprotected intercourse is.

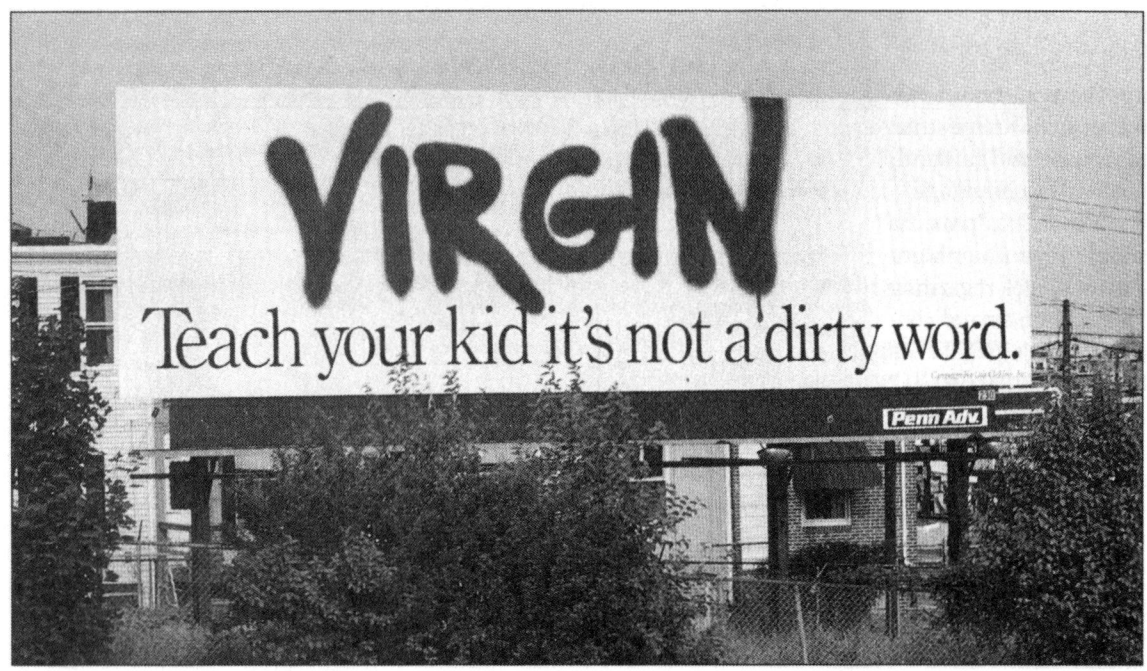

■ *Advertising abstinence:* Various groups and localities have begun to run billboard ads, such as this one in Maryland, promoting abstinence as a way of stemming the STD epidemic.

To liberals, the problem of high STD rates stems from Americans' inability to talk about sexuality and provide factual sex education in the home, school, and health care setting.

Peggy Clarke, president of the American Social Health Association, the only nongovernmental organization devoted to fighting STDs, says that the reason STDs are flourishing is that "we, as a culture, have not been good at dealing with sexuality."

"We need to raise people's skills in talking about sexuality and becoming more comfortable with it," says Kent Klindera, director of the HIV/STD education department at Advocates for Youth. The message that humans are "sexual beings" has to come from all sectors of society, he says, including "schools, churches, the mass media."

For example, Klindera conducts a peer education program through the Episcopal Church. His workshops help young people build better communication skills around their sexuality, whether it be through condom negotiation or abstinence role playing. He says if young people can communicate better about their sexuality, they'll be able to prevent the spread of STDs.

Liberals say that the best way to prevent STDs among the sexually active is to use condoms. They claim that condoms are "very effective" in preventing disease if used correctly every time. Thus, they want condoms to be distributed in schools, and they advocate increased funding for clinics that distribute condoms.

The AGI's Donovan says television networks should air condom ads to educate people about the risks of unprotected sex.

Planned Parenthood sums up the communication and condoms message this way: "Talk with your partners before the heat of passion, and use a condom every time!"

THE VALUES BATTLEFIELD

Conservatives say that the liberal approach is ultimately self-defeating, primarily because the underlying problem of promiscuity is not addressed. They also believe condoms are a poor substitute for true prevention, citing the following reasons:

1. Sending the implicit message that sex outside marriage is permissible will increase the number of people choosing to have sex with multiple partners.

2. Talking explicitly about sexuality piques curiosity and increases the likelihood of sexual experimentation.

3. Condoms provide only partial protection at best. Studies show that condoms have a 12–16 percent failure rate at preventing pregnancy after one year of using the devices. And while pregnancy can only occur a few days during the month, an STD can be transmitted any time a person has sex. Studies also indicate that condoms provide no detectable protection against HPV, genital herpes, or chlamydia.

4. It is unrealistic to expect people to use condoms consistently and correctly with every act of intercourse for a long period of time. McIlhaney says that the highest rate of condom use is a little more than 50 percent, and this was among adults who knew their partners were HIV-positive and whose participation in a research study exposed them to constant encouragement to use condoms. He also cites a 1997 *CDC Update* that said that if people do not use condoms

effectively 100 percent of the time, the outcome would be the same as if they were not using condoms at all.

Liberals say that their approach is superior to the conservatives' for the following reasons:

1. Promiscuity exists, and a "just say no" message is an inadequate and unrealistic response. Conservatives have no response, liberals say, for those who choose to be sexually active outside marriage.

2. Condoms provide very effective protection against STDs. When asked about the 12–16 percent pregnancy failure rate of condoms, liberals respond that such a rate reflects "typical use." Perfect use of condoms, they say, results in an annual pregnancy rate of only 2 percent. They are also adamant about the effectiveness of condoms in preventing STDs. Planned Parenthood says that latex condoms offer "good protection" against many STDs, including gonorrhea, HIV, syphilis, and chancroid, and "some protection" against HPV and genital herpes.

3. Their approach does not impose moral absolutes on people's sexual behavior. Choosing abstinence is just as fine an option as choosing to be sexually active using condoms. It is more important that people be open and comfortable with their own sexuality.

> "Seventy-five percent of women with chlamydia don't have any symptoms. They don't know until . . . 10 years later, when they can't get pregnant," says an Alan Guttmacher Institute official.

In the final analysis, liberals are right in saying that not everyone is going to practice abstinence until marriage and faithfulness within marriage.

Conservatives are also accurate in saying that far from everyone who engages in sex with multiple partners is going to use condoms consistently and correctly 100 percent of the time.

But ultimately, the debate is more about values than science. It's about whose ideas about human sexuality, family, and lifestyle will prevail.

And that is a question only the American public can answer.

Gracie S. Hsu is a policy analyst specializing in adolescent sexuality and life issues at the Family Research Council, a Washington, D.C.-based research and educational organization.

Your Sexual Landscape

For too long, women and doctors have maintained an uneasy silence about what goes on below the beltline. It's time we got comfortable with our own anatomy—

our health depends on it

By Beth Howard

Vagina. There, I've said it. This simple three-syllable word is no tongue twister—but it leaves even the boldest of us sputtering.

And it's not just talking about vaginas that makes women nervous. Many of us can't bear to *look* at our anatomy. The vagina is the locus of our most profound feelings about intimacy. No wonder it's shrouded in mystery and shame, or that the men in our lives often know their way around our bodies better than we do.

Until recently even medicine was guilty of keeping the vagina under wraps. Research on vulvar-vaginal disorders (the vulva is the external genitalia) is nearly nonexistent, says Libby Edwards, M.D., a vulvar-disease specialist at the Carolinas Medical Center in Charlotte, NC. And medical training on the subject is notoriously scanty. Even the obvious specialties limit their scope. Gynecologists tend to focus on the internal reproductive organs; urologists on urinary tract problems. Most dermatologists stop short of the vulva. "Thanks to sexual taboos, this area has been virtually ignored," says Peter Lynch, M.D., chairman of dermatology at the University of California at Davis and one of the field's few specialists in vulvar dermatology.

Medicine may be neglecting women, but we are often our own worst enemies when it comes to vaginal health. "*Vagina* is a dirty word. Women don't think about taking care of their vaginas," says Sharon Hillier, Ph.D., director of reproductive infectious disease research at Magee-Women's Hospital at the University of Pittsburgh. Add the shame factor, and you've got the setup for a stalemate: Doctors don't ask about vaginal problems, and women don't tell.

But times are changing. Spurred by new data about vaginal health, gynecological researchers have begun to advocate a newer, friendlier way of thinking about the vagina. Not simply a place for penises, babies and tampons, this four-inch-deep tunnel is also home to a variety of microscopic organisms that conspire to make it as delicately balanced an ecosystem as a tropical rain forest. When the system is running properly, friendly bacteria called lactobacilli constantly manufacture hydrogen peroxide, in effect churning out tiny bits of bleach to keep not-so-friendly organisms in check. Left to itself, the vagina is one of the cleanest surfaces on the body.

The idea of a naturally clean vagina is so at odds with women's beliefs and society's stereotypes that Dr. Hillier has embarked on a virtual vagina campaign. "The healthy vaginal ecosystem," she declares, "is an endangered habitat."

IRRITANTS AND INFECTION:
Preserving a Pristine Environment

As with other ecological disasters, we can blame ourselves when the vagina's natural balance is upset. We have unsafe sex, take antibiotics (which kill off healthy bacteria) or mistakenly use nonprescription yeast cures when we don't really have yeast infections.

Ironically the primary culprits are often products aimed at helping women feel "fresh." Douches, vaginal deodorants and scented panty liners contain chemicals that can irritate the vaginal walls and disrupt the normal flora. A study of 182 women done at the University of Washington in Seattle found that women who routinely douched for hygiene were four times as likely as those who didn't to lose their healthful lactobacilli. "Douching can upset the ecosystem in much the same way as putting weed killer on the lawn can kill the underlying lawn," Dr. Hillier says. "It has no medical benefits," and it's actually associated with an *increased* risk for pelvic inflammatory disease.

Fortunately tampons seem to have little effect on the vagina. Today's less absorbent, natural-fiber tampons are far safer than the super-absorbent synthetic ones that spurred cases of toxic-shock syndrome in the early 1980s. Researchers reported in the *Journal of Infectious Diseases* last November that tampons did not adversely affect the vaginal ecosystem.

Not only can some vaginal products cause internal trouble, but they also can result in external redness or itching and derail sex. What to do: Stop using the product and let the ecosystem's natural cleanup squad restore things to normal. Vulvar irritation often comes in the form of dermatitis: dry, itchy skin that may be due to tight or chafing clothes combined with the moisture of normal vaginal secretions. The solution: loose-fitting clothes. Your doctor may prescribe a steroid ointment if the problem persists.

BACTERIA, VIRUSES AND YEAST:
Stopping an Ecological Disaster

The good news for women of all ages is that the vagina has a natural tendency to restore itself—to a point: Discharge combined with odor, particularly a fishy odor, is almost always a tip-off to the presence of an infection that can make intercourse painful and require medical attention. "Normal secretions are not foul or fishy," says David E. Soper, M.D., director of the division of benign gynecology at the Medical University of South Carolina in Charleston. The wise course of action is to become familiar with these sex stoppers before they strike. (For a list of common complaints, see "The Infection Connection."

The problem is, some women blame bad hygiene for their symptoms. Doctors are often party to the cover-up: In a recent survey by the National Vaginitis Association, nearly 50% of gynecologists said that even when they found evidence of the

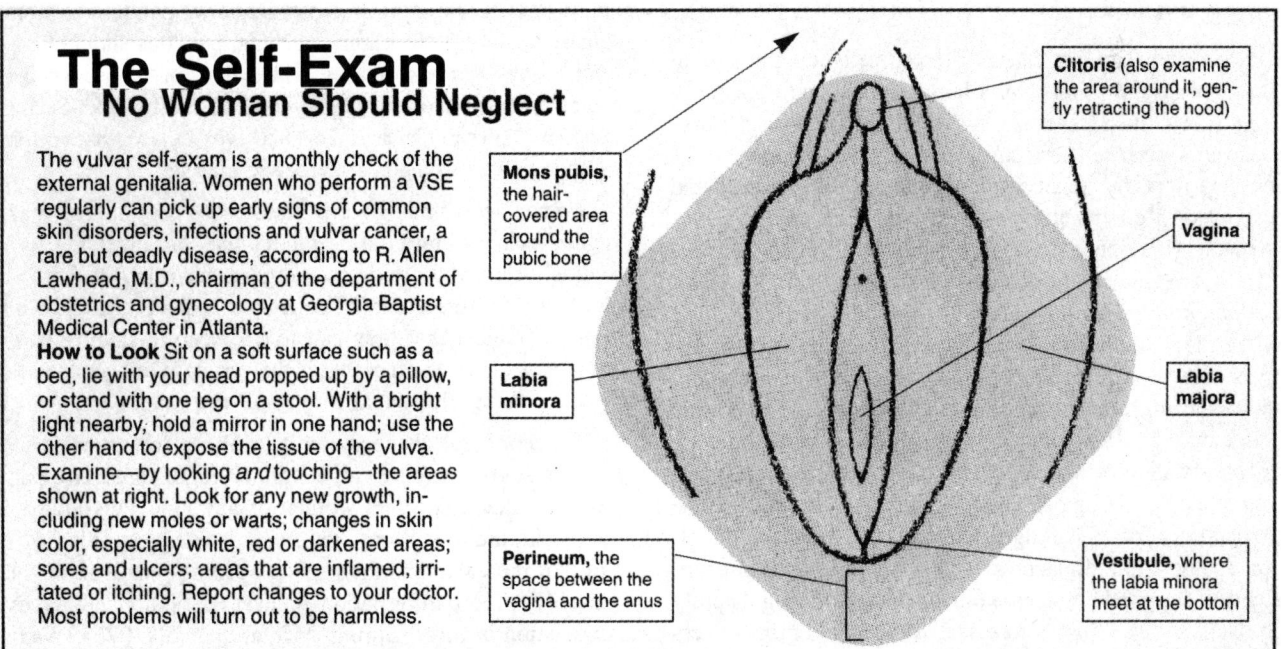

The Self-Exam
No Woman Should Neglect

The vulvar self-exam is a monthly check of the external genitalia. Women who perform a VSE regularly can pick up early signs of common skin disorders, infections and vulvar cancer, a rare but deadly disease, according to R. Allen Lawhead, M.D., chairman of the department of obstetrics and gynecology at Georgia Baptist Medical Center in Atlanta.

How to Look Sit on a soft surface such as a bed, lie with your head propped up by a pillow, or stand with one leg on a stool. With a bright light nearby, hold a mirror in one hand; use the other hand to expose the tissue of the vulva. Examine—by looking *and* touching—the areas shown at right. Look for any new growth, including new moles or warts; changes in skin color, especially white, red or darkened areas; sores and ulcers; areas that are inflamed, irritated or itching. Report changes to your doctor. Most problems will turn out to be harmless.

- **Clitoris** (also examine the area around it, gently retracting the hood)
- **Mons pubis,** the hair-covered area around the pubic bone
- **Vagina**
- **Labia minora**
- **Labia majora**
- **Perineum,** the space between the vagina and the anus
- **Vestibule,** where the labia minora meet at the bottom

most common infection, bacterial vaginosis, they treated it only if patients complained of symptoms.

A vaginal infection won't always be diagnosed during a routine gynecological visit, notes Jill Maura Rabin, M.D., head of urogynecology at Long Island Jewish Medical Center in New Hyde Park, NY. The Pap smear is not designed to detect vaginal infections. That's why it's important to speak up about symptoms such as odor and discharge, especially because unchecked infections now appear to be more dangerous than previously believed. Bacterial vaginosis, for example, has recently been linked to a higher rate of pelvic inflammatory disease, pregnancy complications and postoperative infections.

Viruses present an altogether different threat to vaginal health and sexual pleasure, so it's also crucial to bring any herpes blisters or genital warts to a doctor's attention. (For information about how to examine yourself, see box on previous page.)

AGE-RELATED DRYNESS:
Changes in the Terrain

Sometimes discomfort during intercourse is not a symptom of infection but the primary problem. Its most common cause is vaginal dryness. Some women develop premenopausal dryness due to a drop in estrogen or as a result of hysterectomy, chemotherapy or the use of antidepressants, antihistamines and some hormonal contraceptives. "And after menopause, nearly all women experience dryness," says Geoffrey Redmond, M.D., a Cleveland endocrinologist and author of *The Good New About Women's Hormones*.

When the ovaries stop producing estrogen, the vaginal lining gets drier and thinner, making it vulnerable to irritation, which can result in pain during sex. The vulva and the vagina also become less elastic, although regular stimulation—through either masturbation or intercourse—may reduce this change, according to Beverly Whipple, Ph.D., an associate professor in the department of nursing at Rutgers University in Newark, NJ.

For a quick fix, drugstores display a variety of slippery substances designed to keep your love life gliding happily along. Gels are used just before sex, while liquid moisturizers can be applied as often as needed. Choose a water-soluble product; oil-based ones can upset the vaginal ecology and erode latex used in diaphragms and condoms.

Lack of moisture puts a damper on intimacy. But the right lubricant can keep things gliding along.

The best solution for postmenopausal women, though, is estrogen replacement. "The minimal dose that protects women against heart disease and osteoporosis may not be enough to adequately relieve thin, dry tissue," says Dr. Redmond. You'll have to speak up if you want your doctor to fine-tune treatment. One offbeat solution is the Reality female condom. Anecdotal reports suggest some women are using it to protect thinning tissues during intercourse.

Menopause produces other vaginal changes. The vagina begins to narrow and shorten, and the rugae—tiny ridges that help the vagina expand at childbirth and enhance its gripping effect during sex—gradually disappear. For many women, pelvic muscle strength decreases with age. This may reduce the sensation of friction during intercourse. Some women turn to cosmetic surgery to tighten the vaginal opening, but "this should be a last resort," says Linda Brubaker, M.D., director of urogynecology and reconstructive pelvic surgery at Rush-Presbyterian-St. Luke's Medical Center in Chicago. For most women, exercises or physical therapy can strengthen the pelvic muscle.

Women who undergo a hysterectomy may notice that the vagina feels different during intercourse, because the cervix is routinely removed during the surgery, according to Dr. Whipple. Many doctors don't tell patients to expect this, and women may not realize that they can ask for cervix-sparing surgery. "Studies support the fact that if the cervix is left, women don't report a change in sexual response," she says.

If menopausal changes aren't to blame for sexual discomfort, the source may be vulvodynia or vaginismus, two painful problems that can affect women of any age. Vulvodynia is a set of chronic symptoms—burning, rawness, stinging or irritation of the vulva and the vaginal opening—with an unknown cause. (For more information, contact the National Vulvodynia Association in Silver Spring, MD, at 301–299–0775.) Vaginismus, an involuntary spasm of the vaginal muscles that occurs before or during penetration, also causes extreme pain. It's often related to fear or anxiety about sex.

Finding the Elusive G Spot

The G spot usurped the clitoris as the focus of sensual pleasure in the 1980s, when researchers reported that orgasm often results when a small area beneath the front of the vaginal wall is stimulated. It's easiest to find your G spot when you're kneeling. You or your partner can insert two fingers about halfway into the vagina and explore the front wall until you find a patch of tissue that begins to swell. (Use your other hand to press on the lower abdomen just above the pubic hair.) Stimulation produces a pleasant sensation for most women and often leads to orgasm, reports Beverly Whipple, Ph.D., an associate professor in the department of nursing at Rutgers University in Newark, N.J. Once you've located the G spot, you and your partner can try different positions to improve his contact with the area during lovemaking.

The Infection Connection

Here's how to cope with the most common vaginal infections that strike women in midlife:

The culprit	The symptoms	The cure
Bacterial vaginosis, an overgrowth of normal vaginal bacteria.	Thin grayish or white discharge that has a foul, fishy odor. Possible itching and irritation.	The prescription drugs metronidazole or clindamycin. Avoid nonprescription yeast drugs—they could make matters worse.
Yeast infection, an overgrowth of the *Candida* fungus.	Odorless white, cottage cheese-like discharge and itching.	If you're sure it's yeast, try an over-the-counter yeast fighter; otherwise, see your doctor. Eating yogurt that contains live *Lactobacillus acidophilus* cultures may reduce the risk of future infections.
Trichomonas, a parasite usually transmitted during sex.	Frothy, yellow-green fishy-smelling discharge; itching, painful urination or intercourse.	Prompt treatment with the prescription drug metronidazole for both you and your partner.
Herpes simplex virus, which can be transmitted sexually even in the absence of blisters.	Itching, stinging sores on the vulva or in the vagina.	There is no cure, but prescription antiviral drugs can reduce outbreaks and to some extent protect a partner from infection.
Human papillomavirus, which can be sexually transmitted.	Vaginal warts which may itch or burn after sex.	Certain types of HPV place women at above-average risk of cervical cancer, so most growths are surgically removed.

Whether it's the pain of vaginismus or the annoyance of a yeast infection, doctors are taking vaginal symptoms more seriously. "There is a transition from seeing them as a nuisance to seeing them as a threat to women's health and psychological well-being," says Dr. Hillier. As more physicians fight to clean up the vagina's public image, this under-appreciated part of our anatomy will no doubt be seen as less mysterious—and more marvelous.

Your next step? See the box for advice on how to use vulvar self-exams to get acquainted with your body. Debra Gussman, M.D., a Denver gynecologist, puts it this way: "If you don't know what you look like, how are you going to know everything's okay?"

Beth Howard lives in New York City and is writing a book about sexual wellness for women.

Unit 7

Unit Selections

31. **Family History: What You Don't Know Can Kill You,** Consumer Reports on Health
32. **The Heart Attackers,** Geoffrey Cowley
33. **Heart Disease in Women: Special Symptoms, Special Risks,** Consumer Reports on Health
34. **Beyond Cholesterol,** Judith Mandelbaum-Schmid
35. **Strategies for Minimizing Cancer Risk,** Walter C. Willett, Graham A. Colditz, and Nancy E. Mueller
36. **AIDS, after the "Cure": Amid Setbacks, Search for New Hope,** Laurie Garrett

Key Points to Consider

❖ Do doctors have a right to know if their patients are infected with AIDS? If so, how would you secure this information?

❖ What role can and should education play in combating the spread of AIDS?

❖ What lifestyle changes could you make that would reduce your risk of developing cardiovascular disease, cancer, and AIDS?

❖ What dietary advice would you give someone to reduce his or her risk of cancer?

❖ To what extent should the government be involved in promoting preventative medicine?

❖ Assuming that you live long enough, which chronic disease do you think you are most likely to contract, based on your family history and lifestyle?

❖ How do the risk factors for coronary disease differ for men and women?

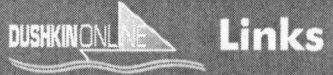 **Links**   www.dushkin.com/online/

25. **American Cancer Society**
    http://www.cancer.org/frames.html
26. **American Heart Association (AMA)**
    http://www.amhrt.org
27. **Body Health Resources Corporation**
    http://www.thebody.com/cgi-bin/body.cgi

These sites are annotated on pages 4 and 5.

Current Killers

Cardiovascular disease and cancer are the leading killers in this country. These diseases, which are termed chronic illnesses, are most likely to afflict people who have made lifestyle choices that disregard their genetic predisposition toward these illnesses. It is not always possible to prevent these illnesses, but your chances of success are much greater if you are aware of any genetic predisposition that you may have inherited. The report "Family History: What You Don't Know Can Kill You" identifies several diseases that have a strong genetic component, and it suggests how to go about constructing a family tree to find out if you are at risk.

Of all the diseases in America, coronary heart disease is this nation's number one killer. Frequently, the first and only symptom of this disease is sudden death. Epidemiological studies have revealed a number of risk factors that increase one's likelihood of developing it. These include hypertension, a high serum cholesterol level, diabetes, cigarette smoking, obesity, a sedentary lifestyle, a family history of heart disease, age, sex, race, and stress. When discussing risk factors, it is important to remember that they are just that, and not absolute predictors of disease. Serum cholesterol is an excellent case in point. No one can deny that having an elevated LDL cholesterol level increases one's risk, but the fact is that most heart attack victims have a cholesterol reading in the normal range. This finding suggests that there other elements operating that have yet to be identified. Recent scientific investigations into serum lipid levels appear to have uncovered some of these elements. "Beyond Cholesterol," by Judith Mandelbaum-Schmid, discusses these newly identified risk factors and suggests that if you have a family history of heart disease it would be a good idea to have them tested.

Unfortunately, as it currently stands we apparently do not know all of the risk factors for coronary artery disease but the scientific community may have uncovered additional ones, such as low birth weight, cytomegalovirus, *Chlamydia pneumoniae*, and *Porphyromonas gingivalis*. "The Heart Attackers" by Geoffrey Cowley discusses the evidence in support of these new risk factors and what you can due to control them. "Heart Disease in Women: Special Symptoms, Special Risks" discusses current findings that suggest that the risk factors for heart disease in women differ from those in men and should be managed accordingly. Fortunately 7 of the 11 risk factors associated with heart disease are controllable and, if controlled properly, can forestall or prevent this deadly disease.

Cardiovascular disease is America's number one killer, but cancer takes top billing in terms of the "fear factor." This fear of cancer stems from an awareness of the degenerative and disfiguring nature of the disease. Today, cancer specialists are employing a variety of complex agents and technologies, such as monoclonal antibodies, interferon, and immunotherapy, in their attempt to fight it. Progress has been slow, however, and the results, while promising, suggest that a cure may be several years away. A very disturbing aspect of this country's battle against cancer is the fact that millions of dollars are spent each year trying to advance the treatment of cancer, while funding for the technologies used to detect cancer in its early stages is quite limited. A reallocation of funds would seem appropriate, given the medical community's position that early detection and treatment are the key elements in the successful management of cancer. The authors of "Strategies for Minimizing Cancer Risk" address the importance of prevention and early detection as our best strategy for reducing the death toll associated with this feared disease.

Of the three diseases discussed in this unit, HIV/AIDS has the potential to become the worst epidemic of this century. As medical researchers intensify their search for an effective HIV/AIDS vaccine, the disease continues to spread and infect countless innocent people. 33.4 million worldwide are living with HIV. Of those diagnosed with AIDS, half are already dead and the rest are dying. Conservative estimates indicate that by the year 2000, between 30 and 110 million people could be infected with the AIDS virus. The World Health Organization estimates that during 1998 5.8 million people were infected with the virus. One of the problems with trying to estimate the exact number of potential AIDS victims is the fact that this disease has an incubation period that may be as long as 10 years.

What is known about AIDS? Researchers have been able to identify the virus that causes AIDS. This virus, termed the HIV virus, has been found in both the blood and body fluids of infected persons, and case studies have documented that the disease can be transmitted through intimate sexual contact and the mixing of blood products. Despite the failure by the scientific community to produce an AIDS vaccine or cure, optimism ran high at the 11th International Conference on AIDS in 1996, based on a newly developed treatment regime that appeared to be very effective in reducing the viral load and thus retarding the progression of HIV into AIDS. The term assigned to this new treatment regime was Highly Active Anti-Retroviral Therapy (HAART). As scientists prepared for the 12th International Conference on AIDS in June of 1998, the optimism regarding HAART therapy turned to pessimism and fear. It had been about 2 years since the first clinical trials with HAART and major problems were starting to surface in a large number of patients. "AIDS, after the 'Cure': Amid Setbacks, Search for New Hope" examines the HAART treatment regime and discusses how this once promising new approach to treating HIV infections has become a source of frustration and fear for both doctors and patients.

Family history: What you don't know can kill you

Your risk of deadly disease can be influenced or even determined by hereditary factors.

Knowing that a specific disease runs in your family can save your life. Depending on the disease, it can allow you to watch for early warning signs, get more frequent screening tests, or change your health habits.

Unfortunately, most doctors pay scant attention to family background. One study of medical records for nearly 9000 patients found that physicians had noted family history in only 4 percent. The recent advances in genetic testing for hereditary disease may force many physicians—and their patients—to attend more closely to family matters. For the vast majority of people, however, there's no need for genetic tests; an old-fashioned family tree will be far more helpful.

Genetic mandate

For certain uncommon diseases, heredity is the primary cause: If your parents gave you the necessary genes, you're almost sure to get the disease. Such disorders include hemophilia, cystic fibrosis, sickle-cell anemia, at least some cases of Alzheimer's disease, certain cancers, and some 4000 other diseases, nearly all of them rare. It's impossible to prevent those disorders, but early detection can allow doctors to prevent or treat the complications that may develop.

In addition, some genetic disorders, while not harmful in and of themselves, can pave the way for disease. For example, familial hypercholesterolemia, an inherited elevation in blood cholesterol, is implicated in one of every five heart attacks that strike before age 60. And about 1 percent of all colorectal cancers evolve from polyps caused by a hereditary disorder known as familial polyposis. Detected early, those conditions can be treated before any disease develops.

Learn from history In one study, doctors noted family history on only 4 percent of all medical records. But virtually all families have some hereditary concerns.

If an uncommon disease appears somewhere in your family tree, you can get valuable information by looking it up in the medical section of your local library. A medical dictionary will usually tell you whether the disease is inherited directly and, if it is, which of the following types of genes transmits it:

■ **Dominant:** If one parent had a disease transmitted by a dominant gene, you have a 50/50 chance of getting the gene. If you carry the gene, you'll probably get the disease. Examples include familial hypercholesterolemia and familial polyposis of the colon.

■ **Recessive:** You'd get the disease only in the unlikely event that both parents carried the gene and both passed it on to you. The most common recessive diseases occur only in certain ethnic groups—such as Tay-Sachs disease, found primarily in Ashkenazic Jews.

■ **X-linked:** Only males get X-linked diseases, but only females transmit the gene. The son of a woman who carries the faulty gene has a 50/50 chance of inheriting the gene and almost as high a chance of getting the disease; daughters will not get the disease but have a 50/50 chance of being carriers. X-linked conditions include hemophilia and color blindness.

Genetic influence

Heredity plays a subtler role in many other diseases, which are caused at least in part by "environmental" influences such as infection, cancer-causing chemicals, or an artery-clogging diet. While your genes alone will not produce those diseases, they can determine how susceptible you are.

Researchers have found a genetic influence in most common disorders, including several major killers—coronary heart disease, diabetes, and cancer of the bladder, breast, colon, lung, ovaries, prostate, skin, or uterus. Heredity also influences susceptibility to many familiar, less deadly disorders, such as allergies, asthma, glaucoma, migraine, osteoporosis, and rheumatoid arthritis. Some psychological or behavioral problems, including depression, schizophrenia, and alcoholism, have a genetic link as well.

Fortunately, many of those diseases, unlike the purely genetic disorders, do have risk factors you can change. People whose relatives had coronary disease or type II diabetes, for example, may lower their risk by eating a low-fat, high-fiber diet, losing excess weight, and exercising regularly.

> **To gauge your true risk, you need to know something about your family's medical history.**

In general, the more relatives who had a genetically transmitted disease and the closer they are to you, the greater your risk. To gauge your true risk, however, you need to know something about your family's medical history. In some cases, nongenetic factors may have been more important than genetic ones in causing their diseases. As a general rule, however, signs of strong hereditary influence include:

■ Early onset of the disease. It generally takes decades for nongenetic factors to produce coronary disease, cancer, and many other disorders. So the earlier the disease strikes, the more likely it is that heredity played a role.

■ Appearance of the disease largely or exclusively on one side of the family.

■ Onset of the same disease at about the same age in more than one relative.

■ Tumors that cropped up independently in more than one place (as opposed to spreading from site to site). The daughter of a woman who had cancer in both breasts, for example, has three times the risk of getting the disease before menopause, compared with someone whose mother had cancer in one breast only.

■ Disease despite good health habits. Coronary disease in a physically fit vegetarian, for example, is more likely to have a genetic influence than the same disease in an unfit relative who ate lots of meat.

Constructing a family tree

You can put together a simple family tree by digging up a few key facts on your closest relatives: siblings, parents, aunts and uncles, and grandparents. Those facts include the date of birth, major diseases, and, for deceased relatives, the date and cause of death. (see the sample tree on the next page.)

Of course, the more you find out about each of your relatives, the more useful your tree will be. So you might want to try collecting at least some of these additional facts, particularly for your parents and grandparents.

■ Age when any disease first started. For cancer, ask whether tumors independently struck different sites.

■ Disabilities or major operations. (Asking may remind your relative of a disease he or she had.)

■ Allergies, including allergic reactions to drugs.

■ Other health-related conditions, notably obesity, hypertension, and high blood cholesterol.

■ Health-related habits, such as excessive consumption of alcohol, smoking, exercise, and general type of diet.

■ Miscarriages, abortions for medical reasons, stillbirths, infant deaths, and birth defects. Those are all possible signs of hereditary problems with the fetus or infant.

■ Psychological or behavioral problems, including alcoholism, anxiety, major depression, schizophrenia, psychiatric treatment or hospitalization, and suicide.

You can also expand your family tree by getting some basic medical information on some of your less-close relatives—your great-grandparents and any cousins, nieces, or nephews. While they're less genetically significant than your closest relatives, they can add weight to a pattern of, say, cancer or coronary disease. Casting a wider net may also allow you to identify a strictly genetic disease, since the genes for a great number of those diseases can be carried through many generations without actually causing the illness to develop. (Note that women can inherit the genes for diseases such as breast or ovarian cancer from their father.)

How to get the facts

Some relatives may be reluctant to divulge all that personal information about their health. So try to explain how important knowing a family health history can be, and promise to keep the information confidential if they wish.

Learn about a deceased relative from several family members, if possible, in order to corroborate their information. If you can't identify a disease from the

---

For more information
■ **Alliance of Genetic Support Groups.** Referrals to organizations providing peer support and education on specific inherited disorders. Call 800-336-GENE. (Internet: http://medhelp.org/www/agsg.htm)

7 ❖ CURRENT KILLERS

description, which may be vague, colloquial, or outdated—"consumption" instead of tuberculosis, for example—jot down the description and ask your physician to help decipher it.

You could also ask whether anyone has a copy of the death certificate. Or request a copy from the department of health in the state where your relative died. If a relative died fairly recently, see whether your doctor can contact the physician or the hospital that treated the person to learn the cause of death as well as any other diseases he or she may have had.

Once you've collected the information you want, plug it all into the tree format, using the example below as a guide. We've included a few basic symbols, which can help you see key facts at a glance.

Summing up

Armed with information about your family medical history, you'll be better able to take steps to safeguard your health—through early warnings, increased screening, or changes in health habits. To get the information you need:

■ Round up the medical facts on your closest relatives, at the very least including any diseases plus date of birth and, for deceased relatives, date and cause of death.

■ Plug all that data into a family tree and bring it to your doctor or a specialist for interpretation.

■ Plan ways to head off or prepare for any genetic risk you uncover.

■ Don't rush to have a genetic test. It often won't lead to actions any different from what would be suggested by family history alone, and testing poses a new set of problems.

How to create a family tree—and what to make of it

To get a full picture of what your family tree means, show it to your family doctor—and possibly to a physician or counselor specializing in genetics. You can also glean a lot of valuable information yourself, if you know what to look for.

In this family tree, the prostate cancer that killed this man's father means that he should be tested for a prostate tumor at a younger age and more frequently than usual. His sisters need to have earlier, more frequent mammograms because of their mother's breast cancer.

One grandmother and one uncle each died of a heart attack. There are several reasons not to worry too much about that: The two relatives were from different sides of the family; both had the attack at a relatively advanced age; both had two other major risk factors for coronary heart disease—smoking and either diabetes or obesity; and neither of the man's parents had any apparent heart trouble. Still, it would be worth checking further to see whether either relative had highly elevated cholesterol levels, which could be a sign of familial hypercholesterolemia.

The colon cancer that struck another grandmother and uncle is a different story. Two factors suggest a possible hereditary link: They were mother and son, and they both developed the disease at a comparatively young age. So the man should be screened early and often for colon cancer.

Finally, alcoholism seems to run in the family. The man should be aware that such a history could indicate a hereditary susceptibility to the problem, though the habit might simply have been passed down by example.

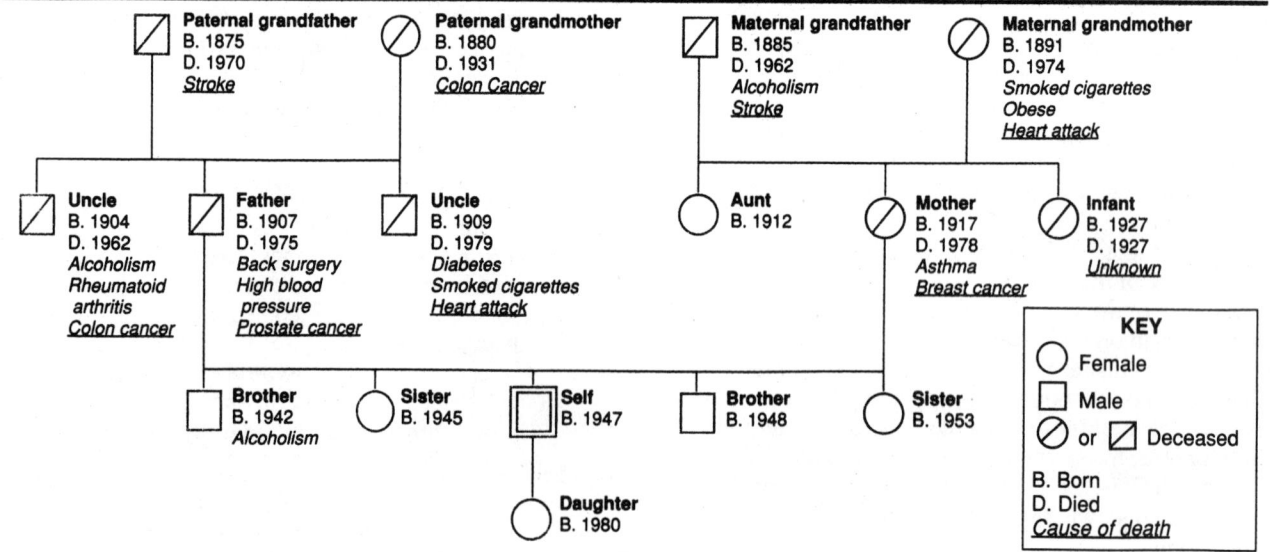

Scientists are finding a slew of new risk factors. Recognizing them could save your life.
BY GEOFFREY COWLEY

The Heart Attackers

IF YOU CARE A WHIT ABOUT YOUR health, you can probably recite your cholesterol level in your sleep. Thanks to the tireless efforts of health officials and drugmakers, Americans can hardly escape the supermarket, let alone the doctor's office, without submitting to a cholesterol check. Five percent of the adult population—some 9 million people—now take cholesterol-lowering drugs in the hope of warding off heart disease, and the potential market swells every time another boomer turns 50. "Cholesterol consciousness is incredibly high," says Dr. James Cleeman, coordinator of the federally sponsored National Cholesterol Education Program. "Fifteen years ago scientists were the only ones who talked about cholesterol. Today you see the word in the funnies."

From Cleeman's perspective, this is excellent news. Heart disease is, after all, the nation's No. 1 killer. It claims a half-million lives every year, and high cholesterol is a well-established risk factor. No one denies that excess LDL (the so-called bad cholesterol) can increase the risk of a heart attack, or that cholesterol-lowering therapy can help reduce the risk. But does one blood component warrant so much attention? The fact is, most heart-attack victims have cholesterol levels that would qualify as normal. Moreover, America's heart-attack rate has fallen by half in recent decades, while average cholesterol levels have declined only slightly (chart). So while monitoring cholesterol may be a worthwhile exercise, there is clearly more to staying healthy.

What else should we worry about? Smoking, obesity and high blood pressure all pose well-known hazards—yet roughly a fourth of all heart attacks occur in people with no known risk factors. Fortunately, researchers are now starting to identify other sources of trouble. An avalanche of new studies suggest that an amino acid called homocysteine (pronounced HO-mo-SIS-teen) plays a critical role in destroying our arteries—perhaps as large a role as smoking or cholesterol. Other research suggests

Contrary to the CW
There's a steady decline in deaths from heart attacks despite the fact that cholesterol levels haven't changed much.

PER 100,000 POPULATION, AGE-ADJUSTED
Heart-attack death rates

ADULTS, AGE 20–74 MG/DL OF BLOOD
Cholesterol levels

SOURCES: AHA, NATIONAL HEALTH & EXAMINATION SURVEYS

that our risk of developing heart disease depends at least partly on the nourishment we receive in the womb and the infections we contract as we age. The most important of the emerging risk factors are subject to our control, and together they could revolutionize the art of prevention.

Arterial disease may kill you in a minute, but it usually develops over a lifetime. And though the root causes are not perfectly understood, the disease process involves several well-known steps. It begins when something injures the lining of an artery and the body tries to repair the damage. Circulating immune cells known as monocytes burrow into the blood-vessel walls, where they mature into macrophages (literally "big eaters"), gorge themselves on oxidized fatty substances and die (diagram). Eventually, this inflammatory process causes a buildup of tough, fibrous scar tissue that can inhibit blood flow and promote the formation of clots.

According to conventional thinking, high-fat diets trigger this process by causing a buildup of LDL cholesterol in the blood. No one has ever demonstrated that circulating cholesterol is what first injures the arterial wall. But because it collects there, experts have been content to think of it as the primary culprit. Dr. Kilmer McCully, a pathologist at the VA Medical Center in Providence, R.I., has spent three decades advancing a different idea. According to McCully, the initial injury is caused not by cholesterol but by homocysteine, a substance derived from the protein in our diets. If McCully is right, this little-known molecule is what makes our blood vessels vulnerable to cholesterol—and disarming it could be as simple as upping our intake of three B vitamins. That may sound outlandish. But after years of neglect, homocysteine is now inspiring a research explosion, and McCully's ideas are looking more credible every day.

Like cholesterol, homocysteine can be useful. Our bodies derive it from methionine, an amino acid that abounds in animal protein, and use it to build and maintain tissues. During normal metabolism, any excess homocysteine is quickly swept away. With the help of vitamins B_6, B_{12} and folic acid, the liver either converts it back into methionine or breaks it down for excretion. But when that process is disrupted, the consequences can be dire. McCully discovered just how dire back in 1968, while studying a rare genetic disorder called homocystinuria.

CHILDREN BORN WITH THAT condition lack proper levels of the liver enzymes required to process homocysteine, so it reaches astronomical levels in their blood. Kids who go untreated often die of strokes and heart attacks before they reach adulthood, even though their cholesterol levels are normal. McCully discovered during autopsy studies that the young victims' arteries looked a lot like those of elderly heart patients, and that finding raised an intriguing possibility. If severe homocysteine overload can destroy a child's arteries, could milder but more chronic elevations—the kind that anyone might develop from a diet low in vitamin-rich plant foods—foster cardiovascular disease in adults?

It was just a hunch, and the research community was too focused on cholesterol to pay it much heed. But as McCully explored the idea, he found that homocysteine could help explain many of the known risk factors for heart attack and stroke. Smoking and inactivity tend to raise homocysteine levels, for example. And when heart disease runs in a family, the victims often share a minor flaw in one of the genes governing homocysteine metabolism. McCully's hypothesis also squares with what we know about the effects of gender and age. During their reproductive years, women's homocysteine levels are roughly 20 percent lower than men's. But after menopause their homocysteine levels, and their heart-disease risk, rise to male levels. Both sexes experience homocysteine increases in old age, as the body grows less efficient at absorbing B vitamins, and their heart-disease rates rise accordingly.

This is all circumstantial evidence, nothing that would send an amino acid to jail. But there is good reason to suspect that the association between homocysteine and heart disease is more than coincidental. In test-tube studies, the substance not only injures blood-vessel linings but accelerates the buildup of scar tissue and promotes the formation of blood clots. Moreover, researchers have known for years that homocysteine injections produce arterial plaques in animals.

You can't inject people that way, but there are other ways to spot patterns. In a 1992 study of 14,000 male physicians, Harvard researchers found that those with homocysteine levels above the 95th percentile had more than three times the heart-attack risk of those in the bottom 90 percent. Likewise, researchers involved in the Massachusetts-based Framingham Heart Study found in 1995 that people with high homocysteine levels are the most likely to suffer from a dangerous narrowing of the carotid artery, the main vessel feeding the brain. A homocysteine level of less than 14 micromoles per liter of blood is considered normal, but the Framingham researchers found that any reading above 11.4 brought an increase in risk. Scores of scientists are now reporting similar findings. In the past month alone, University of Washington researchers have reported that high homocysteine doubles the risk of heart attack in young women. And scientists in Norway have shown that heart patients with elevated homocysteine are the most likely to die.

That's just the bad news. As they confirm homocysteine's hazards, researchers are also identifying simple ways to avoid them. Some of us are more prone to homocysteine buildup than others (roughly one person in eight inherits a gene that slows disposal of the substance). But almost anyone can control homocysteine by getting enough B vitamins. Blood studies have consistently linked low levels of folic acid to high levels of homocysteine. And a recent European study found that people who reported taking B-vitamin supplements had just half the heart-disease rate of those who didn't.

No one yet has taken the final step, showing in a controlled clinical trial that a specific combination of foods or supplements brings a particular benefit. Meir Stampfer, an epidemiologist at Harvard, is now launching one to see whether a daily folic-acid supplement can help prevent strokes. Until the evidence is definitive, your annual physical isn't likely to include blood tests for homocysteine or B vitamins (though commercial labs will soon offer a full battery). And the government's heart-health promoters say they'll continue to ignore homocysteine in favor of cholesterol until the evidence is definitive.

But that doesn't mean you should. The evidence already in hand suggests that we have nothing to lose, and much to gain, by paying more attention to the vitamin levels in our diets. Unless you're a strict vegetarian, chances are you're getting plenty of B_{12}. Vitamin B_6 is also easy to come by, since U.S. food makers pump it into flour. In his new book, "The Homocysteine Revolution" *(242 pages. Keats. $14.95)*, McCully speculates that the B_6 in processed foods may help explain the sharp drop in heart disease since the 1960s. But folic acid is another story. Experts agree that 400 micrograms a day is probably enough to hold homocysteine in check (and to help women of childbearing age prevent neural-tube defects in their babies). The trouble is, folate is found mostly in beans, grains and greens, which are not America's favorite foods. Nearly half of us fall short of the 200-mcg daily allowance, and only a small minority get 400. Megadoses of folic acid are unnecessary and unwise, but a multivitamin and a few ounces of spinach won't hurt you. And over time, they may well save your life.

Kilmer McCully isn't the only maverick whose novel ideas are gaining currency in heart-disease research. Consider the case of David Barker, an epidemiologist at the University of Southampton, in England. Barker has long argued that our chances of developing heart disease and other chronic ills depend to a surprising degree on what happens to us early in life—not just as kids but as fetuses. He reasons that, like a poorly made car, an undernourished fetus is more likely to break down later. "We've been obsessed with the breaking-down bit," he says, "and we've forgotten how easy it is to influence people permanently before they're born."

Barker and others have amassed considerable evidence that smaller-than-average babies run a bigger-than-average risk of developing hypertension, diabetes and heart disease as adults. The possibility first occurred to him back in the early '80s, as he puzzled over Britain's regional disease patterns. Heart-disease mortality is twice as high in some areas as in others, even when dietary and lifestyle differences are taken into account. Looking back in time, Barker noticed that the heart-attack hot spots had been infant-mortality hot spots 70 years earlier. Suspecting that early deprivation might have long-delayed consequences, he gathered data on 16,000 Britons born between 1911 and 1930. His analysis showed that among people who reached full term and weighed from 5.5 to 9.5 pounds at birth, those with the lowest birth weights had the highest average heart-disease rates.

Subsequent studies have brought mixed results, but most tend to support Barker's hypothesis. In the past year alone, he and his colleagues have linked low birth weight to stroke and heart attack in British men, and to cardiovascular disease in men and women from southern India. Large studies conducted in Wales and the United States have turned up the same pattern. When Dr. Gary Curhan of Harvard looked at birth weight and blood pressure in 164,000 female nurses, he found that hypertension was 40 percent more common among those born weighing less than 5 pounds than among those born at 7 to 8.5 pounds. "It really looks like there's something to this," says Harvard epidemiologist Walter Willett.

How could low birth weight foster chronic disease? One theory holds that when a fetus lacks the nutrients it needs, its body resorts to a costly sort of triage. "The first thing it does is alter its metabolism so it can continue to grow," says Barker. That could mean ratcheting up its blood pressure to draw more nutrients through the placenta, or abandoning work on the liver, pancreas and blood vessels to complete construction of the brain. When unborn rats or sheep are deprived of nutrients, they make all these adjustments, and suffer accordingly. Barker draws the lesson that women can protect their kids against heart disease by eating well during pregnancy, but many experts are skeptical. A newborn's size is only modestly related to its mother's diet, says Dr. Nigel Paneth, an epidemiologist at Michigan State University. And even if low birth weight does contribute to heart disease,

---

Bugs in Your Pipes

Does heart disease spread like the flu? Growing evidence suggests that infectious agents play a role. Some suspects:

Chlamydia pneumoniae Causes respiratory illness; may also damage the arteries

Porphyromonas gingivalis People plagued by gum-disease bug have more coronaries

Cytomegalovirus Common herpes virus seems to exacerbate vascular conditions

32. Heart Attackers

Some Keys to Warding Off Heart Disease

It may be the nation's leading cause of death, but it needn't be yours. How to counter the risk factors.

Some cardiovascular risks are impossible to avoid. You can't change your age or your genes, and changing your sex is rarely worth the trouble. But small changes in diet or lifestyle can minimize other hazards. Some—such as smoking, obesity and a lack of physical exercise—are so obvious they hardly bear repeating. Here are some other known or suspected risk factors, and some strategies for avoiding them.

HOMOCYSTEINE
This amino acid can damage arterial walls if it reaches high concentrations in the bloodstream.

YOUR RISK: A routine physical doesn't include a homocysteine check, but you can take a test for $50 to $100. An ideal level is 6 to 10 micromoles per deciliter of blood for premenopausal women and 8 to 12 micromoles for men and postmenopausal women. The lower the better, even in the normal range

WHAT YOU CAN DO: Controlling homocysteine levels requires adequate intake of vitamins B_6, B_{12} and folic acid. Ordinary multivitamins contain all three. You may want to increase vitamin B_6 intake beyond the 2-milligram recommended daily allowance to 4 mg and folic-acid intake beyond the 200-microgram RDA to 400. If you're over 65, you may need more than the standard 5 to 15 micrograms of B_{12}. Of these three nutrients, folic acid is the hardest to get from a typical American diet. Good sources include cooked beans (130 to 180 mcg per half cup), spinach (131 mcg per half cup) and orange juice (109 mcg per half cup).

Heart attackers can be obvious or obscure. Improving your diet and ditching those nasty habits are the best defenses.

CHOLESTEROL
Oxidized LDL is a major component of arterial plaques.

YOUR RISK: Adults should have their cholesterol checked at least every five years. Tests cost $10 to $20. Total cholesterol should be less than 200 milligrams per deciliter of blood. Ideally, LDL (bad) cholesterol should be less than 130 mg/dL, and HDL (good) cholesterol should be at least 35. A good ratio is 3.5 to 1.

WHAT YOU CAN DO: Stay physically active, control weight and cut back on saturated fat. When total cholesterol levels exceed 240, most experts recommend drug treatment.

BLOOD PRESSURE
Hypertension raises your risk of heart attack and stroke.

YOUR RISK: Optimal blood pressure is 120/80 millimeters of mercury. Normal systolic is less than 130, and normal diastolic is less than 85.

WHAT YOU CAN DO: Lose weight, stop smoking, reduce alcohol and salt intake, and increase potassium intake. Hold your sodium intake to 2,400 milligrams (one teaspoon of salt) each day, and get at least 3,500 mg of potassium. One banana contains 500 mg of potassium, one potato with skin contains 850 mg, and a half cup of spinach contains 400. Avoid convenience foods such as frozen pizza, TV dinners and canned or dried soups.

THE WRONG FATS
Fats aren't all bad. The unsaturated oils found in fish, nuts and vegetables may help protect your heart.

YOUR RISK: If you're addicted to deep-fried foods or packaged snacks, you need to change your habits.

WHAT YOU CAN DO: Bacon cheeseburgers are easy to avoid, but bad fat comes in less conspicuous packages. To avoid transfatty acids, which elevate bad cholesterol while suppressing the good, you have to read nutrition labels. Avoid products containing partially hydrogenated oils. Hard margarine and solid Crisco are full of them. So are packaged cakes, pies, cookies, crackers and candy bars.

TOO LITTLE FIBER
Odd as it seems, foods you can't digest are important. Fiber helps you control LDL cholesterol and excrete fat more rapidly.

YOUR RISK: If you're eating processed foods instead of fresh fruits, vegetables and whole grains, you may not get enough fiber.

WHAT YOU CAN DO: Eat foods containing at least 25 to 30 grams of fiber every day. A half cup of bran cereal supplies 12.8 grams, a cup of oatmeal 4.1 grams and a pear 4.6 grams. Eat fewer carbohydrates that have been stripped of their fiber, such as white rice, white bread and plain pasta.

INFECTIONS
Cytomegalovirus, *Chlamydia pneumoniae* and *Pophyromonas gingivalis* (a common cause of gum disease) may promote arterial disease.

YOUR RISK: Everyone encounters these bugs.

WHAT YOU CAN DO: To keep P. gingivalis in check, floss regularly. You may or may not prevent a heart attack, but you'll save some teeth.

LOW BIRTH WEIGHT
Babies born small may be more likely to develop heart disease later.

YOUR RISK: During pregnancy, women should gain 28 to 40 pounds if they're underweight, 25 to 35 pounds if they're normal weight and 15 to 25 pounds if they're overweight. Babies should weigh at least 5.5 pounds at birth.

WHAT YOU CAN DO: Don't smoke or diet during pregnancy. Until the baby is born, a typical woman needs to eat an extra 300 calories each day.

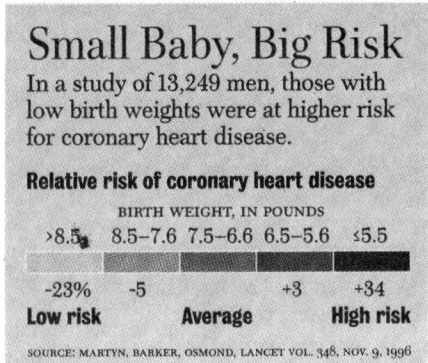

Small Baby, Big Risk
In a study of 13,249 men, those with low birth weights were at higher risk for coronary heart disease.

SOURCE: MARTYN, BARKER, OSMOND, LANCET VOL. 348, NOV. 9, 1996

Barker's own studies show that adult obesity is a stronger predictor.

Low birth weight is fairly rare in this country, but the viruses and bacteria now being linked to arterial disease are not rare at all. Like homocysteine, the infectious suspects have long been eclipsed by cholesterol, but some are starting to look like major offenders. For 17 years, Dr. Joseph Melnick of Houston's Baylor College of Medicine has made a hobby of removing lesions from diseased coronary arteries and testing them for cytomegalovirus (CMV), a common herpes virus. It shows up with surprising frequency—and it's looking less harmless all the time. Scientists have long known that CMV can spell trouble for people receiving heart transplants; infected patients are roughly twice as likely as others to lose their new organs, or their lives, to arterial disease within five years. Transplant patients aren't unique. In a 1996 study, Dr. Stephen Epstein of the National Heart, Lung, and Blood Institute found that CMV infection quintupled the odds that someone having his arteries reamed out by angioplasty would see them close back up within six months. The bug's role is still under investigation, but Epstein says the evidence linking it to cardiovascular disease is as strong today as the evidence for cholesterol was 15 years ago.

The same goes for *Chlamydia pneumoniae*, an airborne bacterium known mainly as a cause of respiratory illness. In recent years, researchers have amassed a boatload of evidence linking C. pneumoniae to arterial disease (NEWSWEEK, April 28). And British researchers have recently shown that treating infected people with antibiotics may reduce their risk of heart attack. In a study involving 213 male heart-attack survivors, Dr. Sandeep Gupta of St. George's Hospital in London found that patients with evidence of C. pneumoniae infection were up to four times more likely than others to suffer further heart problems over an 18-month period. But the disparity vanished when those patients were given a three-day course of the antibiotic azithromycin. "We're not yet in a position to say this could prevent first heart attacks," he says. "We can only say this is interesting."

THERE'S NOT MUCH YOU CAN DO to keep CMV or C. pneumoniae out of your arteries. But a third possible troublemaker—*Porphyromonas gingivalis*—may be easier to control. P. gingivalis is a bug that inflames our gums, and preliminary evidence suggests that it may also gum up our arteries. As part of the VA Normative Aging Study, Dr. Raul Garcia of the Boston VA Outpatient Clinic followed 1,100 men over a 25-year period. They were all basically healthy at the outset, but they had varying levels of gum disease. And over the course of the study, the men with bad gums suffered nearly twice the heart-attack rate of their fresh-mouthed counterparts—and nearly three times the stroke rate. The bottom line, as Garcia puts it half jokingly: "Floss or die." In truth, no one knows whether P. gingivalis can kill you, but the bacterium has been found in diseased carotid arteries. Researchers now hope to see whether treating gum disease can help prevent heart attacks.

Together, these inquiries are painting an ever-richer picture of America's leading killer. None of the new findings imply that cholesterol doesn't matter, but they suggest it's not our only enemy—or even our worst one. As the homocysteine revolution unfolds, it may turn out that we can accomplish more with with nickel-and-dime vitamin supplements than with drugs that cost hundreds of times more. And if the bacterial connections hold up, antibiotics and dental floss may become major weapons in cardiology. But whatever happens, the way we eat and live will count as much as ever.

With KAREN SPRINGEN, MARY HAGER *and* ANNE UNDERWOOD

Heart disease in women: Special symptoms, special risks

Coronary heart disease in women, often overlooked or undertreated, is finally getting its due.

The prevalence of risk factors for coronary heart disease and the death rate from the disease itself have both been dropping steadily in the U.S. for several decades. But those declines have been much less impressive in women than in men. One major reason: Physicians have traditionally regarded coronary disease as mainly a man's disease. So they've diagnosed and treated it less aggressively in women, and they haven't pushed women as hard as men to reduce their risk of the disease by changing their health habits.

Equally important, researchers have traditionally studied coronary disease mainly in men. That has obscured significant differences between the sexes concerning both the symptoms and the causes of the disease—and may have further hindered efforts to prevent or diagnose the disease in women.

The box on the next page focuses on symptoms; here, we tell how the traditional risk factors—and risk-reducing factors—differ in women.

The differences in risk

The female hormone estrogen, abundant in premenopausal women, may protect the heart in at least four ways: It helps lower the "bad" LDL cholesterol, elevate the "good" HDL cholesterol, increase blood flow to the heart, and distribute body fat favorably. That protection helps explain why heart attack rarely strikes women before age 50, the average age of menopause, while it often strikes men in their forties. After menopause, when estrogen levels fall, the protective benefits generally start to fade, and coronary risk starts to rise; by age 60 or so, coronary disease becomes the leading cause of death in women.

Estrogen's benefits may contribute to at least some of the following differences between women's and men's coronary risk factors:

■ **Low HDL cholesterol.** Average levels of the "good" HDL are significantly higher in women than in men. (For unknown reasons, that gap shrinks only slightly after menopause.) So a low HDL level—less than 35 mg/dl—increases a woman's risk more than a man's, possibly because it represents a greater deviation from the norm in women. Further, a North Carolina study suggests that women may be able to raise their HDL level more than men can. The study found that aerobic exercise increased HDL by 20 percent in female coronary patients but by only 5 percent in male patients. (Other steps that can boost HDL include weight loss, smoking cessation, moderate alcohol consumption, and medications that not only lower LDL but also raise HDL, provided the patient needs both benefits.)

■ **High blood pressure.** Women tend to develop hypertension later in life than men do, so the elevated pressure typically has less time to damage a woman's heart. That difference has led some doctors to treat hypertension less aggressively in all women. But when a woman does develop hypertension, it's just as harmful as in a man of the same age.

In addition, women are more likely than men to develop isolated systolic hypertension, or elevation of just the upper blood-pressure number. While doctors used to consider that condition relatively harmless, research has shown that reducing elevated systolic pressure reduces substantially the risk of both coronary disease and stroke. (To lower blood pressure: Lose weight, exercise regularly, don't drink alcohol excessively, reduce stress, restrict sodium intake, and, if necessary, take medication.)

■ **Diabetes.** Diabetes is more likely to damage the arteries, raise blood pressure, and worsen cholesterol levels in women than in men. Further, it can blunt the protective effects of estrogen. Indeed, diabetes multiplies the chance of developing coronary disease substantially more in women than in men.

So it's particularly important for female diabetics to reduce their alterable risk factors for coronary disease, including the ones listed in this story as well as obesity, inactivity, and high levels of the "bad" LDL cholesterol. In addition, postmenopausal women with diabetes should strongly consider hormone replacement therapy and regular aspirin use to further protect the heart.

Women who have had gestational diabetes—high blood sugar during pregnancy—are at high risk for eventually developing type II diabetes, the most common kind; that, in turn, increases their coronary risk. So they need to take protective steps against both diseases, particularly losing excess weight, exercising regularly, and not smoking.

■ **Body-fat distribution.** Fat tends to accumulate around the hips in women, the belly in men. The male pattern poses greater coronary risk; that's mainly because belly fat breaks down more readily than hip fat, causing metabolic changes that push up the "bad" LDL cholesterol, lower the "good" HDL cholesterol, and increase blood pressure.

> Estrogen may protect the heart in at least four ways.

But when women do develop that typically male pattern, it may be even more worrisome than when men do, since it often reflects a disorder dubbed "syndrome X." The disorder involves insulin resistance, probably the underlying cause of diabetes; that resistance leads to increased insulin levels, which may contribute to hypertension. Women with syndrome X also tend to have increased male-hormone levels, which reduce the protective benefits of estrogen.

The waist should be considerably smaller than the hips in women; in men, the waist and hips should be about the same size. Fortunately, the instability that helps make belly fat more dangerous also makes it easier to eliminate than hip fat. (Take the same steps you would to lose weight anywhere in your body: Do regular aerobic and strengthening exercise, and follow a low-fat, moderately low-calorie diet.)

■ **Smoking.** Some women incorrectly believe that smoking is less dangerous to a woman's heart than to a man's heart. Smoking not only damages the lining of the arteries but also lowers levels of the protective HDL and can speed the onset of menopause. Smoking may be particularly bad for the heart in women who take birth-control pills.

How the risk reducers differ

Exercising regularly and eating a low-fat diet can provide broad coronary protection by reducing several risk factors at once. Here are three other broadly protective steps that women may want to consider.

■ **Hormone replacement therapy.** Taking female hormones sharply reduces the risk of coronary disease by restoring the protection that women had before menopause. It also eases menopausal symptoms, slashes the risk of osteoporosis, and may decrease the chance of colon cancer, tooth loss, and possibly osteoarthritis and Alzheimer's disease. For most women, those benefits clearly outweigh the treatment's main drawbacks—renewed menstrual bleeding with some regimens, and possibly a slight increase in the risk of breast cancer and blood clots in the legs and lungs. Potential exceptions include women who have a personal or family history of breast cancer; a low risk of coronary disease and osteoporosis; or large uterine fibroids, active liver disease, or a history of blood clots.

■ **Aspirin.** Regular use of low-dose aspirin clearly lowers the risk of heart attack in men by lowering the risk of blood clots. The available evidence suggests that aspirin may have the same effect in women. However, aspirin can also cause gastrointestinal bleeding and may increase the chance of hemorrhagic stroke, the kind caused by bleeding.

So an aspirin regimen is worth considering only by people who are at increased risk of having a heart attack. That includes anyone with coronary disease; postmenopausal women under age 60 or so who have at least two risk factors for the disease; and postmenopausal women over age 60, as well as men, who have at least one risk factor. (Risk factors include the

Diagnosis in women: Why the delay?

Heart attacks are twice as deadly in women as in men. That's partly because the attacks typically strike women when they're older and in poorer health than men. But it's also because doctors often diagnose and treat the underlying coronary disease in women at a later, more advanced stage.

One reason for the later diagnosis is that women's coronary complaints may be harder to interpret than the usually unmistakable symptoms in men. For coronary disease, the hallmark in men is angina, or central-chest pain that comes on with exertion and subsides with rest; for heart attack, it's crushing chest pain, often spreading to the shoulders, neck, jaw, arms, or upper back.

The same symptoms often signal coronary disease or heart attack in women. But female coronary patients tend to be less physically active than male patients, partly due to age and poorer general health. And the disease is often diagnosed at a later, more advanced stage in women. For both reasons, women are more likely than men to develop chest pain when they're resting.

Further, women with coronary disease are more likely to report vague symptoms that can be caused by many other ailments or even medications. Those symptoms include breathlessness, heartburn, nausea, and severe fatigue for coronary disease; and mild chest pain accompanied by breathlessness, dizziness, heartburn, or nausea for heart attack. Researchers theorize that advanced age, diabetes (which is far more prevalent in female than male coronary patients), and unknown causes may all help produce vaguer coronary symptoms in women.

But vaguer symptoms may not be the only reason for the delayed diagnosis: Some evidence suggests that doctors may take coronary disease less seriously in women. For example, a recent study found that when women come to the emergency room with essentially the same coronary symptoms as men do, they're less likely to receive heart medications, and more likely to be handed drugs for an "anxiety attack." Other studies have shown that even when women have *worse* coronary symptoms than men or are actually having a heart attack, they're less likely to undergo angiography, the definitive diagnostic test.

So if you're a woman, you need to know all the symptoms listed above—the classic complaints as well as the vague ones. And you need to take those symptoms seriously, and make sure that your doctor does the same.

items listed in the preceding section, plus high LDL-cholesterol levels, physical inactivity, and a family history of coronary disease before age 60.)

But those guidelines consider only the general risks of aspirin. Many specific conditions and medications can make aspirin excessively dangerous (see *Consumer Reports on Health* March 1997 issue). So it's essential to consult your doctor before starting to take aspirin regularly.

■ **Alcohol.** Moderate drinking may reduce the risk of coronary disease by up to 40 percent, mainly because it boosts HDL cholesterol and fights blood clots. But even moderate drinking has significant risks, such as an increased chance of alcoholism, auto accidents, falls, and breast cancer. In men, the benefits start to outweigh the risks by age 40 or so. In women, that shift doesn't start until after menopause. However, the same precaution about taking aspirin applies even more strongly to drinking alcohol: Talk with your doctor first.

Note that the definition of moderate drinking differs between the sexes, too: no more than two drinks per day for men, one per day for women. That's because women tend to have smaller amounts of a certain stomach enzyme as well as a smaller liver, both of which help break down the alcohol.

Summing up

The following measures are even more important for women than for men—or apply to women only:

■ Try to boost low HDL, stop smoking, and lose abdominal fat.

■ Be particularly diligent about reducing your overall coronary risk if you have diabetes.

■ Make sure your doctor is aware of—and takes seriously—any coronary risk factors you may have, including isolated systolic hypertension.

■ If you're postmenopausal, talk to your doctor about estrogen therapy and possibly moderate drinking. If you're postmenopausal *and* at increased coronary risk, talk about aspirin therapy as well.

BEYOND Cholesterol

Think About It: Nearly half the people who have chest pain or heart attacks have normal cholesterol levels. **New Tests Can Help Show Who's Really at Risk.** **BY JUDITH MANDELBAUM-SCHMID**

LAST SUMMER Olivia O'Hara,* a healthy 36-year-old management consultant in California's Silicon Valley, had a doctor's appointment she was reluctant to keep. As she sped along the freeway to meet heart specialist Robert Superko, O'Hara wondered if she was rushing off to borrow trouble.

Sure, heart disease ran in her family. Her mother, an aunt, and two uncles all had high blood pressure by the time they reached their forties. One uncle went on to have a heart attack, and her mom, after suffering pangs of angina at 70, underwent a procedure to open clogged arteries.

But O'Hara herself was young and slim, didn't smoke, and rarely got sick. Even juggling the many demands of her job hadn't raised her blood pressure; in fact, she and her husband had recently decided they both at last had a firm enough grip on their careers to consider having a baby. With so much sliding into place, wouldn't it be a mistake to let scolding doctors and their obscure tests thwart her plans? As she turned into the driveway of the Berkeley Heart-Lab, tucked into a commercial corner of San Mateo, O'Hara had nearly talked herself into hightailing it home.

This wasn't the first time a blood test had threatened her world. In 1993, at the repeated urging of her older sister, an obstetrician, O'Hara had gone in for a routine cholesterol check. The results, even O'Hara had to admit, were ominous: Despite her apparent good health, her total cholesterol—a colossal 300—was already higher than her mother's, and levels of worrisome blood fats called triglycerides were stratospheric. Her doctor immediately prescribed a cholesterol-lowering drug, which tugged the values down, though maybe not enough.

Now, amidst all the talk of starting a family, her older sister was sounding alarm bells again. The practice of giving cholesterol-lowering drugs to young women is less than two decades old, and while these medications are an excellent hedge against heart disease, no one is certain they're safe for a developing fetus. Still, if O'Hara were to stop taking the drug and then conceive a child, pregnancy could drive up those blood fats to levels that would

*This name has been changed.

34. Beyond Cholesterol

endanger both her life and the baby's.

It was time to call in experts, everyone agreed, and the name that rose to the top of every list was Robert Superko. His two-year-old clinic, with its affiliated lab, is the brainchild of scientists at the Lawrence Berkeley National Laboratory in Northern California. Widely considered one of the nation's most innovative groups in heart disease research, the LBNL team has spent the last 15 years peering beyond cholesterol, trying to tease apart the more crucial distinctions that determine why one person drops dead of heart disease and another does not. The first fruits of their labor, new diagnostic blood tests, are just coming to market. O'Hara hoped a more precise diagnosis might help her escape the family curse—preferably without drugs.

She arrived early for her appointment. Having imagined Superko as a dry professorial sort, she was relieved when the guy who bustled into the room carrying a thick blue folder was instead athletic and fortyish, with reddish hair curling to his collar. He wore blue jeans and a tie decorated with a fly-fishing scene.

The doctor wasted no time. "You've inherited several genetic traits that make your body exceptionally efficient at transporting fats into your blood," he said. "That's why you're very vulnerable to getting clogged arteries."

"This really *is* serious, isn't it?" O'Hara asked. Superko rushed to reassure her. "There's a lot you can do to keep yourself from getting sick." He'd arranged for her to have blood drawn a few weeks before. Now he handed her results of a long list of tests, including many she'd never heard of: lipoprotein(a), homocysteine, and an analysis of the size of her low-density lipoprotein particles.

Unless you've been boning up on the latest medical literature, those terms probably sound as foreign to you as they did to O'Hara. But it's time to become acquainted, researchers say.

"Total cholesterol has pretty much outlived its usefulness as a way to predict heart disease and follow its progression," says William Castelli, director of the Framingham Cardiovascular Institute. "We've identified more than a dozen kinds of cholesterol or other substances in blood that tell us much more about an individual's risk. These newer tests are just starting to be available, but they'll do a much better job."

CHOLESTEROL TESTING, although a breakthrough in its time, has always been a much blunter tool than doctors would like, because it doesn't identify everyone headed for a heart attack.

Granted, if your total cholesterol is high—above 240—it's likely that bulges of fat and scarred tissue have already begun to thicken the walls of your coronary arteries. With her family history and a cholesterol count of 300, O'Hara seemed ripe for heart disease, no matter how you keep score.

Yet some people at high risk respond better to treatment than others do, and until recently doctors had no idea why. What's more, even a total under 200 is no guarantee of safety. Many studies have found that at least 40 percent of people who experience chest pain or a heart attack have total cholesterol readings that wouldn't raise an eyebrow.

This is why leading cardiologists have been urging doctors to dig a little deeper into the equation by ordering up blood tests that sort HDL (high-density lipoprotein, or good cholesterol) from LDL (low-density lipoprotein, or bad cholesterol). Having very low HDL, it turns out, can presage heart trouble even when total cholesterol is normal. Still, this measure won't turn up everyone at risk. About 75 percent of people diagnosed with heart disease have acceptable levels of HDL.

To understand why cholesterol testing isn't enough anymore, you may have to revamp your ideas about ailing arteries. Most of us mistakenly envision heart disease as essentially a plumbing problem: Eat too much fat and cholesterol, and the goop oozes into your blood vessels, filling them up like so many clogged drains. Fortunately, scientists now have a clearer picture of what happens.

The first stage is often an injury to the inner lining of one of the heart's arteries. The cause of this initial wound probably differs from person to person. One new member of the large cast of likely instigators is homocysteine, a modified amino acid that spills into the bloodstream after a meal rich in animal protein.

Whatever the trigger, the damage builds as the tissue tries to heal itself. Overzealous immune cells mobilize to build a crude patch called a plaque—a fibrous mishmash of overgrown smooth muscle cells, bloated immune cells, and puddled fat that accumulate beneath the vessel's lining, within the artery wall. Bulky plaques threaten life when they either burst through the lining, spurring the formation of a blood clot, or narrow the vessel so much that blood can barely squeeze through. Both scenarios set the stage for a heart attack or stroke.

Of course, those wayward immune cells wouldn't run amok without some encouragement. First, you have to eat the sorts of foods that flood the bloodstream with cholesterol and troublesome fats called triglycerides.

Next, your LDL particles, which serve as dump trucks for those fats, must deliver the nefarious load. Not just the number of particles but also their size and density influence their effectiveness in getting fat beneath the vessel lining. And genes play a big part in determining size.

If you were born with a tendency to have big LDL particles, you are less likely to get heart disease than someone whose LDL bits are generally tiny and dense. And a particular type of LDL, known as lipoprotein(a), or Lp(a), seems to do its dirty work primarily by keeping blood

> If you're feeling safe because the doctor said your bad cholesterol levels are low, take a deep breath. **Several other substances in your blood could be damaging your arteries.**

7 ◆ CURRENT KILLERS

WHAT'S YOUR RISK?

SHORT OF PEERING INSIDE YOUR ARTERIES, a check of your blood for these troublemakers may offer doctors the best measure of how far you've wandered down the path toward a heart attack. The first two tests are widely available. James I. Cleeman, head of the National Cholesterol Education Program in Bethesda, Maryland, calls the other three promising, but says that if and when they pass final muster, it will be several years before they're routine. If a family legacy of heart disease makes you loath to wait, you can get the tests now by having your doctor mail samples of your blood to the Berkeley HeartLab (800/432-7889) for analysis. Tests to consider:

Cholesterol, Good and Bad
DANGEROUS LEVELS OF LDL: above 160
BORDERLINE: 130–160
TARGET FOR PEOPLE AT HIGH RISK: under 95

ADVICE: What boosts your risk, experts now say, is not your total cholesterol but a high ratio of bad to good. Women in general want the good stuff, HDL, to stay above 55; at that level, most excess cholesterol gets trucked out of the body instead of winding up within artery walls. Eating a diet low in saturated fat and getting plenty of exercise should tip your ratio in the right direction; if those moves aren't enough, your doctor may prescribe one of several drugs.

Triglycerides
DANGEROUS LEVELS: above 400
BORDERLINE: 200–400
TARGET FOR PEOPLE AT HIGH RISK: under 70

ADVICE: Doctors used to consider levels of 400 just "borderline high." Now they think less than half that amount can harm arteries when combined with LDL pattern B (see last item) or low HDL. Inactivity, excess weight, and a diet high in refined carbohydrates (alcohol, sweets, pasta, white bread) can send triglycerides soaring. To tug levels down without drugs, watch what you eat, exercise, and shed some flab, especially if it's around your waist.

Homocysteine
DANGEROUS LEVELS: above 14
BORDERLINE: 10–14
TARGET FOR PEOPLE AT HIGH RISK: under 10

ADVICE: The amount of this modified amino acid in your blood rises after you eat a protein-rich meal; consistently high concentrations seem to spell trouble for arteries, although scientists aren't certain why or how. They *do* know that B vitamins, especially folic acid, can bring levels down. Orange juice, broccoli, and beans are good sources, but the folic acid in food isn't easily absorbed, so you may not be getting enough. Many experts now recommend a 400-microgram supplement. And if your homocysteine is abnormally high, your doctor may suggest an even higher dose.

Lipoprotein(a)
DANGEROUS LEVELS: above 25
BORDERLINE: 15–25
TARGET FOR PEOPLE AT HIGH RISK: under 15

ADVICE: This particular form of LDL seems to do its primary dirty work by both preventing clots from dissolving and spurring the overgrowth of smooth muscle cells inside artery walls. The only current treatments: estrogen or prescription doses of niacin.

LDL Pattern
DANGEROUS: pattern B (small dense LDL bits)
BORDERLINE: a mix of sizes
TARGET FOR PEOPLE AT HIGH RISK: pattern A (mostly large LDL particles)

ADVICE: Bad cholesterol comes in shades of evil; the more compact the LDL, the more efficient it is at dumping its fat inside your arteries. Genes influence the size of the particles, but so can exercise and diet. If the test shows you're a pattern B, regular workouts and meals low in refined carbohydrates and saturated fat may be enough to transform you into a pattern A. Prescription doses of niacin or a drug called gemfibrozil can also help. —*J.M.-S.*

clots from dissolving and by stimulating the overgrowth of smooth muscle cells.

Each new piece of evidence, Superko says, tells us we should forget the image of clogged drains. Heart disease, it now appears, is more like a soufflé that requires certain ingredients but can be cooked up with more than one recipe. To get an accurate picture of your risk—as a first step in reducing it—you need to know which "ingredients" you have, and that's where the new generation of tests comes in.

Researchers at Lawrence Berkeley National Laboratory developed several of the diagnostic measures that Superko's clinic offers. For years LBNL used its tests mostly in research, also providing them to a small number of private doctors who put in requests. Then, two years ago, to meet increasing demand, the LBNL scientists decided to go into business.

Their firm, the Berkeley HeartLab, has access to all tests developed at LBNL and in exchange pours back a portion of earnings into research there. "If we find a test that has enough scientific evidence to make it worth using," Superko says, "we can turn around and offer it to the public in 24 hours."

The lab's standard set of tests can be ordered by any doctor (blood samples are shipped overnight) and costs $300. Typically health insurance covers only half that sum, but that could change soon.

"Once commercial labs gear up to offer these tests on a large scale, we hope costs will come down," says Ronald Krauss, chief of molecular medicine at LBNL. "Just a few years ago HDL testing was a really big deal. Now it's routine."

Superko spent more than an hour with O'Hara, going through her test results page by page. He explained that through her mother (who was also tested) she had inherited a powerful risk factor for heart disease: LDL pattern B. "This trait causes you to have small dense particles of LDL that have a special talent for messing up arteries," he said, "and to have more fat in your blood than most people do right after eating, which also helps coronary disease get started."

Recent research indicates that LDL pattern B is one of the heaviest-hitting—if least recognized—triggers of coronary disease. It's beginning to look as though people with pattern B are three times more likely than others to develop clogged arteries, even if they have high HDL cholesterol and low LDL. Other research has suggested that among people with diagnosed heart disease more than 40 percent of men and perhaps 20 percent of women are pattern B types.

The syndrome is also quite common among people who haven't a clue they are vulnerable. In random samplings of healthy people 33 percent of men and up to 20 percent of postmenopausal women (plus 5 to 10 percent of premenopausal women) were LDL pattern B.

GENES ALONE DON'T control the condition. Overeat, spend long hours sitting at a desk or on the couch, and acquire too much flab around your middle, and you could wind up with LDL that is small, dense, and damaging. Luckily, the reverse is also true. If born with the genetic propensity for pattern B, you may be able to enlarge your LDL particles by losing excess girth and becoming more active.

"The good news is, once discovered, pattern B is usually reversible," Superko told O'Hara. "But you'll have to make some serious changes in the way you live. What's your diet like?"

"It's not exactly perfect," O'Hara admitted. "I have a serious sweet tooth—can't resist candy bars."

Superko shook his head. "I'm afraid you'll have to cut that out entirely." No pastries, no pasta, no white bread, no white rice. Such high-sugar, low-fiber foods tend to drive up blood fats in people with pattern B.

This probably sounds different from most dietary prescriptions for heart health you've heard, and indeed it isn't for everyone. For example, people whose main problem is elevated Lp(a)—the form of LDL that keeps clots from breaking up—needn't be so vigilant about carbohydrates. For better and worse, diet does not seem to affect Lp(a) levels.

And while it's safe to say that we could all benefit from winnowing our fat intake to roughly 30 percent of the calories we eat, recent research hints that steeper cuts are, for some people, counterproductive. In a study of 105 men, Krauss found that about 40 percent of those whose LDL size started out pattern A veered into the dreaded pattern B when they further restricted their fat intake to 24 percent. Their levels of protective HDL also took a nosedive. Why that happens and which pattern A's are vulnerable remains to be ascertained, Krauss says.

As a clear pattern B, O'Hara was told to focus on whole grains, vegetables, lean poultry, fish, and fruit. "You shouldn't eat too much fat, but you don't have to go crazy," Superko added. "Getting about 20 percent of your calories from fat is fine, as long as you avoid saturated fat."

Though her weight was all right, regular exercise was crucial, the doctor said. Getting the heart pumping and muscles moving seems to jolt metabolism in a way that pulls blood fats into line. "Exercising every single day for an hour is the single most important thing you can do."

If she hadn't been hoping to become pregnant, Superko would have advised O'Hara to take large doses of niacin (megadoses of the vitamin, available only by prescription, may not be safe for a fetus). Niacin not only tilts the ratio of good and bad cholesterol in the right direction, Superko has found, it also increases the size of LDL particles in people with pattern B. In O'Hara's case, Superko said, pronounced changes in diet and exercise might be enough. "Let's hope you have that baby you want soon. Then we'll see where we are," he said.

Pattern B was O'Hara's main problem but not the only one. "Your homocysteine level is higher than I'd like to see," Superko told her. He prescribed prenatal vitamins, which contain sizable doses of three B vitamins, B-6, B-12, and folic acid. The body needs these to clear homocysteine from the bloodstream; skimp on fruits and vegetables, and you are unlikely to get enough of these B's. Eating heaps of protein is another way to overload your system. Combine the two situations and things can really get nasty.

By the time O'Hara left the clinic her head was a jumble of predictions and percentages. Yet, as she sorted through all that Superko had said, she felt relieved. For the first time in years she had come away from a doctor's visit with a prescription for hope.

She'd had to face the disquieting truth that she might already have some damage. But, as Superko explained, research strongly hints that changes in diet, stepped-up exercise, and the right drug therapy can stop coronary disease in its tracks. Sometimes the condition can even be partially reversed.

> Superko told O'Hara she'd inherited a little-known risk factor for heart disease: **"It causes you to have small dense LDL particles that have a talent for messing up arteries."**

Superko has a lot riding on that bet. Like O'Hara, he has a sobering family history. His father, a career naval officer, started having chest pain at 58 and died from a heart attack at 64. Yet even his dad's untimely death didn't cause Robert Superko profound worry over his own health; he ran fairly regularly, and his cholesterol levels were normal. But a few years later, when his lab needed a blood sample to test its equipment, Superko volunteered. The result was a wake-up call: LDL pattern B.

"I decided then and there that I had to exercise more," he recalls. "I found that by running or doing karate an hour a day, as well as watching my diet, I could bring my LDL around to pattern A."

Now 49 years old and healthy, Superko is optimistic. "We have every reason to believe that at least 80 percent of people who get heart disease have at least one inherited defect that makes them vulnerable," he says. "But we also think that if you identify those vulnerabilities early enough, you can beat the odds."

Judith Mandelbaum-Schmid is a freelance science and medical writer.

Strategies for Minimizing Cancer Risk

Simple, realistic preventive measures could save hundreds of thousands of lives every year in developed countries alone

Walter C. Willett, Graham A. Colditz and Nancy E. Mueller

During 1996, more than 550,000 people will die of cancer in the U.S. In Europe, there will be at least 840,000 cancer fatalities. Yet accumulating evidence indicates that in these two parts of the world, which have relatively high and closely tracked cancer mortality rates, more than half these deaths could theoretically have been prevented.

The notion that we can modify cancer risk emerges from decades of investigation. One laboratory experiment after another has demonstrated that a variety of chemicals and other environmental agents can cause cancer in animals, and studies of people have linked heavy exposure to certain substances in the workplace with high risks of specific types of cancer. Also, international studies of migrants repeatedly confirm that they tend to adopt the cancer pattern of their new country within a period that varies from about a decade (for cancer of the colon and rectum) to a few generations (for breast cancer)—a sign that something in the environment, such as changes in diet or exercise patterns, is implicated. If outside factors can increase cancer risk, avoiding those factors should decrease it.

How did we determine the extent to which mortality can be reduced? We began by identifying the lowest rates for various types of cancer among large international populations that keep reliable figures on death from cancer. The incidence of many of the most common cancers in the U.S. and Europe is much lower in Japan and China. To compile a list of estimated "baseline" cancer incidences, then, we chose the lowest rate for each type of cancer from among the data for the U.S., Japan and China. Then we calculated the difference between the highest rate and the baseline. From these comparisons, we conclude that it should be possible to reduce cancer mortality by approximately 60 percent in the U.S.—perhaps slightly less for black American women, because their incidence rate is already a bit lower. The figures for most Europeans would be similar.

Although we are confident that the death rates of most types of cancer could be substantially cut, there are two notable exceptions. For breast cancer in women and prostate cancer in men, there are no established preventive measures that are likely to have a major impact.

These figures are of interest to more than policy experts and actuaries. For millions of individuals, the results mean that changes in lifestyle can lengthen life—for several years, on average, but several decades for those who would have been stricken in midlife. For most of these people, minimizing the risk of cancer would require a good many changes to address a broad spectrum of causes. For the few people who have inherited mutant genes that dramatically increase the risk of particular types of cancer or for those who have been exposed to unusual occupational hazards, the strategies would be focused mainly on avoiding that specific cancer.

An Ounce of Prevention

A cancer death can be avoided through prevention of cancer, through detection of the disease early enough to treat it successfully, or through a combination of the two (trying to prevent the disease but being vigilant enough to catch it and treat it early if it develops). Examples of prevention strategies include never smoking and, if it is too late for that, giving up the practice. Kicking the habit enables a former smoker to enjoy a nonsmoker's lower risk for lung cancer after about a decade. Another prevention tactic is eating certain vegetables and other foods that counteract the activity of cancer-causing agents (carcinogens) in the body. In theory, vaccination against the various infectious agents that are known to cause cancer could help as well, although at the moment the only vaccine that can serve this purpose prevents hepatitis B infections.

Early detection relies on the diagnosis of disease at a more treatable stage, before the onset of symptoms that would bring the patient to medical attention. This approach has been applied to some cancers, such as cervical and colorectal cancer. Epidemiologic studies indicate that death rates from these

35. Minimizing Cancer Risk

two diseases could be reduced by at least 50 percent if screening were widely applied, making it possible to remove precancerous growth and to detect malignancies earlier. The test for cervical cancer is the well-known Pap smear; the most effective procedures for detecting cancer of the colon and rectum are sigmoidosocopy and colonoscopy.

No matter how effective they may be, early detection and treatment are less desirable than primary prevention, for many reasons. Most obviously, prevention avoids the shock and pain of being diagnosed and treated for cancer. In addition, many methods for cancer prevention, such as regular exercise and a sensible diet, have side benefits, such as reducing the risk of cardiovascular and other diseases—which makes them even more cost-effective in comparison with treatment. Moreover, the ability of medical science to treat many forms of cancer is limited by the disease's tendency to spread to other parts of the body, the phenomenon of metastasis. And of course, the failure of prevention still leaves treatment as a last resort.

These advantages notwithstanding, the power of prevention as a defense against cancer has never been fully appreciated by the public at large, if the widespread persistence of unhealthy habits is any indication. This disappointing observation is perhaps understandable. It is, after all, impossible to tell whether a healthy lifestyle warded off cancer in an individual. Conversely, successful treatment invariably becomes a landmark event. Moreover, the results of effective treatment become apparent quickly, whereas the impact of a prevention regime—quitting smoking, say—may take years to emerge.

As in our colleagues' article on causes of cancer, we focus here on fatal kinds of cancer rather than all cases to avoid distortions introduced by the large number of highly localized cancers and those forms of skin cancer that are seldom fatal. For each major cause, we estimate how much mortality could be reduced for people living in the U.S. or a similar developed country.

Potent Mix: Tobacco and Alcohol

Most cancer prevention campaigns rightly focus on controlling the tobacco smoking epidemic. But the goal has proved to be an elusive one. The decline of smoking in most developed countries has been more than offset in recent years by a rapid increase elsewhere in the world. Small-scale programs and traditional health education efforts are no match for the addictive power of nicotine and the marketing clout of the tobacco industry.

In democratic societies, three complementary approaches appear most promising: improved general education, taxation, and cultivation of an antismoking social ethos. The strong inverse association between educational achievement and smoking reinforces the importance of health education for all segments of society. High taxes on tobacco products, as well as social disapproval or regulation of smoking in office buildings, airplanes and public places, have been shown to reduce smoking rates.

Perhaps, too, we could do more to bring people's perceptions of risk in line with reality. It is not uncommon to meet heavy smokers who are genuinely concerned about the health effects of unproved or possibly trivial environmental agents, such as magnetic fields or chlorinated water.

Tobacco smoking cannot be completely eradicated; hardly any vices ever have been. But on the basis of the dramatic decline in smoking among the more educated adults in the U.S. over the past few decades and the increasingly pervasive sentiments against smoking, it would not be unrealistic to hope that tobacco smoking—and, eventually, deaths related to tobacco—can be reduced by about two thirds within a few

REALISTIC GOAL for reducing the chances of being stricken with any kind of cancer during a normal life span is, for white women, about one third (*right*). The corresponding goal for black women is less because their rates are already lower than those of white women. Men should be able to cut their risk at least in half (*next page*). Almost anyone can achieve such a reduction in cancer risk by adopting prudent habits, such as not smoking, exercising regularly, eating plenty of fruits, vegetables and whole grains and by avoiding animal fats, red meat, refined starches and alcohol. That such reductions in risk are realistic is supported by the fact that they have already been largely achieved by Seventh-Day Adventists, many of whom follow these practices. As the incidence of many cancers declines, the proportion of breast and prostate cancer cases will increase, because no established preventive measures are likely to have a major impact in the near future.

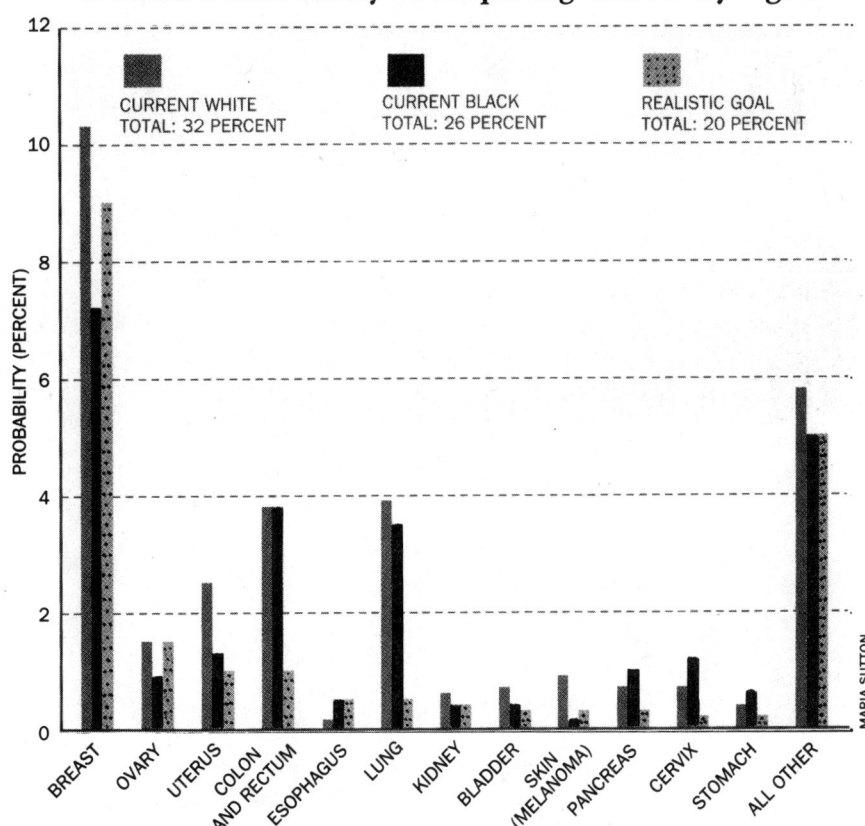

decades. Such a reduction would of course require that the trend not only continue but also spread to less educated groups.

The moderate intake of alcoholic beverages, at about one or two a day, reduces mortality from cardiovascular causes. At the same time, alcohol has been linked with several forms of cancer. Effects of alcohol consumption and tobacco smoking are also believed to interact to cause cancer in the upper respiratory and gastrointestinal tracts.

Clearly, on many grounds, heavy alcohol consumption should be avoided. Anyone considering drinking moderately for the good of the heart should consult a physician and take into account any family history of alcoholism while weighing the risk of cancer against that of cardiovascular disease. Also, for women younger than 50 years, who are at relatively low risk of cardiovascular disease, there does not appear to be any reduction in mortality from moderate alcohol use. Overall, alcohol-related cancer mortality could probably be decreased by about one third if a realistically smaller number of people had more than two drinks a day.

Preventing Diet-Related Cancer

Although we know little about the specific beneficial or harmful constituents of food, we have a good idea of what people should eat if they want to improve their odds of avoiding cancer. Their diet should be high in vegetables, fruits and legumes (such as peas and beans) and low in red meat, saturated fat, salt and sugar. Carbohydrates should be consumed as whole grains—whole-wheat bread and brown rice as opposed to white bread and rice, for example. Added fats should come mainly from plants and should be unhydrogenated; olive oil, especially, appears potentially beneficial.

Everyone should work assiduously to avoid being overweight, ideally in part through physical activity. In addition to helping to control weight, exercise reduces the incidence of colon cancer and, perhaps, of other types as well. Regular physical activity during childhood and adolescence may also slow down excessive growth and avoid an early onset of menstrual cycles, both of which have been implicated in malignancy.

Some evidence links increased risk of breast and prostate cancer with high birth weight and other factors dating to around the time of birth. Although this information is of interest to scientists, it does not readily translate into practical means of prevention. This situation contrasts with that in most other forms of cancer, for which prevention strategies became apparent when causes were established. The implication is that in the near future, in developed countries, the incidence of cancers of the breast and prostate will prove more difficult to reduce—and that, therefore, these cancers could be responsible for an increasing percentage of all cancer mortality as deaths from many other kinds of cancer decline [*see illustrations on this and previous pages*].

Although the benefits of exercise and dietary moderation have been known for decades, the proportion of overweight Americans has been increasing. Between 1980 and 1991 the prevalence of obesity rose by 33 percent in the U.S. Nevertheless, many people, particularly those with higher education and income, have learned how to avoid age-related weight gain, so it is not unrealistic to hope for some improvement among other groups in the foreseeable future.

Similarly, modest shifts toward more healthy habits by the population as a whole should be possible. If a majority of people were to make two or more wise changes—exercising vigorously for 20 minutes a day, eating one more serving of leafy vegetables each day or consuming no more than one serving of red meat a week, for example—both diet-related and sedentary-life-related cancer mortality might be reduced by about one quarter. Taken together, such changes could prevent an estimated 40,000 premature cancer deaths annually in the U.S. The same measures would also lessen the incidence of cardiovascular disease, saving additional lives. Further knowledge of the specific cancer-fighting components of vegetables and fruits, which scientists are now striving to uncover, could allow more focused and effective dietary strategies

A great deal of evidence already suggests that most Americans do not get enough folic acid in their diets. Lack of this nutrient may contribute to colon cancer and heart disease, so multivitamins that include folic acid, also called folate, might prove beneficial. Regard-

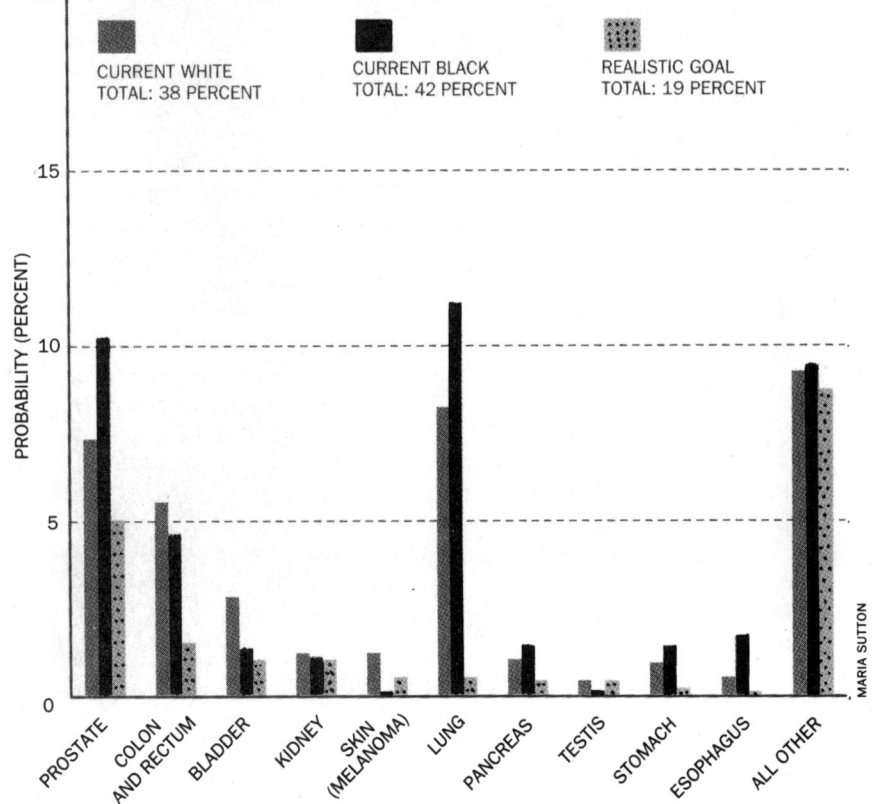

ing so-called megavitamins, little reliable research indicates that these highly concentrated supplements are any more protective against cancer than plain old multivitamins (and even for these, a benefit has not been established).

Avoiding Viruses

The human papillomavirus is the most common cancer-causing infection in the U.S. The sexually transmitted strains, which can lead to cervical cancer, are the most lethal. They can be combated, however, by the same measures directed against transmission of the AIDS-causing human immunodeficiency virus (HIV)—such as delaying initial sexual activity, reducing casual sexual contact and using latex condoms. More widespread application of these precautions could lead to a further modest decline in deaths from cervical cancer and from other genital tumors traceable to papillomavirus. Pap screening, which enables doctors to detect incipient tumors early enough to cure them, has contributed over the past few decades to the dramatic decline in deaths from cervical cancer. Greater use of this technique could enhance this decrease.

In the U.S., the hepatitis B and C viruses cause a minority of the cases of hepatocellular carcinoma, a form of liver cancer. The recently introduced vaccines against the hepatitis B virus, improved screening of blood and blood products and more pervasive use of disposable syringes and needles by intravenous drug abusers are all expected to help reduce the spread of the viruses. Although common, the Epstein-Barr virus causes relatively few American cancer deaths. No immunization for this large, complex virus is available yet.

Mortality from stomach cancer in the U.S. has been declining for the past half century. A partial explanation may be that improved sanitation has delayed infection by *Helicobacter pylori*, a bacterium causing chronic stomach inflammation that can become cancerous. Later infection by this prevalent microbe gives the disease less time to develop. Also, people now tend to consume less salt and more fruits and vegetables that contain vitamin C than was common years ago; these dietary improvements also seem to interfere with the infection's ability to induce cancer. Use of antibiotics to treat the infection may lead to further reductions.

Barring a breakdown of the measures and policies currently in force, mortality from cancers of infectious origin is likely to decline over the next few decades in the U.S., and most other advanced countries, probably by about one fifth. In less developed countries, however, infections are likely to continue causing substantial cancer deaths.

Reproductive Factors

Considerable evidence links certain reproductive behavior with cancer, particularly for cancer of the breast or ovaries in women. Unfortunately, as with many other findings about the causes of breast cancer, the insights have not led to effective prevention strategies. Part of the problem is that reproductive behavior is driven mainly by social and economic forces, so that modifying it to prevent cancer is for the most part unrealistic.

Birth-control pills cause a small increase in breast cancer rates while they are being used, but this excess risk declines rapidly after their use is discontinued. Use before 35 years of age, when the incidence of breast cancer is low, has minimal impact on breast cancer mortality. On the other hand, use of oral contraceptives for five or more years substantially reduces the lifetime risk of ovarian and endometrial cancer. Thus, the overall impact on cancer mortality—

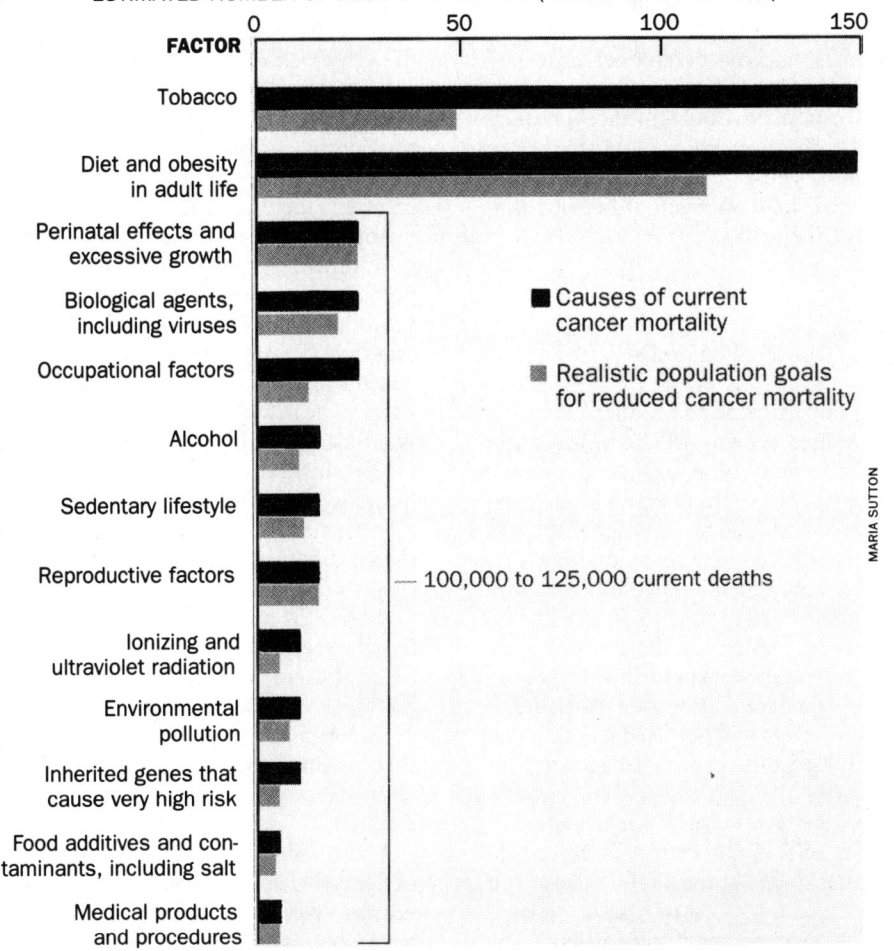

Realistic Goals for Reducing Cancer Mortality

TOBACCO AND DIET, including the latter's effects on obesity, account for about 300,000 cancer fatalities every year in the U.S.—or about 60 percent of the country's annual cancer mortality. Researchers hope these numbers, particularly those for tobacco-caused cancer deaths, can be significantly reduced. Other factors, however, such as those dating to around the time of birth (perinatal factors) or those related to reproduction, are expected to be much more resistant to improvement.

if pill use is limited to earlier reproductive life—is beneficial. Some evidence suggests that tubal ligation may also reduce ovarian cancer risk but that vasectomy may increase risk of prostate cancer in men.

Hormonal contraceptives that simulate early pregnancy in women in their teens or early twenties—or an early menopause in women in their thirties or forties—could potentially reduce the risks for breast cancer. A modest amount of research and development is being done on such contraceptives. Although the first early-menopause preparations may be available within a decade, another 10 years or more may be needed for investigators to assess their effects on breast cancer risk.

Environment and Pollution

Over the past 20 years, no field of cancer epidemiology has seen as many new hypotheses as that concerned with environmental pollution. The candidate carcinogens are diverse enough to include extremely low frequency magnetic fields from electric power lines, radio-frequency electromagnetic radiation used in cellular telephones, proximity to nuclear plants or chemical-waste dumps, water fluoridation and even unseen, unspecified sources responsible for "clusters" of cancer cases within small geographic regions. Few of these hypotheses have been corroborated. But they all serve an important function: preserving the necessary vigilance in the face of the exploding pace of technological change.

With respect to radiation from nuclear or x-ray sources and workplace carcinogens, all any one citizen can do is demand that the authorities enforce regulations. Technological progress resulting in a shift away from traditional industrial employment, fewer workers in relatively high cancer risk jobs, and the phasing out of asbestos use in buildings justify an expectation that deaths from job-related cancers can be cut by about one half over the next several decades.

In addition, greater awareness of the risks of being in the sun between 11 A.M. and 3 P.M. and more widespread use of sunscreens could reduce deaths from melanoma, the most lethal form of skin cancer, by one half. The reduction will be less, however, if the depletion of the earth's ozone layer continues, allowing more of the sun's ultraviolet rays through. Part of the ultraviolet spectrum is responsible for most skin cancers.

Air pollution has declined over the past 30 years in the U.S. Although the measures that brought about the reduction were mostly aimed at short-term goals, such as providing relief for those suffering from asthma, some drop in pollution-related cancer mortality may occur. Yet any such benefit will be as difficult to document as the existence of the original link itself. A decline of one quarter in pollution-related cancer, corresponding to less than 1 percent of all cancer deaths, may be possible.

Mammography, menopausal estrogens and tamoxifen for preventing breast cancer have also come under scrutiny as possible cancer-causing agents. It is now generally recognized that mammography conveys a negligible risk and a substantial benefit. Menopausal estrogens can cause cancer of the endometrium and the breast, although preparations that include progestin are safer in relation to endometrial cancer.

Tamoxifen, a valuable drug for treating breast cancer, is now being evaluated to determine whether it can prevent breast cancer among healthy women who are at high risk for the disease. The catch is that considerable evidence indicates that tamoxifen can cause endometrial cancer. No doubt, medical products and procedures will continue to cause a small proportion of all cancers, but in general, their substantial benefits outweigh their risks.

What to Do

In sum, anyone can reduce his or her chances of being afflicted with cancer by following some sensible guidelines: eat plenty of vegetables and fruits; exercise regularly and avoid weight gain; and avoid tobacco smoke, animal fats and red meats, excessive alcohol consumption, the midday sun, risky sexual practices and known carcinogens in the environment or workplace. Of course, not everyone will follow this advice, and many others will not heed it consistently. Taking this reality into account, we estimate [*see illustration on previous page*] that a reasonable medium-term objective of prevention programs in the U.S. or any other economically advantaged population is a reduction of cancer mortality by about one third, even without new discoveries or technological developments. This reduction is far less than the almost two thirds that is theoretically possible, but it is still considerable. With further research and new information about the causes of cancer, more reductions are likely.

For a small group of people, prevention strategies will be much more customized. Individuals born with mutant genes for various cancers, which greatly increase the probability that they will be afflicted, are commonly offered genetic counseling that focuses on preventing the kind of cancer they are facing. Assuming that such mutations are uncommon, that some high-risk births might be avoided and that prophylactic measures are taken in affected persons, it might be possible to reduce mortality from inherited cancer by about one half. Still, this is a very speculative estimate in a field that is rapidly changing and in which any impact would not be measurable for many years.

Because most of the actions to prevent cancer must be taken by individuals, the distribution of accurate information, together with peer support for the elimination of bad habits and for other behavioral changes, is critical. But effective cancer prevention requires activities at other levels, too, including counseling and screening by health care providers. At this level, dissemination of scientifically sound information to the providers themselves is crucial.

Another level involves regulation by government agencies to minimize the public's exposure to harmful agents, promote healthier products and ensure that industry provides safe working environments. In some cases, officials will have to deal with the displacement of workers whose livelihood depends on the production of toxic products. For example, the costs of subsidizing tobacco farmers to grow something other than tobacco may help avoid higher costs in the future if fewer people need to be treated for lung cancer. An additional level involves the implementation of policies to improve public health. Examples include providing community facilities for safe physical activity, such as bikeways for commuting and after-school gymnasium programs for children.

At the international level, the actions of developed countries affect cancer prevention worldwide. Unfortunately, tobacco exports are often promoted, and hazardous manufacturing processes are moved to unregulated Third World countries. Both trends will contribute to rising rates of cancers worldwide.

Most types of cancer are to a large extent preventable, even with today's knowledge and technologies. The "war on cancer," primarily fought by searching for improved cancer treatments, has met with limited success and should be better balanced by more extensive efforts in prevention.

The Authors

WALTER C. WILLETT, GRAHAM A. COLDITZ and NANCY E. MUELLER are colleagues at Harvard University. Willett is chairman of the department of nutrition and professor of epidemiology in the School of Public Health, professor in the Medical School and associate physician at Brigham and Women's Hospital in Boston. Colditz is associate professor in the Medical School and associate director for education at the Harvard Center for Cancer Prevention. Mueller is professor of epidemiology in the School of Public Health and a member of the board of scientific advisers for the National Cancer Institute.

Further Reading

THE TREATMENT OF DISEASES AND THE WAR AGAINST CANCER. John Cairns in *Scientific American,* Vol. 253, No. 5, pages 51–59; November 1985.

SMOKING AND HEALTH: A 25-YEAR EXPERIENCE. Kenneth Warner in *American Journal of Public Health,* Vol. 79, No. 2, pages 141–143; February 1989.

TOWARD THE PRIMARY PREVENTION OF CANCER. Brian E. Henderson, Ronald K. Ross and Malcolm C. Pike in *Science,* Vol. 254, pages 1131–1138; November 22, 1991.

THE CAUSES AND PREVENTION OF CANCER. Bruce N. Ames, Lois Swirsky Gold and Walter C. Willett in *Proceedings of the National Academy of Sciences,* Vol. 92, No. 12, pages 5258–5265; June 6, 1995.

AVOIDABLE CAUSES OF CANCER. Special issue of *Environmental Health Perspectives,* Vol. 103, Supplement 8; November 1995.

AIDS, After the 'Cure' / Amid setbacks, search for new hope

Laurie Garrett
STAFF WRITER

Combinations of drugs that revolutionized treatment of people infected with the AIDS virus over the past two years are now proving too toxic for many to take, too difficult for others to take and too weak to eliminate the virus altogether.

It's been two years since the hopeful pronouncements about protease inhibitors were made at the 11th International Conference on AIDS in Vancouver. Within days after that meeting more than 100,000 Americans are estimated to have gone on a combination of three drugs in a treatment program referred to by caregivers as HAART, highly active anti-retroviral therapy. Since then, as about a million more followed onto the therapy, HIV death rates plummeted in the United States, Canada and Western Europe.

But now, as scientists, doctors and patients prepare for this year's 12th International Conference on AIDS, which begins June 26 in Geneva, they say the latest results on the HAART therapy are no longer rosey. The drug miracle of 1996 is rapidly unraveling, many insist, and there are few viable alternatives on the near horizon.

Huge numbers of patients who began HAART therapy at about the same time are now beginning to face new problems simultaneously, doctors say, including drug resistance prompted partially by the difficulty of following the therapy's complicated drug regimen, toxicity and an inability to properly metabolize fat. And that, the experts say, suggests a grim future in which many of the successful numbers of the past suddenly spike downward.

"We've been discussing this since right after the Vancouver conference, and we looked at two scenarios: eradication versus a collective crash," said Dr. Peter Piot, director of the United States AIDS program. "The question is how soon it [a crash] might happen. I am usually optimistic, but I do think it's inevitable."

Dr. David Katzenstein, a Stanford University virologist who uses sophisticated laboratory tests to spot emerging resistant viruses in his patients, says the complexity of the therapy is definitely a problem. "There are now some 250 combinations of anti-HIV cocktails," he explained. "How can we tell which one is best for whom? We're doing that study, if you will, now on a random basis on our own patients."

"The question to the patients who are asymptomatic and have some virus [in their bodies] is this: Is the deterioration of your immune system worse than the 5 to 10 percent risk annually of severe side effects? That's the toss up," he said. "It's still an old-fashioned doctor thing, deciding what's best for you."

But deciding what's best for individual patients is becoming increasingly complicated and downright chancy in some cases, according to experts scheduled to convene later this month at the AIDS conference in Geneva. A new sense of urgency has risen as physicians see increasing numbers of their patients failing the treatments.

The issues include both drug resistance and increasingly bizarre side effects. And everything is complicated by the difficulties of the rigorous three-drug regimen required to gain full benefit from the protease inhibitors.

For Spencer Cox, a 30-year-old AIDS activist in Manhattan, these complications have proven perilous.

Always au courant on the newest HIV drugs, Cox says now, "I probably took AZT/3TC at the worst possible time. Why did I do it? Because it was the recommended therapy at the time."

The viruses in Cox's body mutated, developing resistance to not only AZT and 3TC, longtime AIDS drugs, but the entire class of drugs that target reverse transcriptase, a key HIV protein. When protease inhibitors came along, Cox added one of them, ritonavir, to his daily drug regimen. The ritonavir nearly killed him, Cox

36. AIDS, after the Cure

Global Epidemic

A look at the spread of HIV/AIDS around the world:

Worldwide HIV and AIDS estimates as of December 1996:

New HIV infections in 1996:

Total	3.1 million
Adults	2.7 million
Children	.4 million

People living with HIV/AIDS:

Total	22.6 million
Adult males	12.6 million
Adult females	9.2 million
Children	.8 million

HIV/AIDS-associated deaths in 1996

Total	1.5 million
Adult males	.65 million
Adult females	.47 million
Children	.35 million

Cumulative HIV infections:

Total	29.4 million
Adult males	15.5 million
Adult females	11.3 million
Children	2.6 million

Cumulative AIDS cases:

Total	8.4 million
Adult males	3.9 million
Adult females	2.8 million
Children	1.7 million

Cumulative HIV/AIDS deaths:

Total	6.4 million
Adult males	2.9 million
Adult females	2.1 million
Children	1.4 million

NOTE: Because of rounding, figures may not add up to total

---

and AIDS research. "But what happens when I break through with highly resistant strains?

"I don't know how many people can take these drugs unfailingly for years," he added. "It may be a disaster waiting to happen."

"Drug resistance is now the No. 1 problem we face in dealing with HIV infection," says Dr. John Coffin of Tufts University School of Medicine in Boston. He and others say they've been shocked at the virus's capacity to outmaneuver even the newest drugs, capacities that well exceed forecasts made by the manufacturers just two years ago. Any lapse in taking the drugs, or problems in absorbing them, can further improve the virus's odds of acquiring resistance.

And the new combination therapy isn't easy. It involves complex schedules of several pills taken at various times throughout the day. A recent study sponsored by DuPont Merck—a drug company that makes the protease inhibitor indinavir—found that 54 percent of patients cannot keep up the regimen.

Physicians at Cook County Hospital in Chicago reported last month that their patients often can't recall the names of all their drugs and dangerously confuse two of them—nevirapine and nelfinavir. The first inhibits the virus's reverse transcriptase molecule; the latter is a protease inhibitor. One is taken once a day, the other three times a day. Confusion could, in this case, promote resistance.

Activists say that while health care providers and drug company representatives often throw up their hands in frustration at such reports, the studies serve only to highlight the inadequacy of current care.

"I'm sick of this we had the cure and they just didn't want to take their pills' stuff," says David Barr, director of the Washington, D.C.–based Forum for Collaborative HIV Research, a private organization. "This is just the demonization of the patients. The boys who are in charge are not taking some of this stuff seriously enough. The transfer of their work into the real world is a rocky, rocky road."

says, causing profound toxic side effects including liver damage.

He switched to other protease inhibitors, his viruses developed resistance, and now Cox is back to square one. For him, it might as well be 1985, an era in which no drugs had been developed for HIV.

What's happened to Cox is a crisis faced by thousands of HIV-positive people. They've run through the list of available drugs, but their viruses have developed resistance and there is nothing they can take.

"I've been on these drugs 2½ years, and I've been fine," said Gregg Gonsalves, of the New York-based Treatment Action Group, an organization that has played a fundamental role in speeding up drug development

7 ❖ CURRENT KILLERS

The percent of global HIV infection in each major region compared to the percent of total world population that region represents.

	% of Global HIV (est.)	% of World Population
E. Asia and Pacific (including China)	0.2	28.9
E. Europe and Central Asia	0.1	7.2
N. Africa and Middle East	0.9	8.3
Australasia (Australia, New Zealand, and South Pacific)	0.1	0.5
S. And S. East Asia	23	25.8
North America	3.7	5.3
Latin America	6	7.8
Caribbean	1.3	0.5
Sub-Saharan Africa	63	9

And experts preparing for this month's Geneva conference say all evidence indicates therapy options are likely to get more complex before they get easier, as drug companies release medicines that offer small permutations of the same basic categories of compounds.

Even without such new challenges, doctors are having a tough time. A survey of physicians released last week by a group of leading AIDS doctors and conducted by the Lou Harris poll shows that one out of every four American doctors who treated an HIV patient last year wrote inappropriate prescriptions. And 60 percent of physicians who handle fewer than 10 HIV patients a year incorrectly medicated their cases.

Top viral resistance researcher D. Douglas Richman of the University of California in San Diego concludes, "We need better drugs."

Several drug companies and biotechnology firms are now hard at work on chemicals that target other HIV proteins—such as integrase, cell receptors and fusion-related compounds—but none are expected to be available for at least eight years. In the meantime drug companies are cranking out new versions of the current drugs, the most promising of which appears to be DuPont Merck's Sustiva. Like so many of the available drugs, it targets the virus's reverse transcriptase molecule, but its advantage is it only needs be taken once daily, simplifying the regimen.

All of which means, says Dr. Neal Nathanson, newly appointed director of the National Institutes of Health's Office of AIDS Research, that "we're going to be in for a long siege."

Further complicating matters is the emergence of new side effects of current protease inhibitors related to fat metabolism. Large numbers of patients—anywhere from 10 percent to 65 percent—on protease inhibitors are developing "protease paunches," buffalo humps, diabetes and heart diseases because their bodies no longer process fats properly.

Most HIV doctors didn't see the distended, hard fat bellies, bulging fat deposits on the neck, soaring cholesterol and triglyceride counts and diabetes until early this year. And even as recently as February, the disorders appeared to be rarities—or if not rare, harmless. Physicians widely believed the changes were largely just vanity concerns.

By February, 11 percent of New York Hospital's HIV patients had the enlarged torsos, dubbed "protease paunch." Australian physicians saw changes in cholesterol counts and insulin use in 64 percent of patients. And doctors in Ottawa said the "buffalo hump" fatty neck deposits were found in one in eight patients.

The Food and Drug Administration issued warnings to physicians this spring on diabetes and fat disorders.

At the State University at Stony Brook, Dr. Roy Steigbigel has seen many such patients, one of whom stopped taking her anti-HIV drugs, prompting a strong rebound by the virus.

"The thing is, we've got to be sure that people don't discontinue drugs because of this. The alternative is obviously worse," Steigbigel said.

Jeffrey Reynolds, policy director of the Long Island Association for AIDS Care, says the problem is particularly acute in the suburbs, where neighbors' eyes feel forbidding and distances to doctors can be quite long.

"To try to take these drugs, see doctors all the time, suffer these side effects," says Reynolds. "People are saying, 'Maybe I should never have taken these proteases in the first place. Is this what living is about?'"

Last week one of internist Dr. Doug Ward's Washington, D.C., patients survived a massive heart attack. The 39-year-old HIV patient had, as a result of protease inhibitor treatment, a cholesterol count of 400 and triglycerides above 1,000. (Cholesterol levels half that high in uninfected patients are considered dangerous enough to warrant treatment.)

"I will admit that in terms of triglycerides and cholesterol, I was sort of sticking my head in the sand," Ward now says. "And this heart attack woke me up last week. I'm sort of beginning to think that we may not be able to give protease inhibitors for more than three years. The body changes one year ago were very rare. And now they are very common."

"If people are going to live for a long time because of the therapy," asked Steigbigel, "is that going to lead to a societal increase in cardiovascular disease?"

None of this was in the cards at the last international AIDS conference two years ago in Vancouver. Indeed, few scientists then imagined that patients would take these drugs long enough to contract such serious side effects. Then, the word "eradication" was spoken, and leading AIDS researchers predicted that just two or four years of combination therapy would be necessary to kill off every single HIV in a person's body.

Nobody is saying that anymore.

Many scientists have found viruses hidden deep in tissues in patients "successfully" treated. Physicians now define success using sophisticated tests that measure the presence of HIV genetic material, or RNA, in the patients' blood. Patient treatment is dubbed successful when no viral RNA can be detected.

But there are two problems.

First, most tests can detect only when the amount of virus exceeds 100 viruses per milliliter of blood. Dr. Steven Wolinsky of Northwestern University Medical School in Chicago has shown that more precise blood tests usually can detect some tiny amounts of HIV in those "zero detectable" patients.

The second problem is more profound, involving latent, hidden viruses.

HIV is capable of infecting T-cells of the immune system, inserting itself inside the cells' DNA and, for all intents and purposes, being invisible. It will hide in these cells until something else—flu, malaria and some other infection—triggers the usually quiet T-cell into action. Then the virus commandeers the T-cells' machinery to produce thousands more viruses that flood the bloodstream.

If patients on combination therapy stop taking the drugs, HIV viral loads swiftly jump from zero detectable to 10,000 or more per milliliter of blood. Two years ago most AIDS researchers agreed with Dr. David Ho's assessment that such T-cells would soon die out, having reached their normal life expectancies, and all the latent HIV would disappear.

But Ho, director of the Aaron Diamond AIDS Research Center in Manhattan, then participated in further research showing that some infected T-cells can live in numerous sites in the body, notably the lymph nodes—hiding the virus—for 20 or 30 years.

"Trying to rid the body of a virus whose genome [DNA] is incorporated into the host genome may be impossible," Dr. Harold Varmus, director of the National Institutes of Health and a Nobel Laureate, said in a recent interview.

Dr. Anthony Fauci, who heads the NIH's infectious diseases institute, showed this year that there is a massive hidden viral reservoir in T-cells in the bodies of all HIV-positive individuals, regardless of whether they are on combination therapy.

"Even if you look at people with acute primary treatment—treated early after infection—they still have a reservoir," Fauci said in an interview.

Several researchers—notably Dr. William Paul, the former director of the Office of AIDS Research—are also convinced HIV is still multiplying copies of itself and infecting neighboring immune cells in seemingly well-treated patients.

Dr. James Mullins of the University of Washington has found reproducing viruses in combination therapy patients whose blood viral load is zero, and shown the virus is evolving and gaining resistance capacities while hidden away in reservoirs.

"So we need to examine, are there ways of eliminating or keeping suppressed that body of reservoir cells," Fauci says.

Next month Ho will embark on a bold experiment addressing just that issue. It will be composed of "one [dozen] to two dozen patients," he says, who will be immunized with a complex new HIV vaccine.

"The idea is this reservoir pool has decreased to a small size [on combination therapy], so now we want to enhance their immune response," Ho says, hoping the patients' own antibodies will wipe out hidden viruses.

Barring that, Plan B is to deliberately make some HIV patients ill, giving them a strong immune system stimulant called anti-CD3. This would activate the patients' latent T-cells, causing the virus to reproduce and therefore, in theory, be killed by the combination therapy. Unless these hidden T-cells are activated, the viruses within will never be released into the bloodstream where they can be destroyed by HAART drugs.

Mark Harrington, of the Treatment Action Group, is a prime example of the benefits of HAART therapy. He has no viruses detectable in his blood, a drop from 196,000 per milliliter two years ago. And his body is now making far more immune system cells—in all important classes—than before HAART, resulting in improved immune responses to such things as tetanus.

Harrinton believes that "some hightech immunology" is necessary to tackle the problem. "For the first time ever, clinical immunology is way out ahead of basic [laboratory] immunology," he said.

In recent months, several sacred cows of immunology have fallen. For example, all medical students have been taught that the thymus produces T-cells in infants but is a useless dormant organ for adults. Yet Dr. Joseph McCune of the University of California in San Francisco has shown that young HIV-positive adults with high viral HIV loads have abnormally large thymuses that crank out T-cells which serve as targets for HIV. The older patients are, the less likely they are to have active thymuses. And patients who are doing well on triple therapy have thymuses of normal sizes.

"There's a lot we don't know about the immune system," Ho says. "We don't have fundamental information about T-cell turnover in the human being."

Or as immunologist Fauci puts it, "You need to continue to try to hark back to classical immunology. When you read a paper you say, 'My goodness! that could be relevant to HIV.'"

Unit 8

Unit Selections

37. **Health Unlimited,** Willard Gaylin
38. **Your Hospital Stay: A Guide to Survival,** Consumer Reports on Health
39. **Choose Treatments You Believe In,** Peter Jaret
40. **Alternative Medicine—The Risks of Untested and Unregulated Remedies,** Marcia Angell and Jerome P. Kassirer

Key Points to Consider

❖ Is health care just another commodity? Should it be treated differently from other consumer services?

❖ Is quality health care a right or a privilege? Defend your answer.

❖ How have third-party payments contributed to the rising cost of health care in America?

❖ What can you as an individual do to help reduce health care costs? Give specific actions that can be taken.

❖ What steps can you take to reduce your risk of injury during hospitalization?

❖ How could outcomes assessment help reduce health care costs? Do you think there is likely to be much resistance to such efforts? Why?

❖ Should medical insurers provide reimbursement for nonorthodox treatments? If so, are there any limitations that you would place on reimbursements?

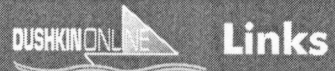 **Links**   www.dushkin.com/online/

28. **Agency for Health Care Policy and Research**
    http://www.ahcpr.gov
29. **American Medical Association (AMA)**
    http://www.ama-assn.org

These sites are annotated on pages 4 and 5.

America's Health and the Health Care System

Americans are healthier today than at any time in this nation's history. Americans suffer more illness today than at any time in this nation's history. Which statement is true? They both are, depending on the statistics you quote. According to longevity statistics, Americans are living longer today and, therefore, must be healthier. Still other statistics indicate that Americans today report twice as many acute illnesses as did our ancestors 60 years ago. They also report that their pain lasts longer. Unfortunately, this combination of living longer and feeling sicker places additional demands on a health care system that, according to experts, is already in a state of crisis.

Despite all the clamor regarding the problems with our health care system, if you can afford health care, the American health care system is one of the best in the world. However, being the best does not mean that it is without its problems. Each year over 1 million Americans are injured or die due to preventable mistakes made by medical care professionals. In addition, countless unnecessary tests are performed that not only add to the expense of health care but may actually place the patient at risk. Reports such as this fuel the fire of public skepticism regarding the quality of care Americans receive. While these aspects of our health care system indicate a system in need of repair, they represent just the tip of the iceberg when it comes to the problems plaguing our health care system. The article "Your Hospital Stay: A Guide to Survival" presents several steps that patients can take to protect themselves from the hazards of hospitalization.

Another indication of America's dissatisfaction with the current health care system is the number of visits made by individuals seeking health care from unorthodox medical practitioners. Unorthodox in this context refers to the use of alternative healing strategies that do not conform to the Western medical model as practiced by licensed physicians. The most popular of these alternative healing therapies include herbalists, accupuncturists, chiropractors, and homeopaths. To fully comprehend the extent to which Americans have accepted the practice of nontraditional healing methodologies, consider the following: (1) Estimates suggest that as many as one in three Americans made use of some form of alternative therapy last year; (2) More visits were made to alternative health care practitioners than to all primary care physicians combined; (3) We spend almost $14 billion for nonorthodox treatments, and most of this money comes directly from the pockets of consumers since reimbursement for this type of health care is rare. This figure amounts to more money than is spent out-of-pocket on all of our hospital bills combined; (4) Perhaps the most remarkable statistic regarding unorthodox medical practices is the expanding rate at which medical insurers are reimbursing consumers for payments made for such services. This change in policy on the part of medical insurers has served to legitimize and strengthen an already thriving business despite the fact that many of the nontraditional therapies are currently unlicensed and unregulated. Many questions still remain, however, concerning the actual benefits that can be derived from many of these therapies. Peter Jaret's article, "Choose Treatments You Believe In," examines the acceptance of alternative healing therapies by physicians as well as by the general public and concludes that, for many of these therapies the benefits experienced are largely the result of the placebo effect. "Alternative Medicine—The Risks of Untested and Unregulated Remedies" takes a critical look at this form of medicine and suggests that what really sets alternative medicine apart from conventional medicine is that it has not had to withstand the rigorous scientific testing that conventional medicine has. The author argues that if alternative medicine were scientifically tested we could do away with the terms *conventional* and *alternative* and instead differentiate medical practices into those that work and those that don't.

Why have health care costs risen so high? The answer to this question is multifaceted and includes such factors as physicians' fees, hospital costs, insurance costs, pharmaceutical costs, and health fraud. It could be argued that while these factors operate within any health care system, the lack of a meaningful form of outcomes assessment has permitted and encouraged waste and inefficiency within our system.

Ironically, another factor driving up the cost of health care is an ever-expanding aging population that is the direct result of improved health care within this country. This is obviously one factor that we hope will continue to rise. Yet another factor that is often overlooked is the constantly expanding boundaries of what is considered within the domain of health care. "Health Unlimited," by Willard Gaylin, addresses how our success in treating various disorders has expanded the domain of health care into areas where health care once had little or no involvement. His discussion is both insightful and pragmatic in asking how far do we go, and on what criteria do we base our rationing of health care?

Traditionally, Americans have felt that the state of their health was largely determined by the quality of the health care available to them. This attitude has fostered an unhealthy dependence upon the health care system and contributed to skyrocketing costs. It should be obvious by now that while there is no simple solution to our health care problems, we would all be a lot better off if we accepted more personal responsibility for our health. While this shift would help ease the financial burden of health care, it may necessitate more responsible coverage of medical news to educate and enlighten the public on personal health issues.

Health Unlimited

Willard Gaylin

WILLARD GAYLIN, M.D., *is professor of psychiatry at Columbia University Medical School and cofounder and president of the Hastings Center, an institution devoted to bioethical research. His most recent book, with Bruce Jennings, is* The Perversion of Autonomy, *published by the Free Press.*

The debate over the current crisis in health care often seems to swirl like a dust storm, generating little but further obfuscation as it drearily goes around and around. And no wonder. Attempts to explain how we got into this mess—and it is a mess—seem invariably to begin in precisely the wrong place. Most experts have been focusing on the failures and deficiencies of modern medicine. The litany is familiar: greedy physicians, unnecessary procedures, expensive technologies, and so on. Each of these certainly adds its pennyweight to the scales. But even were we to make angels out of doctors and philanthropists out of insurance company executives, we would not stem the rise of healthcare costs. That is because this increase, far from being a symptom of modern medicine's failure, is a product of its success.

Good medicine keeps sick people alive. It increases the percentage of people in the population with illnesses. The fact that there are proportionally more people with arteriosclerotic heart disease, diabetes, essential hypertension, and other chronic—and expensive—diseases in the United States than there are in Iraq, Nigeria, or Colombia paradoxically signals the triumph of the American healthcare system.

There is another and perhaps even more important way in which modern medicine keeps costs rising: by altering our very definition of sickness and vastly expanding the boundaries of what is considered the domain of health care. This process is not entirely new. Consider this example. As I am writing now, I am using reading glasses, prescribed on the basis of an ophthalmologist's diagnosis of presbyopia, a loss of acuity in close range vision. Before the invention of the glass lens, there was no such disease as presbyopia. It simply was expected that old people wouldn't be able to read without difficulty, if indeed they could read at all. Declining eyesight, like diminished hearing, potency, and fertility, was regarded as an inevitable part of growing older. But once impairments are no longer perceived as inevitable, they become curable impediments to healthy functioning—illnesses in need of treatment.

To understand how the domain of health care has expanded, one must go back to the late 19th century, when modern medicine was born in the laboratories of Europe—mainly those of France and Germany. Through the genius of researchers such as Wilhelm Wundt, Rudolph Virchow, Robert Koch, and Louis Pasteur, a basic understanding of human physiology was established, the foundations of pathology were laid, and the first true understanding of the nature of disease—the germ theory—was developed. Researchers and physicians now had a much better understanding of what was going on in the human body, but there was still little they could do about it. As late as 1950, a distinguished physiologist could tell an incoming class of medical students that, until then, medical intervention had taken more lives than it had saved.

Even as this truth was being articulated, however, a second revolution in medicine was under way. It was only after breakthroughs in the late 1930s and during World War II that the age of therapeutic medicine began to emerge. With the discovery of the sulfonamides, and then of penicillin and a series of major antibiotics, medicine finally became what the laity in its ignorance had always assumed it to be: a lifesaving enterprise. We in the medical profession became very effective at treating sick people and saving lives—so effective, in fact, that until the advent of AIDS (acquired immune deficiency syndrome), we arrogantly assumed that we had conquered infectious diseases.

The control of infection and the development of new anesthetics permitted extraordinary medical interventions that previously had been inconceivable. As a result, the traditional quantitative methods of evaluating alternative procedures became outmoded. "Survival days," for example, was traditionally the one central measurement by which various treatments for a cancer were weighed. If one treatment averaged 100 survival days and another averaged 50 survival days, then the first treatment was considered, if not twice as good, at least superior. But today, the new antibiotics permit surgical procedures so extravagant and extreme that the old standard no longer makes sense. An oncologist once made this point using an example that remains indelibly imprinted on my mind: 100 days of survival without a face, he observed, may not be superior to 50 days of survival with a face.

Introducing considerations of the nature or quality of survival adds a whole new dimension to the definitions of sickness and health. Increasingly, to be "healthy," one must not only be free of disease but enjoy a good "quality of life." Happiness, self-fulfillment, and enrichment have been added to the criteria for medical treatment. This has set the stage for a profound expansion of the concept of health and a changed perception of the ends of medicine.

I can illustrate how this process works by casting stones at my own glass house, psychiatry, even though it is not the most extreme example. The patients I deal with in my daily practice would not have been considered mentally ill in the 19th century. The concept of mental illness then described a clear and limited set of conditions. The leading causes of mental illness were tertiary syphilis and schizophrenia. Those who were mentally ill were confined to asylums. They were insane; they were different from you and me.

Let me offer a brief (and necessarily crude) history of psychiatry since then. At the turn of the century, psychiatry's first true genius, Sigmund Freud, decided that craziness was not necessarily confined to those who are completely out of touch with reality, that a normal person, like himself or people he knew, could be partly crazy. These "normal" people had in their psyches isolated areas of irrationality, with symptoms that demonstrated the same "crazy" distortions that one saw in the insane. Freud invented a new category of mental diseases that we now call the "neuroses," thereby vastly increasing the population of the mentally ill. The neuroses were characterized by such symptoms as phobias, compulsions, anxiety attacks, and hysterical conversions.

In the 1930s, Wilhelm Reich went further. He decided that one does not even have to exhibit a neurosis to be mentally ill, that one can suffer from "character disorders." An individual could be totally without symptoms of any illness, yet the nature of his character might so limit his productivity or his pleasure in life that we might justifiably (or not) label him "neurotic."

Still later, in the 1940s and '50s, medicine "discovered" the psychosomatic disorders. There are people who have no evidence of mental illness or impairment but have physical conditions with psychic roots, such as peptic ulcers, ulcerative colitis, migraine headache, and allergy. They, too, were now classifiable as mentally ill. By such imaginative expansions, we eventually managed to get some 60 to 70 percent of the population (as one study of the residents of Manhattan's Upper East Side did) into the realm of the mentally ill.

But we still were short about 30 percent. The mental hygiene movement and preventive medicine solved that problem. When one takes a preventive approach, encompassing both the mentally ill and the potentially mentally ill, the universe expands to include the entire population.

Thus, by progressively expanding the definition of mental illness, we took in more and more of the populace. The same sort of growth has happened with health in general, as can be readily demonstrated in surgery, orthopedics, gynecology, and virtually all other fields of medicine. Until recently, for example, infertility was not considered a disease. It was a God-given condition. With the advances in modern medicine—in vitro fertilization, artificial insemination, and surrogate mothering—a whole new array of cures was discovered for "illnesses" that had to be invented. And this, of course, meant new demands for dollars to be spent on health care.

One might question the necessity of some of these expenditures. Many knee operations, for instance, are performed so that the individual can continue to play golf or to ski, and many elbow operations are done for tennis buffs. Are these things for which anyone other than the amateur athlete himself should pay? If a person is free of pain except when playing tennis, should not the only insurable prescription be—much as the old joke has it—to stop playing tennis? How much "quality of life" is an American entitled to have?

New technologies also exert strong pressure to expand the domain of health. Consider the seemingly rather undramatic development of the electronic fetal monitor. It used to be that when a pregnant woman in labor came to a hospital—if she came at all—she was "observed" by a nurse, who at frequent intervals checked the fetal heartbeat with a stethoscope. If it became more rapid, suggesting fetal distress, a Caesarean section was considered. But once the electronic fetal monitor came into common use in the 1970s, continuous monitoring by the device became standard. As a result, there was a huge increase in the number of Caesareans performed in major teaching hospitals across the country, to the point that 30 to 32 percent of the pregnant women in those hospitals were giving birth through surgery. It is ridiculous to suggest that one out of three pregnancies requires surgical intervention. Yet technology, or rather the seductiveness of technology, has caused that to happen.

Linked to the national enthusiasm for high technology is the archetypically American reluctance to acknowledge that there are limits, not just limits to health care but limits to anything. The American character is different. Why this is so was suggested some years ago by historian William Leuchtenberg in a lecture on the meaning of the frontier. To Europeans, he explained, the frontier *meant* limits. You sowed seed up to the border and then you had to stop; you cut timber up to the border and then you had to stop; you journeyed across your country to the border and then you had to stop. In America, the frontier had exactly the opposite connotation: it was where things began. If you ran out of timber, you went to the frontier, where there was more; if you ran out of land, again, you went to the frontier for more. Whatever it was that you ran out of, you would find more if you kept pushing forward. That is our historical experience, and it is a key to the American character. We simply refuse to accept limits. Why should the provision of health care be an exception?

To see that it isn't, all one need do is consider Americans' infatuation with such notions as "death with dignity," which translates into death without dying, and "growing old gracefully," which on close inspection turns out to mean living a long time without aging. The only "death with dignity" that most American men seem willing to accept is to die in one's sleep at the age of 92 after winning three sets of tennis from one's 40-year-old grandson in the afternoon and making passionate love to one's wife twice in the evening. This does indeed sound like a wonderful way to go—but it may not be entirely realistic to think that that is what lies in store for most of us.

During the past 25 years, health-care costs in the United States have risen from six percent of the gross national product to about 14 percent. If spending continues on its current trajectory, it will bankrupt the country. To my knowledge, there is no way to alter that trajectory except by limiting access to health care and by limiting the incessant expansion of the concept of health. There is absolutely no evidence that the costs of health-care services can be brought under control through improved management techniques alone. So-called managed care saves money, for the most part, by offering less—by covert allocation. Expensive, unprofitable operations such as burn centers, neonatal intensive care units, and emergency rooms are curtailed or eliminated (with the comforting, if perhaps unrealistic, thought that municipal and university hospitals will make up the difference).

Rationing, when done, should not be hidden; nor should it be left to the discretion of a relative handful of health-care managers. It requires open discussion and wide participation. When that which we are rationing is life itself, the decisions as to how, what, and when must be made by a consensus of the public at large through its elected and other representatives, in open debate.

What factors ought to be considered in weighing claims on scarce and expensive services? An obvious one is age. This suggestion is often met with violent abuse and accusations of "age-ism," or worse. But age *is* a factor. Surely, most of us would agree that, *all other things being equal,* a 75-year-old man (never mind a 92-year-old man) has less claim on certain scarce resources, such as an organ transplant, than a 32-year-old mother or a 16-year-old boy. But, of course, other things often are not equal. Suppose the 75-year-old man is president of the United States and the 32-year-old mother is a drug addict, or the 16-year-old boy is a high school dropout. We need, in as dispassionate and disinterested a way as possible, to consider what other factors besides age should be taken into account. Should political position count? Character? General health? Marital status? Number of dependents?

Rationing is already being done through market mechanisms, with access to kidney or liver transplants and other scarce and expensive procedures determined by such factors as how much money one has or how close one lives to a major healthcare center. Power and celebrity can also play a role—which explains why politicians and professional athletes suddenly turn up at the top of waiting lists for donated organs. A fairer system is needed.

The painful but necessary decisions involved in explicit rationing are, obviously, not just medical matters—and they must not be left to physicians or health-care managers. Nor should they be left to philosophers designated as "bioethicists," though these may be helpful. The population at large will have to reach a consensus, through the messy—but noble—devices of democratic government. This will require legislation, as well as litigation and case law.

In the late 1980s, the state of Oregon began to face up to the necessity of rationing. The state legislature decided to extend Medicaid coverage to more poor people but to pay for the change by curbing Medicaid costs by explicitly rationing benefits. (Eventually, rationing was to be extended to virtually all Oregonians, but that part of the plan later ran afoul of federal regulations.) After hundreds of public hearings, a priority list of services was drawn up to guide the allocation of funds. As a result, dozens of services became difficult (but not impossible) for the poor to obtain through Medicaid. These range from psychotherapy for sexual dysfunctions and severe conduct disorder to medical therapy for chronic bronchitis and splints for TMJ Disorder, a painful jaw condition. Although the idea of explicit rationing created a furor at first, most Oregonians came to accept it. Most other Americans will have to do the same.

Our nation has a health-care crisis, and rationing is the only solution. There is no honorable way that we Americans can duck this responsibility. Despite our historical reluctance to accept limits, we must finally acknowledge that they exist, in health care, as in life itself.

Your hospital stay: A guide to survival

A hospital stay can be as perilous as the illness that sends you there. Here's how to protect yourself.

Early this year, the perils of hospitalization made headlines when a surgeon at University Community Hospital in Tampa amputated the wrong foot of a patient with diabetes. In the wake of that fiasco, some medical experts seriously suggested that surgery patients ask their doctor to mark the surgery site with a pen or even write "no" on the limbs they hoped to keep.

Since then, such blunders have been much in the news. In March, for example, investigators learned that a Boston Globe health columnist who died at the renowned Dana-Farber Cancer Institute had actually been killed by a chemotherapy overdose, which had been overlooked by at least a dozen doctors, nurses, and pharmacists. In May, surgeons at the equally renowned Memorial Sloan-Kettering Cancer Institute in New York City operated on the wrong half of a cancer patient's brain.

Potentially dangerous hospital errors are indeed alarmingly common. One Harvard study of some 30,000 hospital charts found that nearly 3 percent of patients are injured by some preventable mistake. Another 1 percent are harmed by the inevitable hazards of hospitalization, such as infection and adverse reactions to anesthesia or medications. Nationwide, those rates translate into more than a million injuries each year.

This report describes what you can do to prevent mistakes and minimize the risks.

Make surgery safer

To protect yourself when you're scheduled to go under the knife:

■ **Check out the surgeon.** If you or a friend knows someone who works at the hospital of a surgeon you're considering, ask about his or her reputation. If you can't do that, at least check the hospital's reputation (see box, page 177), since better hospitals tend to have better surgeons. And find out whether the surgeon teaches at the hospital or at a medical school, an indication that he or she probably keeps up with the latest practices.

The American Board of Medical Specialties (800-776-CERT) will tell you whether a physician is board certified; certification means that the surgeon has completed an approved residency program and passed a detailed written exam. In addition, find out whether the surgeon belongs to a professional organization, such as the American College of Surgeons, by calling the county medical society or consulting the medical directories in the library. (Note that none of those sources verifies all the information provided by physicians.) While requirements for joining professional groups vary, membership at least suggests that the surgeon has some interest in keeping up with the latest research. Finally, check the surgeon's experience by asking how many of the operations he or she has performed and what the success and complication rates have been.

■ **Limit preoperative tests.** Surgery patients often undergo a smorgasbord of standard preoperative tests, many of them unnecessary. Those procedures, while generally harmless in themselves, can not only create needless costs but also yield falsely positive results that can trigger other, sometimes hazardous, tests.

Adults younger than age 40 generally need nothing more than a simple blood count and, for sexually active women, a pregnancy test. Healthy people older than 40 may need only a few additional tests, such as an electrocardiogram plus blood tests for diabetes, liver disease, and kidney disease. Ask your doctor which preoperative tests, if any, you truly need. And ask your doctor to check whether you've had any of those tests recently enough to skip them.

■ **Bank your blood.** If you're likely to need a blood transfusion during an upcoming operation, ask your surgeon about banking your own blood supply ahead of time, to eliminate the slight risk of receiving tainted blood.

38. Your Hospital Stay

KNOW YOUR RIGHTS

When you check into a hospital, you should receive a copy of the Patient's Bill of Rights, a nationally recognized code of conduct published by the American Hospital Association. The code expresses firmly established law on patients' rights in all states. Here are six of your most important rights:

- To receive complete, understandable information about your diagnosis, treatment, and expected outcome.
- To review your medical records. Such records can be difficult to decipher, so don't hesitate to ask your physician to explain anything you can't make out.
- To refuse any treatment or test. All procedures require your consent, unless you're unconscious or require emergency care. Major procedures require your informed, written consent—doctors must explain the benefits and risks to your satisfaction before you sign on the dotted line.
- To refuse to let anyone stay in your room who is not directly involved in your care (except, of course, your roommate and anyone seeing your roommate). For example, you don't have to allow medical students to watch while doctors examine you.
- To have the details of your condition, treatment, and medical records kept confidential from anyone in the hospital who is not directly involved in your care.
- To receive reasonable responses to your reasonable requests for the services of doctors, nurses, and other staff members.

Your right to nursing care

As hospitals cut costs by cutting staff, it's becoming increasingly difficult to get those reasonable responses to your requests, particularly from the overworked nursing staff. Indeed, minor delays and other inconveniences are practically inevitable during a hospital stay. Complaining or calling for help too often or too aggressively may only make things worse, by convincing the hospital staff that you're a malcontent.

But that doesn't mean you have to tolerate rudeness, consistently burnt, uncooked, or cold food, or long waits for pain killers or a bedpan. If your nurse ignores your reasonable requests, speak to the head floor nurse or to your doctor. If that doesn't work, ask to see the patient advocate, a specially trained person who will intervene on behalf of patients whose legitimate complaints—about nurses, doctors, or any other hospital employee—are being ignored. Hospitals that don't have a patient advocate often have social workers who can help you get what you need.

- **Get antibiotics on time.** Taking antibiotics at the right time—no more than two hours before major surgery—can slash the risk of developing a wound infection. But surgery patients often receive those drugs too early or too late. Make sure your doctor gives the necessary orders and that your nurse carries them out. (And make sure the nurse checks your wound and changes the dressing regularly after the operation.)

- **Prepare for anesthesia.** In rare cases, general anesthesia can cause devastating complications, including brain damage and death. One cause of such catastrophes is vomiting while you're unconscious. To reduce the risk, refuse any food or drink that the hospital staff may mistakenly offer you in the eight hours before surgery. If anesthesia has nauseated you in the past, ask for antinausea medication before the operation.

Having weak lungs sharply increases the risks from anesthesia. People who smoke, who are older than age 65 or so, or who have recently had a debilitating illness should ask their doctor to check their lungs before surgery and, if necessary, teach them deep-breathing exercises to strengthen their lungs. Smokers should stop smoking for as long as possible before surgery; even stopping for as little as 24 hours can help.

- **Ease the pain.** Postoperative pain can keep you from moving around in bed, breathing deeply, moving your bowels, or even coughing; that can delay recovery and increase the risk of complications. Many physicians and nurses are still reluctant to give morphine, the most potent pain killer, even though the chance of addiction during a hospital stay is minuscule. And they dole out even the weaker pain killers "as needed," which means you get a dose only when you complain.

Ask to receive intravenous morphine after major surgery, at least at first. Better yet, ask whether the hospital offers patient-controlled intravenous analgesia, which lets you administer your own medication by pushing a button on a computerized pump.

- **Fend off complications.** Surgery patients can help reduce their risk of three common postoperative complications:

Pneumonia. The bacteria that cause pneumonia are so abundant in hospitals that an estimated 4 percent of all patients develop the infection. The risk is particularly high following chest, back, or abdominal surgery, since weakness and pain may discourage the deep breathing that ordinarily helps clear the lungs of harmful bacteria. The same breathing exercises that can strengthen the lungs before surgery can reduce the risk of pneumonia after surgery.

Phlebitis. Lying in bed for long periods can lead to inflammation of the leg veins, usually accompanied by potentially dangerous blood clots. To cut the risk, ask the nurse to help you walk as soon as possible after surgery. If you're overweight or have varicose veins, wear special elastic stockings.

Urinary tract infections. These infections often develop because a doctor or nurse failed to remove a catheter soon enough. If 48 hours have passed since your operation and you're still using a catheter, find out whether it's there by design or neglect.

Get the right drugs

Hospital patients receive an average of 10 different drugs. Each patient is typically seen by several different physicians, who may order medications without knowing what other doctors have ordered. And both the pharmacists and the nurses have to decipher the doctors' handwriting and follow their prescriptions accurately.

A study published in July in the Journal of the American Medical Association found that about 7 percent of hospital patients experience some adverse drug reaction. Other studies have found adverse-reaction rates as high as 15 percent, up to half of them caused by errors—giving the wrong drug or the wrong dose, overlooking an allergy, or failing to spot a potentially dangerous interaction with another medication.

The following precautions can help prevent those potential errors:

■ **Check your drugs.** Bring to the hospital a list of all the medications you've been taking at home, including the dosages, so the physician who admits you can order those drugs. Further, ask your doctor whether there will be any additions, deletions, or other changes in your usual drug regimen. The doctor should add that information to your list, including the name, purpose, dosage instructions, and, if possible, the color and shape of any new pills. Use that list to check all the drugs your nurse brings. (If you don't feel well enough, have a friend or relative check for you.) In addition, have your doctor review all your medications at least once every 72 hours.

One other precaution: Ask your doctor to leave standing orders for medications to treat insomnia or constipation. Otherwise, you may face a long, uncomfortable wait for the appropriate order to be written and filled if the need arises.

■ **Check your IV.** Many drugs are started intravenously, then switched to an oral version. If you're getting IV drugs, ask your doctor when you'll start getting pills instead. If you're eating solid foods and drinking fluids but are still receiving drugs intravenously, a doctor or nurse may have forgotten to make the change.

HOW GOOD IS YOUR HOSPITAL?

Long before you need hospital care, you should investigate the hospitals located near you. Then try to choose doctors who have admitting privileges at one or more desirable hospitals in your area.

First, make sure the hospital is accredited by the Joint Commission on Accreditation of Healthcare Organizations (JCAHO), which monitors the nation's hospitals. About 80 percent of all hospitals apply for accreditation. While the JCAHO approves nearly all of them, it has recently started to issue detailed rating reports on all hospitals that have applied. The reports are already available for about one-third of those hospitals, and the rest should be ready by the end of next year. You may be able to get a report by calling a hospital's office of public information. Alternatively, the JCAHO will mail you a copy for $30. (Write to One Renaissance Blvd., Oakbrook Terrace, Ill. 60181, or call 708-916-5600.)

Next, check the quality of the medical staff. The hospital's public relations department or medical-staff office should be willing to answer the following questions over the phone:

■ **Is it a teaching hospital?** Such hospitals, affiliated with a medical school, tend to attract better doctors and to offer the most advanced and widest range of services.

■ **What percentage of the staff physicians are board certified?** Nationally, about 65 percent of all physicians are certified. At a good hospital in a large urban center, that figure may reach 80 percent or more. Smaller, more rural communities typically have fewer certified physicians.

■ **Are there doctors available in most specialties and subspecialties?** The more serious the ailment or the more complex the operation, the greater the need to have a full range of physicians on hand who can treat any unexpected problems.

■ **Do the major clinical departments have full-time chiefs?** Full-time status allows the chiefs to spend more of their time overseeing the department. It also reduces their financial dependence on referrals from other doctors in the department, leaving them freer to discipline the doctors when that becomes necessary.

■ **What percentage of the nurses are RNs?** Registered nurses have substantially more training than the other main type, licensed practical nurses (LPNs). About 70 percent of the nurses in the average hospital are RNs.

■ **How many patients does each RN care for?** Ideally, there should be one RN for every one or two patients in an intensive-care unit and for every six patients or so in most other areas of the hospital.

Does the hospital care?

Hospitals that follow a progressive philosophy that's strongly concerned with satisfying the patient tend to:

■ Use primary nursing, in which nurses are assigned to particular patients rather than to particular tasks (such as giving medications or examining patients).

■ Offer self-administered pain medication (see story).

■ Employ a full-time patient advocate and provide full information on patients' rights (see box, previous page).

■ Employ social workers who counsel patients or who help them obtain various rehabilitative, social, or financial services.

■ Have a hospice program for dying patients and encourage the use of living wills.

■ Have a birthing center, allow a woman to deliver and recuperate in the same room, and employ midwives.

■ Run community-outreach programs, such as support groups for breast-cancer or diabetes patients.

■ Have reasonable, flexible visiting hours.

■ Allow friends and relatives to bring food to patients who aren't on a special diet, or have kitchens where those patients can prepare their own food.

38. Your Hospital Stay

■ **Check your wristband.** Make sure the wristband correctly lists your name and any drug allergies you have. And make sure the nurse checks the band each time he or she brings you any drugs.

Summing up

On average, you face a 4 percent chance of being injured during a hospital stay. Keeping alert and being assertive—or having someone do that for you—can substantially reduce the likelihood of harm.

What to do
- Check the credentials and reputation of the surgeon and the hospital.
- Make sure your personal physician is overseeing your care.
- Keep track of your medications and tests.
- Get ready for the anesthesia.
- Demand adequate pain control.
- Become active as soon as you can after surgery.
- Know your rights and stand up for them.

Testing: Don't just take it

Hospitalized patients may sometimes be given tests that are unnecessary or even meant for someone else. To reduce the risk of that happening to you:

■ **Question the tests.** Medical tests are sometimes risky, painful, or expensive. The following questions can help you determine whether a test ordered for you is really necessary: What are the odds that the test will actually find something wrong? What would happen if you waited, and took it only if the condition got worse? Will the test actually affect treatment? How likely are inconclusive or falsely positive results, and would such results lead to further tests or treatment?

■ **Know what's coming.** Find out what tests your doctor plans for you while you're in the hospital. Refuse to be wheeled off to unexpected or unexplained tests.

In addition, patients often spend extra time in the hospital because staff members failed to withhold food, administer an enema or laxative, or make other preparations for a scheduled test. To avoid needless delays, find out what preparations you'll need, and see that they get done on time.

Even the most skeptical doctors now agree that hope has tremendous healing power. And it's true whether the remedy is homeopathy—or heart surgery.

CHOOSE TREATMENTS YOU BELIEVE IN

By Peter Jaret

BY ALL RIGHTS THEY SHOULD have been banished to the dusty attic of medicine's fanciful past. Herbal remedies, healing crystals, homeopathic potions containing the tiniest bits of belladonna and Saint-John's-wort. Ten years ago, in fact, if medical researchers regarded such quaint relics of a less enlightened age at all, it was usually to scoff.

No longer. In a shift that's taken nearly everyone by surprise, treatments such as herbal medicine and acupuncture, even New Age approaches like guided imagery, are being embraced not just by alternative practitioners but by many medical doctors as well.

The signs of change are unmistakable. In 1992 the National Institutes of Health, a bastion of established science, created an Office of Alternative Medicine to study popular techniques that lie outside the realm of accepted treatment. But by then remarkable numbers of us were experimenting on our own. In a landmark report published in the *New England Journal of Medicine,* Harvard Medical School researchers estimated that one in three Americans had used some form of alternative therapy during the previous year. Astonishingly, we made more visits to herbalists, acupuncturists, chiropractors, homeopaths, and other alternative healers than to all primary care physicians

6 Alternative Therapies

That Came in From the Fringe

WHAT A LONG, STRANGE TRIP IT'S BEEN: Touted during the sixties, then vilified by a medical establishment that couldn't believe anyone could ever fall for mind-body hype, alternative therapies are now edging into the mainstream. How come? Skeptical scientists did some studies—and were surprised by what they found.

Meditation

BREAKOUT In 1967, eight years after Maharishi Mahesh Yogi first promoted transcendental meditation to westerners, the Beatles joined up. "We don't need [drugs] anymore," said Paul McCartney.
BACKLASH TM was attacked as a cult while meditation was marginalized into a hippie excuse to avoid facing real life.
WHAT SCIENCE SAYS NOW Regular sessions of meditation can lower blood pressure and help alleviate insomnia, headaches, and other chronic pain.

Herbal Remedies

BREAKOUT Bumped from medicine cabinets for 40 years by commercial drugs, herbs—ginger tea to fight off colds, chamomile lotion to treat skin problems—made a resurgence during the back-to-nature 1960s.
BACKLASH The Food and Drug Administration to this day warns consumers that homespun remedies are mostly untested and potentially dangerous.
WHAT SCIENCE SAYS NOW Herbal compounds are active ingredients in many FDA-approved drugs. A handful of remedies sold in health food stores have also been shown to have therapeutic value.

Prayer

BREAKOUT In 1966 Pat Robertson debuted "The 700 Club" on national television, praying for audience members. "I have a word of knowledge that someone is having trouble with a tracheotomy," he proclaimed. "God is miraculously healing it!"
BACKLASH In 1968 the Amazing Randi exposed TV healers on "The Tonight Show." He showed a video of a healer bringing a woman out of her wheelchair with his detailed knowledge of her illness—as his wife surreptitiously fed him the information.
WHAT SCIENCE SAYS NOW Praying lowers blood pressure, and worshipers live longer than nonreligious people. In a tantalizing study, heart patients were less likely to die when designated well-wishers prayed for them—though the patients didn't know the experiment was going on.

Megavitamins

BREAKOUT Impressed by the research of unknown scientist Irwin Stone, Nobel Prize-winner Linus Pauling in 1970 penned the best-selling *Vitamin C and the Common Cold*. Pauling advised taking 5,000 milligrams of vitamin C a day, 80 times the daily allowance. Soon two other nonphysicians, Durk Pearson and Sandy Shaw, recommended huge doses of many vitamins as part of their *Life Extension* program.
BACKLASH Many considered Pauling a crackpot. Life magazine condemned "vitamin cultists": "Every age has had its panaceas but none has triggered as much speculation or *has* been insinuated into as many gullets as has vitamin C."
WHAT SCIENCE SAYS NOW Vitamin C can lessen cold symptoms, and experts haven't ruled out claims that as an antioxidant it impedes tumor growth and protects blood vessels. Vitamin E has passed muster: Taking 400 international units a day, 13 times the RDA, lowers heart disease risk.

Acupuncture

BREAKOUT In 1971 *New York Times* reporter James Reston, on a trip with Henry Kissinger to China, had acupuncture following an emergency appendectomy and wrote a glowing article about the 5,000-year-old technique.
BACKLASH The National Council Against Health Fraud lamented that Reston's tale had evolved into a wild rumor of acupuncture's power. Contrary to the public impression, Reston was anesthetized with standard drugs; acupuncture was used only to treat his postoperative cramps.
WHAT SCIENCE SAYS NOW Acupuncture relieves a variety of complaints, perhaps by triggering pain-blocking endorphins. Last year the FDA decreed acupuncture needles safe and effective. More than 3,000 physicians practice the technique nationally.

Chiropractic

BREAKOUT B.J. Palmer spent decades pushing the therapy that his father, a fish peddler, invented when he cured a man's deafness with a blow to his back. The shift came in 1963 when the country's most populous state, New York, licensed chiropractors. By 1973 visits had nearly doubled nationwide.
BACKLASH Also in 1963, the American Medical Association's Committee on Quackery declared war on what it called an "unscientific cult." Tactics in a 25-year effort included lying about studies and deleting chiropractic from career guidance literature.
WHAT SCIENCE SAYS NOW Chiropractors ease back pain better than doctors, especially in the first month.

combined. We plunked down almost $14 billion for untested treatments—mostly from our own wallets, since such therapies aren't usually covered by insurance. That's more than we spent out of pocket on all of our hospital bills combined. And now, in the most startling change of all, one medical insurer after another has decided to pay for acupuncture, chiropractic, or other therapies once considered dubious or downright daffy.

Purveyors of these therapies couldn't be happier, naturally. They say the official recognition their treatments have received is proof of their effectiveness. Skeptical scientists, meanwhile, insist that when these remedies work it's usually only by way of the placebo effect: Even a sugar pill will bring many people relief if they believe it will.

It's a withering charge. Modern medicine, after all, has always staked its claim to authority on its ability to offer more than psychological soothing. To obtain approval, a new drug or therapy must perform better than a sugar pill; otherwise it's quickly abandoned. Any treatment that offers nothing but a placebo, in the view of Western medicine, is no treatment at all.

Or so we've been taught. But now some maverick physicians are turning the debate on its head. The fact is, they say, placebos do work. A pill whose only active ingredient is hope *can* make many people feel better. And when it comes to healing, the new thinking suggests, that's really what matters.

Howard Spiro, a professor of medicine at Yale University, first put forth this bold idea in the 1986 book *Doctors, Patients, and Placebos*. Instead of deriding the placebo effect, he wrote, we should understand and respect it for what it is: proof of the remarkable healing influence of belief. Rather than dismissing the uncanny power of mind over malady, all of us, patients and doctors alike, should try to tap it.

"Some alternatives may in fact offer nothing more than placebos," says Spiro. "All the same, they can be remarkably effective. And as I tell medical students, even the treatments mainstream doctors offer depend in large part for their effectiveness on the power of belief."

EVER SINCE MEDICINE became a science, researchers have grappled with the discomfiting fact that almost any treatment—a saltwater injection, a sugar pill, a reassuring prognosis—will make a sizable percentage of people improve. Give a sugar capsule to patients with moderate depression, tell them it's the latest antidepressant, and two-thirds will find they feel better.

The placebo-controlled study was devised for exactly that reason—to distinguish between high hopes and a "real" effect. Since 1962, when the Food and Drug Administration began to require them for new-drug approval, placebo studies have helped elevate medicine from art to science. They're why we can be sure a drug that's been approved by the FDA really does what it's supposed to—because it proved more effective than a placebo.

But along the way, placebos have also led scientists smack into the mystery that still lies at the heart of healing.

Consider a classic experiment in the 1960s to test a cholesterol-lowering drug. At first, the drug looked effective. Patients who took their pills regularly were half as likely to die of a heart attack over five years as were those who didn't stick to the regimen as carefully. But a look at the placebo group told another story: Those who had taken their *sugar* pills exactly as ordered also were half as likely to be felled by a heart attack as those who hadn't followed the instructions. Researchers had to conclude that the drug was no better than a placebo. Still, believing in a treatment had protected patients from heart attacks.

Similar puzzles abound in the scientific literature. In one early experiment researchers gave two women who were suffering bouts of nausea a promising antinausea drug. Or so they said. The drug was actually ipecac, which is widely used to induce vomiting. No matter: It relieved symptoms in both women within a half hour. In another experiment a placebo pill caused stomach contractions, prevented them, or had no effect at all, depending on what patients were informed the drug would do before they took it.

The more elaborate the dosage regimen, the better placebos seem to work. Two sugar pills, for instance, usually get better results than one. Researchers can enhance the power of the placebo by instructing volunteers to return all of the unused pills at the completion of the study, thus underscoring how valuable the medicine is. Even the color of a phony tablet can make a difference in how well it works.

A pill isn't the only form of placebo that doctors have found can do wonders. Sham injections are even more potent. And surgery appears to produce the strongest placebo effect of all. Back in the 1950s doctors began performing a simple operation believed to ease the chest pain caused by angina. To test it out, researchers carried off an elaborate deception (one that medical ethics boards would nix in a heartbeat these days, needless to say). They put a group of patients under anesthesia, made an incision, then stitched them back up without actually performing the surgery. Over half said that they felt significantly better afterward.

How powerful can placebos be? To find out, Alan Roberts, a psychologist at the Scripps Clinic and Research Foundation in La Jolla, California, looked at five treatments that were once highly regarded. Three were said to fight herpes infections (one with fluorescent lights, a second with organic solvents), and another was an operation to relieve bronchial asthma. The fifth involved freezing the stomach lining to treat ulcers. Enthusiasm ran high when each was introduced. Experiments have since proved that none of them worked better than placebos—the reason all were abandoned.

Still, they worked. Reviewing studies done at the time, Roberts found that only 30 percent of patients were disappointed by the results. An astonishing 70 percent reported a good or excellent outcome.

ARE WE REALLY SO SUGGESTIBLE that a few shakes of a wand, a magic pill, even a bit of hocus-pocus will make us well? Is most of what ails us really just in our heads?

Of course not. A sugar pill can't fix a ruptured appendix. An acupuncture session can't set a broken bone. A shot of salt water can't protect against diphtheria or whooping cough or polio.

But the complaints that typically bring us to the doctor's office tend to be subjective in nature—back pain, headaches, muscle sprains, insomnia, fatigue, stomach upset, anxiety. The symptoms are real enough, but the way we view them—casually or with alarm, as fleeting problems or as certain evidence of something serious—shapes the way we experience them. It's for these kinds of symptoms that placebos are most effective. It's for these complaints, too, that most of us seek alternative therapies, the Harvard study found.

39. Choose Treatments You Believe In

Some alternatives clearly act directly on our bodies. Acupuncture's success in alleviating chronic pain, for instance, has many researchers convinced that some process beyond the placebo effect is at work. And some herbal remedies contain potent active ingredients; a few, such as the antidepressant Saint-John's-wort, have consistently outperformed placebos in blind studies.

But as with conventional medicine, some therapies may help patients mend simply because a little hope is all they need. Herbert Benson, president of the Mind/Body Medical Institute of Harvard Medical School and Boston's Beth Israel Medical Center, estimates that as many as 90 percent of all the visits we make for medical care are for stress-related conditions like back pain and insomnia. "So it's not surprising that just having someone say there's nothing seriously wrong with you, that this or that treatment will help, goes a long way toward making people better," he says.

Over the past decade several studies have shown that life's stresses (the anxiety of exams, the pain of a troubled marriage, the grief of losing a loved one) can undermine the body's immune system, making us vulnerable to illness. Therefore treatment that eases our fears just might bolster our immune defenses. And researchers have discovered that chemical signals used by brain cells are shared by immune cells, suggesting a common language linking a person's state of mind to her state of health. Scientists haven't deciphered the language entirely. But many suspect that optimism triggers healing processes yet to be explored.

There's a telling irony in all of this. Just as medical science uncovers evidence of the power of faith and hope, doctors on the front lines find both in short supply. For many reasons, we no longer regard physicians as all-knowing. A dose of skepticism about our medical care can be healthy, of course. But when it diminishes trust and confidence it may jeopardize our ability to heal.

Even the best doctors often find they can't combine the science of medicine with the art of healing. "Getting to know patients, listening to their stories, counseling and reassuring, instilling a sense of trust takes time," says Spiro. "Unfortunately, more and more doctors claim they just don't have it."

So we turn to alternative practitioners in part because they seem to have more time to care for us. Massage therapy is by its nature hands-on, intimate. Acupuncture involves listening to patients, talking over their lives, and touching them to sense the flow of energy in their bodies. Even herbalists usually base their remedies on the premise that we're more than the sum of our parts—that health is more than findings from a blood test and a hastily written prescription.

Wisely, we haven't abandoned Western-style scientific medicine. The Harvard survey found that many people who use unconventional therapies are also being treated by medical doctors. That's as it should be. When a proven treatment exists, and you and your doctor both believe in it, there's almost no limit to how powerful that treatment can be.

Howard Spiro knows this. Three years ago, at the age of 70, Spiro started to experience chest pains so severe they forced him to give up the brisk walks he loved. His doctor—a former student of his—recommended that he have coronary bypass surgery. Spiro knew that studies show drugs like beta-blockers are as effective as such surgery. But he decided to follow the advice. "I welcomed the surgery," Spiro remembers, "because I thought it gave me the best chance of doing the things I'd been able to do before, and because it was advised by a physician I trusted." Once the decision was made, he says, "I felt enveloped in a chrysalis of certainty."

Today, back to walking as far and as fast as he wants, Spiro admits that he doesn't know how much of his recovery was the result of his surgery and how much stemmed from the confidence he felt. He suspects it was a little of both. "Of course I'm very grateful to have had specialists taking care of me," he says. "But after becoming a patient I'm more convinced than ever of the power of faith, and hope, and the expectation that all will be well."

(Continued)

> Spiro put forth a bold, new idea: Instead of deriding the placebo effect, patients and doctors alike should be trying to tap it.

Peter Jaret has been a contributing editor since 1989 and helped edit this special issue.

Is Negative Thinking Harming Your Health?

YOU AND A FRIEND have both been prescribed a regimen of exercise, stretching, and acupuncture for your aching backs. You feel confident that the treatment will work, and indeed you start feeling better within a couple of weeks. Your friend, on the other hand, is skeptical from the start and doesn't notice any change. You wonder: Is that a self-fulfilling prophesy?

It could be, says Martin Seligman, a prominent psychologist and expert on how the mind influences health. Seligman's research suggests that feeling hopeful about a particular treatment actually makes it more likely to work. (Scientists call this the placebo effect.) Generally optimistic people, of course, will probably adopt a positive attitude toward their prospects of healing.

Take this quiz to see how you rate on Seligman's optimism scale. Read each hypothetical situation, and mark the explanation you'd be most likely to give. When you're done, add up your points to find out whether a pessimistic view of life might be putting your health at risk—and what you can do to change.

YOU FORGET YOUR PARTNER'S BIRTHDAY.
A. I'm not good at remembering birthdays. 1
B. I was preoccupied by other things. 0

YOU OWE THE LIBRARY TEN DOLLARS FOR AN OVERDUE BOOK.
A. When I am really involved in a book, I often forget when it's due. 1
B. I was so involved in writing a report on the book that I forgot to return it. 0

YOU LOSE YOUR TEMPER WITH A FRIEND.
A. She is always nagging me. 1
B. She was in a hostile mood. 0

YOU ARE PENALIZED FOR NOT RETURNING YOUR INCOME TAX FORMS ON TIME.
A. I always put off doing my taxes. 1
B. I was lazy about doing my taxes this year. 0

YOU'VE BEEN FEELING RUN-DOWN LATELY.
A. I never get a chance to relax. 1
B. I was exceptionally busy this week. 0

A FRIEND SAYS SOMETHING THAT HURTS YOUR FEELINGS.
A. She always blurts things out without thinking of others. 1
B. She was in a bad mood and took it out on me. 0

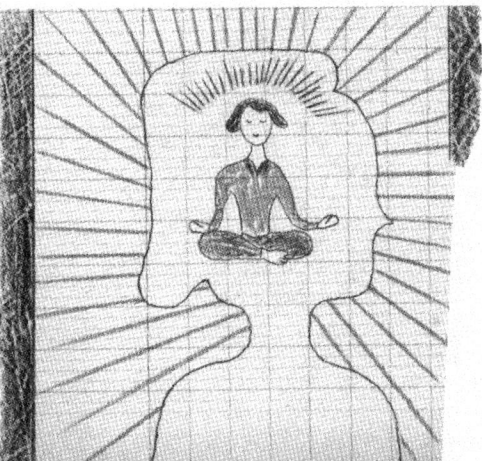

YOU FALL DOWN A GREAT DEAL WHILE SKIING.
A. Skiing is difficult. 1
B. The trails were icy. 0

YOU GAIN WEIGHT OVER THE HOLIDAYS AND CAN'T LOSE IT.
A. Weight-loss plans don't work in the long run. 1
B. The strategy I tried didn't work. 0

.................................Total

If you scored **ZERO OR ONE**, you are very optimistic. Research suggests you may have feistier immune defenses than a pessimist. **TWO TO FOUR** is a fairly optimistic score. Anything **OVER FOUR** is quite pessimistic. To safeguard your health, try nudging your thoughts in a more upbeat direction.

Learning to Be Optimistic

View setbacks as temporary. Seligman notes that if you tend to think that unpleasant events will last a long time, perhaps even a lifetime, you will feel helpless to change them. Rather than explaining misfortunes to yourself with words like *never* and *always*, think of specific causes that would lend themselves to specific solutions.

Don't take everything personally. You may be blaming yourself for events you can't control. If you ask someone to a dinner party and are turned down, for example, it may be just that the other person doesn't like parties.

Recognize that beliefs aren't facts. One mistake many people make, Seligman says, is to assume that whatever they think about themselves—no matter how negative—must be true. But consider the way you react when someone accuses you of something you believe is unfounded. It's easy to disregard, right? Well, why not take the same attitude toward self-recriminations? You can't change a pessimistic outlook until you realize that it's not set in stone.

Play detective with yourself. When you notice that you're anxious or glum, ask yourself, "What is the evidence for this belief? Is there an alternative way to look at this?" "In most cases," Seligman says, "negative thoughts are distortions. Challenge them."

But don't be a Pollyanna. Sometimes pessimists are just more realistic than optimists; low expectations may turn out to be justified. That's why Seligman says he's not encouraging blind optimism but rather what he calls "flexible optimism, or optimism with its eyes open." When something goes wrong, don't despair *or* gloss over it; focus on why it happened and what you can do to make it better.

This quiz is adapted from *Learned Optimism: How to Change Your Mind and Your Life*, by Martin E. P. Seligman. The book has a chapter on changing a pessimistic style to one of flexible optimism.

Alternative Medicine — The Risks of Untested and Unregulated Remedies

WHAT is there about alternative medicine that sets it apart from ordinary medicine? The term refers to a remarkably heterogeneous group of theories and practices — as disparate as homeopathy, therapeutic touch, imagery, and herbal medicine. What unites them? Eisenberg et al. defined alternative medicine (now often called complementary medicine) as "medical interventions not taught widely at U.S. medical schools or generally available at U.S. hospitals."[1] That is not a very satisfactory definition, especially since many alternative remedies have recently found their way into the medical mainstream. Medical schools teach alternative medicine, hospitals and health maintenance organizations offer it,[2] and laws in some states require health plans to cover it.[3] It also constitutes a huge and rapidly growing industry, in which major pharmaceutical companies are now participating.[4]

What most sets alternative medicine apart, in our view, is that it has not been scientifically tested and its advocates largely deny the need for such testing. By testing, we mean the marshaling of rigorous evidence of safety and efficacy, as required by the Food and Drug Administration (FDA) for the approval of drugs and by the best peer-reviewed medical journals for the publication of research reports. Of course, many treatments used in conventional medicine have not been rigorously tested, either, but the scientific community generally acknowledges that this is a failing that needs to be remedied. Many advocates of alternative medicine, in contrast, believe the scientific method is simply not applicable to their remedies. They rely instead on anecdotes and theories.

In 1992, Congress established within the National Institutes of Health an Office of Alternative Medicine to evaluate alternative remedies. So far, the results have been disappointing. For example, of the 30 research grants the office awarded in 1993, 28 have resulted in "final reports" (abstracts) that are listed in the office's public on-line data base.[5] But a Medline search almost six years after the grants were awarded revealed that only 9 of the 28 resulted in published papers. Five were in 2 journals not included among the 3500 journal titles in the Countway Library of Medicine's collection.[6-10] Of the other four studies, none was a controlled clinical trial that would allow any conclusions to be drawn about the efficacy of an alternative treatment.[11-14]

It might be argued that conventional medicine relies on anecdotes, too, some of which are published as case reports in peer-reviewed journals. But these case reports differ from the anecdotes of alternative medicine. They describe a well-documented new finding in a defined setting. If, for example, the *Journal* were to receive a paper describing a patient's recovery from cancer of the pancreas after he had ingested a rhubarb diet, we would require documentation of the disease and its extent, we would ask about other, similar patients who did not recover after eating rhubarb, and we might suggest trying the diet on other patients. If the answers to these and other questions were satisfactory, we might publish a case report — not to announce a remedy, but only to suggest a hypothesis that should be tested in a proper clinical trial. In contrast, anecdotes about alternative remedies (usually published in books and magazines for the public) have no such documentation and are considered sufficient in themselves as support for therapeutic claims.

Alternative medicine also distinguishes itself by an ideology that largely ignores biologic mechanisms, often disparages modern science, and relies on what are purported to be ancient practices and natural remedies (which are seen as somehow being simultaneously more potent and less toxic than conventional medicine). Accordingly, herbs or mixtures of herbs are considered superior to the active compounds isolated in the laboratory. And healing methods such as homeopathy and therapeutic touch are fervently promoted despite not only the lack of good clinical evidence of effectiveness, but the presence of a rationale that violates fundamental scientific laws — surely a circumstance that requires more, rather than less, evidence.

Of all forms of alternative treatment, the most common is herbal medicine.[15] Until the 20th century, most remedies were botanicals, a few of which were found through trial and error to be helpful. For example, purple foxglove was found to be helpful for dropsy, the opium poppy for pain, cough, and diarrhea, and cinchona bark for fever. But therapeutic successes with botanicals came at great human cost. The indications for using a given botanical were ill defined, dosage was arbitrary because the concentrations of the active ingredient were unknown, and all manner of contaminants were often present. More important, many of the remedies simply did not work, and some were harmful or even deadly. The only way to separate the beneficial from the useless or hazardous was through anecdotes relayed mainly by word of mouth.

All that began to change in the 20th century as a result of rapid advances in medical science. The emergence of sophisticated chemical and pharmacologic methods meant that we could identify and purify the active ingredients in botanicals and study them. Digitalis was extracted from the purple foxglove, morphine from the opium poppy, and quinine from cinchona bark. Furthermore, once the chemistry was understood, it was possible to synthesize related molecules with more desirable properties. For example, penicillin was fortuitously discovered when penicillium mold contaminated some bacterial cultures. Isolating and characterizing it permitted the synthesis of a wide variety of related antibiotics with different spectrums of activity.

In addition, powerful epidemiologic tools were developed for testing potential remedies. In particular, the evolution of the randomized, controlled clinical trial enabled researchers to study with precision the safety, efficacy, and dose effects of proposed treatments and the indications for them. No longer do we have to rely on trial and error and anecdotes. We have learned to ask for and expect statistically reliable evidence before accepting conclusions about remedies. Without such evidence, the FDA will not permit a drug to be marketed.

The results of these advances have been spectacular. As examples, we now know that treatment with aspirin, heparin, thrombolytic agents, and beta-adrenergic blockers greatly reduces mortality from myocardial infarction; a combination of nucleoside analogues and a protease inhibitor can stave off the onset of AIDS in people with human immunodeficiency virus infection; antibiotics heal peptic ulcers; and a cocktail of cytotoxic drugs can cure most cases of childhood leukemia. Also in this century, we have developed and tested vaccines against a great many infectious scourges, including measles, poliomyelitis, pertussis, diphtheria, hepatitis B, some forms of meningitis, and pneumococcal pneumonia, and we have a vast arsenal of effective antibiotics for many others. In less than a century, life expectancy in the United States has increased by three decades, in part because of better sanitation and living standards, but in large part because of advances in medicine realized through rigorous testing. Other countries lagged behind, but as scientific medicine became universal, all countries affluent enough to afford it saw the same benefits.

Now, with the increased interest in alternative medicine, we see a reversion to irrational approaches to medical practice, even while scientific medicine is making some of its most dramatic advances. Exploring the reasons for this paradox is outside the scope of this editorial, but it is probably in part a matter of disillusionment with the often hurried and impersonal care delivered by conventional physicians, as well as the harsh treatments that may be necessary for life-threatening diseases.

Fortunately, most untested herbal remedies are probably harmless. In addition, they seem to be used primarily by people who are healthy and believe the remedies will help them stay that way, or by people who have common, relatively minor problems, such as backache or fatigue.[1] Most such people would probably seek out conventional doctors if they had indications of serious disease, such as crushing chest pain, a mass in the breast, or blood in the urine. Still, uncertainty about whether symptoms are serious could result in a harmful delay in getting treatment that has been proved effective. And some people may embrace alternative medicine exclusively, putting themselves in great danger. In this issue of the *Journal*, Coppes et al. describe two such instances.[16]

Also in this issue, we see that there are risks of alternative medicine in addition to that of failing to receive effective treatment. Slifman and her colleagues report a case of digitalis toxicity in a young woman who had ingested a contaminated herbal concoction.[17] Ko reports finding widespread inconsistencies and adulterations in his analysis of Asian patent medicines.[18] LoVecchio et al. report on a patient who suffered central nervous system depression after ingesting a substance sold in health-food stores as a growth hormone stimulator,[19] and Beigel and colleagues describe the puzzling clinical course of a patient in whom lead poisoning developed after he took an Indian herbal remedy for his diabetes.[20] These are without doubt simply examples of what will be a rapidly growing problem.

What about the FDA? Shouldn't it be monitoring the safety and efficacy of these remedies? Not any longer, according to the U.S. Congress. In response to the lobbying efforts of the multibillion-dollar "dietary supplement" industry, Congress in 1994 exempted their products from FDA regulation.[21,22] (Homeopathic remedies have been exempted since 1938.[23]) Since then, these products have flooded the market, subject only to the scruples of their manufacturers. They may contain the substances listed on the label in the amounts claimed, but they need not, and there is no one to prevent their sale if they don't. In analyses of ginseng products, for example, the amount of the active ingredient in each pill varied by as much as a factor of 10 among brands that were labeled as containing the same amount.[24] Some brands contained none at all.[25]

Herbal remedies may also be sold without any knowledge of their mechanism of action. In this issue of the *Journal*, DiPaola and his colleagues report that the herbal mixture called PC-SPES (PC for prostate cancer, and *spes* the Latin for "hope") has substantial estrogenic activity.[26] Yet this substance is promoted as bolstering the immune system in patients with prostate cancer that is refractory to treatment with estrogen.[27] Many men taking PC-SPES have thus received varying amounts of hormonal treatment without knowing it, some in addition to the estrogen treatments given to them by their conventional physicians.

The only legal requirement in the sale of such products is that they not be promoted as preventing or treating disease.[28] To comply with that stipulation, their labeling has risen to an art form of doublespeak (witness the name PC-SPES). Not only are they sold under the euphemistic rubric "dietary supplements," but also the medical uses for which they are sold are merely insinuated. Nevertheless, it is clear what is meant. Shark cartilage (priced in a local drugstore at more than $3 for a day's dose) is promoted on its label "to maintain proper bone and joint function," saw palmetto to "promote prostate health," and horse-chestnut seed extract to "promote . . . leg vein health." Anyone can walk into a health-food store and unwittingly buy PC-SPES with unknown amounts of estrogenic activity, plantain laced with digitalis, or Indian herbs contaminated with heavy metals. Caveat emptor. The FDA can intervene only after the fact, when it is shown that a product is harmful.[28]

It is time for the scientific community to stop giving alternative medicine a free ride. There cannot be two kinds of medicine — conventional and alternative. There is only medicine that has been adequately tested and medicine that has not, medicine that works and medicine that may or may not work. Once a treatment has been tested rigorously, it no longer matters whether it was considered alternative at the outset. If it is found to be reasonably safe and effective, it will be accepted. But assertions, speculation, and testimonials do not substitute for evidence. Alternative treatments should be subjected to scientific testing no less rigorous than that required for conventional treatments.

MARCIA ANGELL, M.D.
JEROME P. KASSIRER, M.D.

REFERENCES

1. Eisenberg DM, Kessler RC, Foster C, Norlock FE, Calkins DR, Delbanco TL. Unconventional medicine in the United States — prevalence, costs, and patterns of use. N Engl J Med 1993;328:246-52.
2. Spiegel D, Stroud P, Fyfe A. Complementary medicine. West J Med 1998;168:241-7.
3. Cooper RA, Stoflet SJ. Trends in the education and practice of alternative medicine clinicians. Health Aff (Millwood) 1996;15(3):226-38.
4. Canedy D. Real medicine or medicine show? Growth of herbal remedy sales raises issues about value. New York Times. July 23, 1998:D1.
5. National Institutes of Health, Office of Alternative Medicine. Grant award and research data. Bethesda, Md.: Office of Alternative Medicine. (See: http://altmed.od.nih.gov/oam/research/grants.)
6. Chou CK, McDougall JA, Ahn C, Vora N. Electrochemical treatment of mouse and rat fibrosarcomas with direct current. Bioelectromagnetics 1997;18(1):14-24.
7. Olson M, Sneed N, LaVia M, Virella G, Bonadonna R, Michel Y. Stress-induced immunosuppression and therapeutic touch. Alternative Ther Health Med 1997;3(2):68-74.
8. Shaffer HJ, LaSalvia TA, Stein JP. Comparing Hatha yoga with dynamic group psychotherapy for enhancing methadone maintenance treatment: a randomized clinical trial. Alternative Ther Health Med 1997;3(4):57-66.
9. Walker SR, Tonigan JS, Miller WR, Corner S, Kahlich L. Intercessory prayer in the treatment of alcohol abuse and dependence: a pilot investigation. Alternative Ther Health Med 1997;3(6):79-86.
10. Richardson MA, Post-White J, Grimm EA, Moye LA, Singletary SE, Justice B. Coping, life attitudes, and immune responses to imagery and group support after breast cancer treatment. Alternative Ther Health Med 1997;3(5):62-70.
11. Reid SA, Duke LM, Allen JB. Resting frontal electroencephalographic asymmetry in depression: inconsistencies suggest the need to identify mediating factors. Psychophysiology 1998;35(4):389-404.
12. Crawford HJ, Knebel T, Kaplan L, et al. Hypnotic analgesia. 1. Somatosensory event-related potential changes to noxious stimuli and 2. Transfer learning to reduce chronic low back pain. Int J Clin Exp Hypn 1998;46:92-132.
13. Shannahoff-Khalsa DS, Beckett LR. Clinical case report: efficacy of yogic techniques in the treatment of obsessive compulsive disorders. Int J Neurosci 1996;85:1-17.
14. Prasad KN, Hernandez C, Edwards-Prasad J, Nelson J, Borus T, Robinson WA. Modification of the effect of tamoxifen, cis-platin, DTIC, and interferon-α2b on human melanoma cells in culture by a mixture of vitamins. Nutr Cancer 1994;22:233-45.
15. Brody JE. Alternative medicine makes inroads, but watch out for curves. New York Times. April 28, 1998:F7.
16. Coppes MJ, Anderson RA, Egeler RM, Wolff JEA. Alternative therapies for the treatment of childhood cancer. N Engl J Med 1998;339:846-7.
17. Slifman NR, Obermeyer WR, Aloi BK, et al. Contamination of botanical dietary supplements by *Digitalis lanata*. N Engl J Med 1998;339:806-11.
18. Ko RJ. Adulterants in Asian patent medicines. N Engl J Med 1998;339:847.
19. LoVecchio F, Curry SC, Bagnasco T. Butyrolactone-induced central nervous system depression after ingestion of RenewTrient, a "dietary supplement." N Engl J Med 1998;339:847-8.
20. Beigel Y, Ostfeld I, Schoenfeld N. A leading question. N Engl J Med 1998;339:827-30.
21. Wittes B. FDA exemption sought for self-help medicines. The Recorder. October 7, 1994:2.
22. Dietary Supplement Health and Education Act of 1994. (Public Law 103-417.)
23. Wagner MW. Is homeopathy 'new science' or 'new age'? Sci Rev Alternative Med 1997;1(1):7-12.
24. Herbal roulette. Consumer Reports. November 1995:698.
25. Cui J, Garle M, Eneroth P, Björkhem I. What do commercial ginseng preparations contain? Lancet 1994;344:134.
26. DiPaola RS, Zhang H, Lambert GH, et al. Clinical and biologic activity of an estrogenic herbal combination (PC-SPES) in prostate cancer. N Engl J Med 1998;339:785-91.
27. Anticancer botanicals that work supportively with chemotherapy: PCSpes. Alternative Medicine Digest. November 1997:84-5.
28. Love LA. The MedWatch Program. Clin Toxicol 1998;36:263-7.

Unit 9

Unit Selections

41. **How Health Savvy Are You?** *Consumer Reports on Health*
42. **Nutrition in the News: What the Headlines Don't Tell You,** *Environmental Nutrition*
43. **The Switch to OTC: No Prescription, No Protection?** *Consumer Reports on Health*
44. **The Doctor Is On,** Katie Hafner
45. **Nature's Pharmacy,** Burkhard Bilger
46. **An FDA Guide to Dietary Supplements,** Paula Kurtzweil

Key Points to Consider

❖ Why should one question the validity of health-related information reported by the media?

❖ Is the government doing enough to protect the consumer? If not, what recommendations would you make for changes?

❖ Is the switch from prescription to OTC drugs good or bad? Why?

❖ Just how safe are dietary supplements? What regulations and restrictions should there be governing their use?

❖ What factors should one be on the lookout for to avoid falling victim to fraudulent products being marketed as dietary supplements?

❖ What are the pros and cons of going online in search of health-related information? What suggestions would you make to someone who was about to make such a search?

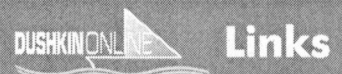 **Links** www.dushkin.com/online/

30. **Alt-MEDMarket**
    http://alt.medmarket.com/indexes/indexmfr.html
31. **HealthyWay/Sympatico**
    http://www1.sympatico.ca/healthyway/
32. **Mental Health Net**
    http://www.cmhc.com/selfhelp.htm

These sites are annotated on pages 4 and 5.

Consumer Health

For many people the term "consumer health" conjures up images of selecting health care services and paying medical bills. While these two aspects of health care are consumer health issues, the term consumer health encompasses all consumer products and services that influence the health and welfare of people. A definition this broad suggests that almost everything we see or do may be construed to be a consumer health issue. In many ways consumer health is an outward expression of our health behavior and decision-making processes and as such is based on both our desires to make healthy choices and to have accurate information on which to base our decisions. In the past most of us have relied on newspapers, magazines, and television for this information, but today, with the widespread use of personal computers and the World Wide Web, it is possible to access vast amounts of health information without ever leaving one's home. Unfortunately, quantity does not necessarily translate into quality. While there is no simple solution to this issue, the following suggestions serve as a general guideline for evaluating health-related information: (1) Does the information appear to be based on logical principles consistent with current thinking on the subject? (2) Is the information based on empirical data rather than testimonials? (3) Is the information coming from a reliable source that has a proven track record in such matters? (4) Can the information be substantiated by other reliable sources? Because health is an area in which new discoveries are constantly taking place what was once considered gospel might at a later date be termed fallacy or myth. "Nutrition in the News: What the Headlines Don't Tell You" examines the impact media coverage of health issues has on our health behavior. This article also provides useful information to consider as part of your decision-making process as you sort through the quagmire of health-related articles vying for your attention.

Suppose that you read the newspaper every day and watch the nightly news religiously. You also subscribe to several magazines, one of which is a health magazine. How much do you really know about health? "How Health Savvy Are You?" examines 20 questions to test your knowledge of nutrition, fitness, and medicine.

When it comes to information about health issues, millions of Americans are turning to the World Wide Web. On the positive side, there are newsgroups where people can turn for emotional support and advice from others suffering with similar illnesses. In addition to the newsgroups, there are also home pages that deal with practically any disease known to humankind. These home pages provide a virtual medical library of the most current information available on a given disease. Obviously, with millions of people logging onto the Web every day in search of answers to health-related issues and concerns, the Web has become fertile ground for charlatans and purveyors of fraudulent claims. Given the free access to all of this information, how is a consumer to judge the quality of the information given? The best answer appears to be simply to consider the source. The information is only as good as the credibility of the provider of that information. Katie Hafner, in "The Doctor Is On," presents the pros and cons of seeking health information from the World Wide Web.

Have you ever wished that you could get the medication you want without first going to see your physician? Each year the number of medications being made available without prescription is growing. The main reason for this shift from prescription to nonprescription is economic. When a patent is about to run out on a prescription medication, the patent will be extended another 3 years if it becomes an over-the-counter medication. While this is good for the pharmaceutical company, it can be bad for the consumer because it removes the safeguards that were deemed necessary when this drug was originally approved for use with humans. The potential hazards for the consumer associated with this switch are discussed in "The Switch to OTC: No Prescription, No Protection?"

One area in particular that has stirred considerable interest in the past few years has been the use of dietary supplements to treat both minor and major health problems. Just how safe and effective are these products? In 1993, the FDA pushed to have some herbs and vitamins exceeding 150 percent of the RDA be treated as prescription medications. Urged by enraged constituents, the U.S. Congress pushed through the Dietary Supplement Health and Education Act, which for all practical purposes thwarted any restrictions from being placed on the sale of not only vitamins and herbs but also amino acids and some hormones. With the FDA out of the picture, supplement manufacturers are not bound to meet any standards regarding the purity and potency of their products. The only restrictions that remain on these preparations are that they bear the words "dietary supplement" on the product label and that they not make specific medical claims or suggest medical warnings on their labels. To do otherwise would constitute an acknowledgment that the product was in fact a drug and would be subjected to the same FDA regulations as all other drugs. Without this information printed on the label, it is up to the consumer to know how and when a product should and should not be used. In "Nature's Pharmacy," Burkhard Bilger examines the self-prescribed use of herbs and extracts and provides a guide to the 10 top natural remedies being sold today. "An FDA Guide to Dietary Supplements" sheds additional light on the labeling laws as they apply to nutritional supplements.

How Health Savvy Are You?

20 questions to test your knowledge of nutrition, fitness, and medicine.

In our five-plus years of publishing Consumer Reports on Health, we've covered some varied—and changing—ground. When we published our first issue back in September 1989, oat bran (remember oat bran?) was the nutritional wonder of the day; now it's beta-carotene (or is it?). Exercise authorities still demanded a vigorous workout every other day for at least 20 minutes a pop; now it almost seems that just getting up to change the channel is a healthful improvement over using the remote.

Since our first issue, we've seen a wide range of genuine medical breakthroughs, including a blood test to detect early prostate cancer, antibiotic treatment to cure ulcers, life-saving therapy for diabetes, and improved drug treatment for heart failure, among many others. And we've witnessed a fair share of medical charades—such as the introduction of several "new" over-the-counter pain relievers no better than the old ones.

It's hard for a health-conscious consumer to keep up. To help you assess your grasp of the field, here are 20 questions on a variety of topics that we've explored over the past five years. You'll find the answers, along with a brief discussion of each topic, on the following pages. We surveyed some 400 readers at random last summer on the same questions, so you'll see how many of your peers knew the right answers.

This isn't an easy quiz. None of the readers we tested got all the answers right. So if you miss a lot of questions, don't get discouraged; just wait five years and check again. Maybe an answer that's wrong now will be right then.

Multiple choice: Take your best guess

1. **Which of the following factors can increase your risk of catching cold?**
   a. Exposure to cold, wet weather.
   b. Lack of rest.
   c. Psychological stress.
   d. All of the above.

2. **Studies suggest that vitamin C:**
   a. Can ease cold symptoms.
   b. Can help prevent a cold.
   c. Can cure the common cold.
   d. None of the above.

3. **Which of the following can harm your eyesight?**
   a. Wearing contact lenses overnight.
   b. Reading in dim light.
   c. Wearing off-the-rack reading glasses.
   d. All of the above.

4. **Eating sugar can:**
   a. Make children hyperactive.
   b. Cause tooth decay.
   c. Increase the risk of diabetes.
   d. All of the above.

Continued on next page

41. Health Savvy

HEALTH QUIZ *Continued*

5. Which can raise your level of "good" HDL cholesterol?
   a. Aerobic exercise.
   b. Strength training.
   c. Low-fat diet.
   d. Eating eggs.

6. Fish may be good for the heart because:
   a. It is low in saturated fat.
   b. It contains omega-3 fatty acids.
   c. It replaces fatty meals in the diet.
   d. All of the above.

7. The strongest evidence on dietary measures to prevent cancer is on:
   a. Beta-carotene.
   b. Fruits and vegetables.
   c. Low-fat diet.
   d. Vitamin E.

8. Vitamin E is plentiful in which foods?
   a. Fruits and vegetables.
   b. Plant fats such as vegetable oils.
   c. Dairy products.
   d. All of the above.

9. The single most powerful measure for preventing osteoporosis in women is:
   a. Calcium supplements.
   b. Estrogen replacement therapy.
   c. Weight-bearing exercise.
   d. Vitamin-D supplements.

10. The single most important thing to do for a muscle sprain is:
    a. Elevate the injury.
    b. Rest the joint.
    c. Apply ice.
    d. Compress the injured area.

True or false: A 50/50 shot

11. Frozen vegetables are usually less nutritious than fresh vegetables.
    True ____ False ____

12. Most people should cut back on salt to ward off hypertension.
    True ____ False ____

13. Exercise and diet are usually enough to control mild hypertension.
    True ____ False ____

14. You should brush your teeth after every meal.
    True ____ False ____

15. Total impotence (erectile dysfunction) usually reflects a psychological problem.
    True ____ False ____

16. Dry-roasted nuts have less fat than oil-roasted nuts.
    True ____ False ____

17. One way to reduce the fat in ground meat is to rinse the meat after cooking.
    True ____ False ____

18. Dark sunglasses help prevent cataracts better than lighter lenses do.
    True ____ False ____

19. Snoring may signal coronary heart disease.
    True ____ False ____

20. Sit-ups are dangerous.
    True ____ False ____

Here are the correct answers to our 20 questions—and a look at how many readers guessed right.

1. Which of the following factors can increase your risk of catching cold?
☑ **c. Psychological stress.** (10% of the readers we tested answered correctly.)

Apparently, not many readers realize that exposure to the elements and lack of rest don't boost your odds of getting sick—despite what your mother told you. Studies have shown that getting chilly or damp doesn't even increase the severity or duration of a cold. Colds are probably more common in cool weather because people spend more time together indoors, where viruses can spread more easily. In addition, the heated indoor air is drier, which leaves the nasal membranes more susceptible to infection. As for lack of rest, that may make you feel worse when you have a cold, but it won't make you more likely to catch cold in the first place.

Psychological stress, on the other hand, may indeed weaken a person's defenses against the common cold. In a recent study of volunteers deliberately infected with a cold virus, stress level made the difference between those who got sick in response to the infection and those who shook it off without developing symptoms.

2. Studies suggest that vitamin C:
☑ **a. Can ease cold symptoms.** (38% correct)

The most enduring legacy of Linus Pauling, who died last year at the age of 93, may be the unflagging popular enthusiasm for vitamin C to ward off the common cold. Unfortunately, there's no convincing scientific support for that practice—although a few studies have suggested that taking extra vitamin C regularly may *slightly* diminish the severity of symptoms after a cold develops.

3. Which of the following can harm your eyesight?
☑ **a. Wearing contacts overnight.** (41% correct)

Half of our readers believe that reading in dim light or using cheap, off-the-rack reading glasses can also damage vision. They can't. Reading in dim light is no more injurious to the eyes than straining to hear a whisper is to the ears. Store-bought reading glasses are perfectly safe and work fine for most people with presbyopia (farsightedness due to aging eyes). The fact is, poor lighting and the wrong lenses—whether off-the-rack or prescription—can cause eyestrain, but they won't harm your eyesight.

Wearing "extended-wear" contact lenses overnight, on the other hand, does threaten eyesight. Even a single night increases the risk of a potentially blinding corneal infection. Closely following the manufacturer's sterilizing regimen doesn't eliminate that risk.

4. Eating sugar can:
☑ **b. Cause tooth decay.** (34% correct)

Nine out of 10 readers know that sugar can cause tooth decay. But 6 of those 9 also believe that sugar makes kids hyper and promotes diabetes. Trust us; it doesn't (see CRH, 10/94). To minimize the cavity risk from sugar, wait for mealtime to eat carbohydrates, including sweets and starchy foods (which contain complex sugars). That way, the other foods will boost saliva, which neutralizes the tooth-dissolving acids that stem from sugar and helps to clear food particles and sugar from the mouth.

Don't fall for the notion that "natural" sweeteners like fruit sugar, honey, and molasses are somehow gentler on the teeth. They all contain fructose, glucose, sucrose, or other sugars that can cause decay. In fact, because syrupy sweeteners like honey tend to stick to the teeth, they may actually be more harmful than refined sugar.

5. Which can raise your level of "good" HDL cholesterol?
☑ **a. Aerobic exercise.** (62% correct)

A low-fat diet tends to lower the "good" along with the "bad" (LDL) cholesterol, so other steps must be taken to boost HDL. The most effective nondrug measure is aerobic exercise. Strength-training exercise doesn't do much for HDL—though unlike aerobics, it does reduce LDL. Other ways to boost HDL without resorting to drugs include losing excess weight and quitting smoking.

6. Fish may be good for the heart because:
☑ **d. All of the above.** (59% correct)

Back in September 1989, the lead story in our first issue asked, "Is fish oil more than snake oil with gills?" At the time, the answer was an unequivocal "maybe." Mixed evidence suggested that the omega-3 fatty acids in fish oil might have cardiovascular benefits. So we recommended "fish, the food" over "fish oil, the capsule." Since then, further research has shifted that "maybe" closer to a tentative "yes." But we still favor fish over fish oil—because those apparent benefits of fish go beyond its omega-3 fatty acids: Low in saturated fat and calories, fish is a healthful alternative to red meat and other fatty meals. We recommend eating fish at least twice a week. (For ways to minimize the risk from potentially contaminated fish, see CRH, 6/94.)

7. The strongest evidence on dietary measures to prevent cancer is on:
☑ **b. Fruits and vegetables.** (47% correct)

About a third of our readers chose c, a low-fat diet. As we noted back in June 1990, however, "Many believe the link is solid, but enthusiasm may have outrun the evidence." Then as now, the closest thing to a clear fat-cancer connection involved colon cancer. Some studies also implicate fat in the progression of prostate cancer. Meanwhile, any link between fat and breast cancer looks increasingly less likely.

Antioxidant nutrients like beta-carotene and vitamin E have been much in the news for their supposed cancer-fighting abilities. In our reader survey, votes of confidence for beta-carotene topped vitamin E by a margin of 20 to 1. But the strength of the actual anti-cancer evidence on the two nutrients is comparable. The jury is still out on those nutrients and other individual antioxidants, such as vitamin C. However, as nearly half of our readers know, there's a clear verdict in support of fruits and vegetables. (Mom got that one right.) Numerous studies have found a connection between a produce-rich diet and reduced rates of various cancers, including cancers of the bladder, breast, colon, lung, mouth, stomach, throat, and prostate.

8. Vitamin E is plentiful in which foods?
☑ **b. Plant fats like vegetable oils.** (32% correct)

About half our readers believe that a low-fat diet rich in fruits and vegetables provides lots of vitamin E—as it does the other two main antioxidant nutrients, beta-carotene and vitamin C. But vitamin E is different from those nutrients. The foods that are highest in E are concentrated plant fats like vegetable and seed oils, as well as vegetable-oil products such as margarine and salad dressing.

Since it's hard to get large quantities of vitamin E through diet alone, many people hedge their bets with supplements. That appears to be safe enough, if you stay within a modest range. The usual multivitamin provides 30 mg of vitamin E (sometimes listed as 45 IU, or International Units). If you choose a supplement containing only vitamin E, stick with a relatively low dosage of 65 to 260 mg (100 to 400 IU).

9. The single most powerful measure for preventing osteoporosis in women is:
☑ **b. Estrogen replacement.** (15% correct)

For maintaining healthy bones after menopause, when the risk of osteoporosis is highest, nothing is more effective than replacing lost estrogen. An adequate intake of calcium (including calcium supplements, if necessary) is also essential—especially when estrogen replacement therapy is not an option. All adults should consume at least 1000 mg of calcium a day. Postmenopausal women who are not on estrogen and men over 65 should get at least 1500 mg. (Vitamin D helps the body absorb calcium, but most people get enough vitamin D from exposure to sunlight and from their diet.)

Regular weight-bearing exercise helps preserve bone, too. Recent research suggests that strength-training workouts may provide the maximum benefit—and without the jarring of high-impact exercise, such as running.

10. The single most important thing to do for a muscle sprain is:
☑ **c. Apply ice.** (59% correct)

All four strategies help heal a sprain, as summed up by the acronym RICE: Rest, Ice, Compression, Elevation. But the most important step to minimize the damage and speed recovery is to apply ice immediately. Cold constricts blood vessels and thus helps limit bleeding and prevent swelling. If you don't have a flexible ice pack, use a bag of frozen vegetables. (Crushed ice soon turns into a solid block.) Ice the injury for 10 to 20 minutes every hour or two for the first 6 to 12 hours—at least until the swelling is no longer increasing. If swelling resumes, apply ice again. After a day or two of RICE, gently stretch the muscle throughout the day for several days.

11. Frozen vegetables are usually less nutritious than fresh vegetables.
☑ **False.** (18% correct)

That's generally true only if you buy your vegetables fresh off the farm—or if you grow your own. Most people eat "fresh" vegetables that have been hauled across the country and displayed for a few days in the supermarket. That leaves plenty of time for air, heat, and light to break down vitamins. Frozen vegetables are especially likely to beat fresh vegetables that are out of season or that sit in the refrigerator for more than a couple of days. For maximum nutrition, don't thaw frozen vegetables before cooking. (Vegetables clumped together in the bag indicate thawing somewhere along the line.)

Canned vegetables don't stack up to fresh or frozen vegetables. Much of the vitamin content (not to mention taste) is destroyed by high processing temperatures or lost to water in the can.

12. Most people should cut back on salt to ward off hypertension.
☑ **False.** (28% correct)

Some people with hypertension do need to restrict their sodium intake to keep their blood pressure under control. But for everyone else, salt is simply not the health threat it's made out to be. To find out if you're in the salt-sensitive minority, see our April 1994 report for a dietary test you can take at home.

13. Exercise and diet are usually enough to control mild hypertension.
☑ **False.** (8% correct)

Those "lifestyle" measures are a good place to start, but they're usually not enough, even for mild hypertension—typically defined as a systolic reading (the upper number) of 140 to 160 mm Hg or a diastolic reading (the lower number) of 90 to 105 mm Hg. And there's now strong evidence that reducing even such borderline elevations in blood pressure helps prevent more serious disease.

Of course, nondrug measures to lower blood pressure are still valuable. Even if such therapy doesn't eliminate the need for medication altogether, it can enable many patients to use lower drug doses, thereby cutting down on possible side effects. Before starting on medication, people with mild hypertension should at least give nondrug therapy a fair trial. That means getting regular exercise (especially aerobic exercise), losing weight, reducing stress, and cutting down on alcohol and (possibly) sodium. If blood pressure does not decline after six months, antihypertensive medication may well be necessary—particularly if you have other risk factors for coronary heart disease.

14. You should brush your teeth after every meal.
☑ **False.** (19% correct)

There's really no need to brush every time you eat. It takes 16 to 24 hours for the bacteria fueled by food residues left on the teeth to produce plaque, which can eventually cause cavities and gum disease. If you brush properly in the morning and in the evening, and floss on one of those occasions, there won't be time for the bacteria to cause a problem. In fact, it's possible to get too much of a good thing: Brushing too often or too vigorously can irritate or even damage the gums.

15. Total impotence (erectile dysfunction) usually reflects a psychological problem.
☑ **False.** (61% correct)

Until recently, impotence was almost always blamed on psychological factors, such as stress, anxiety, or depression. Although such factors can contribute to impotence, they're usually not the primary cause. (Occasional difficulty achieving or maintaining an erection, which becomes increasingly frequent with age, is not considered true impotence.) The problem is much more likely to stem from medical factors, such as drug side effects, impaired circulation, neurological problems, or hormonal imbalance. If psychological factors really are to blame, counseling by a sex therapist or treatment for depression may help. When physiological or psychological treatment fails to correct the underlying problem, men can try a number of mechanical techniques for creating an erection, including drug injections, vacuum pumps, and surgical implants.

16. Dry-roasted nuts have less fat than oil-roasted nuts.
☑ **False.** (26% correct)

You'll save virtually no fat at all by choosing dry-roasted nuts over the usual oil-roasted kind. That's because oil-roasted nuts are not immersed in the boiling oil long enough to absorb any of it. And the excess oil is drained off afterward.

17. One way to reduce the fat in ground meat is to rinse the meat after cooking.
☑ **True.** (21% correct)
Here's the simplest technique: Brown ground meat in a nonstick pan, drain off the fat, pour hot water over the meat, and drain it again. That can rinse away as much as three-quarters of the fat. Of course, some of the flavor gets drained off with it. And the meat doesn't hold together well. So rinsed meat is best reserved for spaghetti sauce, casseroles, chili, and other seasoned dishes.

18. Dark sunglasses help prevent cataracts better than lighter lenses do.
☑ **False.** (57% correct)
Darkening the lenses blocks visible light, but has no effect on ultraviolet light, the end of the spectrum that contributes to cataracts. Plastic lenses—even clear ones—block most UV light, and glass lenses block some. Special coatings increase UV absorption. Darker lenses may help protect against a potential though unproved hazard from visible light: There's some evidence that lifetime exposure may damage the part of the retina that distinguishes fine detail.

19. Snoring may signal coronary heart disease.
☑ **True.** (50% correct)
Not all snorers have coronary disease, but the disease is more common among people who snore than among those who don't. More important, snoring may do more that just *signal* coronary disease; that's because the irregular airflow may actually *contribute* to the development of the disease. Those at greatest risk have a severe condition known as sleep apnea, in which the snorer actually stops breathing repeatedly throughout the night. There are various ways to help remedy snoring and apnea, ranging from changes in sleep position to surgery. A sleep specialist can help diagnose the problem and recommend a solution. . . .

20. Sit-ups are dangerous.
☑ **True.** (45% correct)
Done in the traditional fashion—lifting the upper body into the sitting position with hands clasped behind the head, and legs straight or bent at the knee—sit-ups strain the back. That's especially a problem for older exercisers and people with a history of back trouble (which includes most adults). Moreover, much of the sit-up motion is unnecessary, since the abdominal muscles are used to lift the upper body just the first few inches off the floor.

Partial sit-ups, a modified version of the original, are safer and more efficient for strengthening the abdominal muscles: Lying on your back with knees bent and with your arms crossed in front of your chest or hands clasped loosely behind your head, lift your head, shoulders, and upper back (not your entire upper body) off the floor.

RATING YOURSELF

The scoring guide below is based on the performance of the 400 readers who took the quiz as part of our monthly survey of randomly selected subscribers.
18 - 20 correct: Are you sure you didn't cheat?
15 - 17 correct: We have a staff opening for you.
10 - 14 correct: More than respectable.
5 - 9 correct: Graded on a curve, you should give yourself a solid "B."
0 - 4 correct: Start boning up on those back issues. But don't despair. You have lots of company.

Nutrition In The News: What The Headlines Don't Tell You

It just doesn't make sense. For years, you've been told that to live a long, healthy life, you've got to eat right and take care of yourself. So you cut down on fat, take vitamins and exercise regularly. Then one morning you glance at the headlines and learn that antioxidants may not be so effective in preventing cancer after all. Later, you hear that a low-fat diet may not be as heart-healthy as you were led to believe. How can nutrition experts change their minds so suddenly and so often? Frustrated and confused, you throw your hands in the air and race to the nearest fast-food joint for a cheeseburger and fries.

But before you take that first bite, there are some things you should know about nutrition research and how it is reported in the media. It's seldom as simple and straightforward as it seems.

At Cross Purposes. Much of the confusion exists because researchers and reporters speak different languages. Reporters spotlight unique or unusual findings of scientific studies in order to grab your attention. Scientists, on the other hand, prefer to wait for consensus opinions that are built slowly but surely over time.

"First-time findings are not the most interesting, nor are they necessarily true," says Jo Freudenheim, Ph.D., nutritional epidemiologist at the State University of New York at Buffalo. But they make great headlines.

The media often report on studies published in medical journals as the latest thinking. But scientists look at published studies as "works in progress" that serve either to support or refute existing research. Before a finding becomes fact, it must be confirmed repeatedly. That's why researchers are almost always ultraconservative about recommending changes in diet or lifestyle on the basis of a single study. "More research is needed" is a virtual mantra in scientific circles.

Limited By Design. Scientists conduct studies using a variety of methods, each with its own advantages and limitations. Only when results from all types of studies are viewed collectively can scientists put the pieces of the puzzle together to form a clearer picture of the link between diet and disease.

Epidemiological studies, or population studies, observe large numbers of people to see if there's a link between specific dietary or lifestyle habits and disease in a population. Since these studies observe people's behavior—say, how much fish Eskimo eat per week—it's always possible that unknown factors, like unreported foods or genetics, can influence findings.

For example, many epidemiological studies have found that people who eat diets rich in fruits and vegetables have lower cancer rates. But, people who eat fruits and vegetables may have other healthy habits—like not smoking or not drinking alcohol—that protect them from cancer. Since epidemiological studies do not provide proof of a direct cause and effect relationship, scientists turn to experimental studies with animals or humans to build a stronger case.

Such experiments allow researchers to manipulate the effect of a specific factor (what researchers call a variable), like a vitamin or drug, under tightly controlled conditions. But even experiments have limitations. For example, findings from *animal studies*, while one step beyond epidemiological studies, will not necessarily produce the same results when tested in people.

Human clinical trials offer strongest proof of cause and effect, especially if the studies are *randomized, placebo-controlled* and *double blind*. This means that participants are randomly assigned to a treatment group. One group receives, for example, a vitamin under study. A control group receives a placebo, or dummy pill, and neither subject nor researcher knows who got what until the results are in. However, clinical trials also have shortcomings.

> "It is the totality of evidence, not the latest headlines, that should influence you."

Take last year's highly publicized study showing beta-carotene and vitamin E did not reduce lung cancer in male Finnish smokers. The study was criticized for being too short, providing insufficient amounts of vitamins to show any positive effect and applying only to smokers. It was also suggested that the unexpected results could have been a fluke, due purely to chance.

Since these results went against the accumulating body of evidence, it became a classic example of why you should not change your dietary habits on the basis of a single study. As researchers like to point out, it is the totality of evidence, not the latest headlines, that should influence you.

Risky Business. Understanding risk also helps keep research results in perspective. Since nothing in life is risk-free, changing your lifestyle or eating habits almost always means trading one risk for another. It's important to consider how risky something is and question whether the alternative is actually better. For example, you give up snacking on fruit to avoid pesticides, but you replace it with fat-free cookies. Not only do you lose out on the health benefits of fruit, you've added what is probably a high-calorie, low-nutrient food to your diet—a potentially bigger risk than a small pesticide residue.

That's why it's important to look at the bigger picture and decide how relevant the findings of a study are to you.

Ask yourself if the condition being studied is a rare or common occurrence. How likely is it to affect you? If a study on women showed that eating food X increased the risk of breast cancer by 10%, and eating food Y increased the risk of bladder cancer by 50%, should you give up food Y? Food X? Both? There's no way to know how you personally will be affected, but women in general would probably benefit more by dropping food X from their menus first. That's because breast cancer is so much more common in women than bladder cancer, that even a small increase in risk affects more women. Men should be more concerned about food Y since bladder cancer is three times more common in men than in women.

The point? Getting a sense of the potential risk prevents overreacting to frightening headlines.

Making Sense of It All. Keep these tips in mind when you're alerted to "breaking nutrition news."

❖ Read beyond the headlines. You'll often find practical advice and a broader perspective on the study near the end of an article or TV report.

❖ Consider the source. View industry-funded reports with some caution; corporate profits may be riding on the results. However, much solid research has been funded by industry. Research published in scientific journals like the *Journal of the American Medical Association* and *The New England Journal of Medicine,* which depend on experts to critically review research before publication, are safe bets.

❖ Look at the bigger picture. It makes more sense to stop smoking, lose weight and exercise than to rely primarily on the latest antioxidant research to reduce heart disease risk.

❖ Remember that there are few true breakthroughs in nutrition research. Be skeptical of claims to the contrary.

—*Adrienne Forman, M.S., R.D.*

The switch to OTC: No prescription, no protection?

More and more drugs are going over the counter. That increases your control—but it also increases your risk.

In the past 18 months, the U.S. Food and Drug Administration has approved the over-the-counter sale of four heartburn drugs formerly available by prescription only. Since receiving approval, the drug makers have poured roughly half a billion dollars into dueling ads, each claiming that their cure acts faster, lasts longer, or provides more protection than the others.

Actually, none of the four drugs—cimetidine (*Tagamet HB*), famotidine (*Pepcid AC*), nizatidine (*Axid AR*), and ranitidine (*Zantac 75*)—works any better than the others. In many cases, ordinary antacids are preferable to any of the new drugs (see box "Heartburn: How to quench the flames"). A federal judge, unable to stomach the ads, has ordered two of the combatants to stifle several of their claims and stick to the facts.

The heartburn slugfest highlights the potential problems created by the growing trend toward over-the-counter drugs. While direct access to those drugs increases your ability to manage your own health, it also increases the risk of misuse—a risk compounded by the marketers' claims.

Why the switch?

The FDA must approve the shift of a drug to over-the-counter status. But it's the drug maker, not the agency, that initiates the process. Most companies apply because their patent on a prescription drug is about to expire; going over the counter typically extends patent protection for another three years. Other companies apply simply because they think the drug will sell better without a prescription.

A drug's switch to OTC status sometimes offers little or no benefit to the consumer. The recently switched pain relievers naproxen (*Aleve*) and ketoprofen (*Actron, Orudis KT*) for example, are neither safer nor more effective than the related drug ibuprofen (*Advil, Motrin IB*), long available in cheaper, generic form without a prescription. More important, eliminating the need for a prescription eliminates two major safeguards—the guidance provided by a physician and a pharmacist.

Buyer beware

Here are some of the potential pitfalls you face when you use drugs on your own:

■ **Misdiagnosis.** Proper self-treatment starts with proper self-diagnosis, which can sometimes be dauntingly difficult. Consider vaginal yeast infections. Several antiyeast drugs formerly available only by prescription are now available over the counter. Those include butoconazole (*Femstat 3*), clotrimazole (*Gyne-Lotrimin, Mycelex-7*), and miconazole (*Monistat 3; Monistat 7*). Recent studies have shown that many women who treat themselves with such medications actually have a more serious bacterial infection, such as vaginosis or gonorrhea.

Misdiagnosis can be especially unfortunate if a drug controls symptoms for weeks or months on end while the underlying disease goes untreated. Pain that you think is heartburn, for example, may actually stem from ulcers or even esophageal cancer.

■ **Side effects.** FDA approval for over-the-counter sale simply means that the agency believes the benefits of increased accessibility outweigh the risks of unsupervised use; it doesn't mean the drug is harmless. For one thing, OTC drugs can cause unpleasant or, in rare cases, potentially dangerous side effects, even at the recommended doses. For example, the newly nonprescription versions of ketoprofen and naproxen, like all OTC pain killers except acetaminophen (*Actamin, Tylenol*), can upset the stomach. The decongestant pseudoephedrine, contained in several products, such as *Efidac/24* and *Sudafed*, can cause insomnia and irritability. And the maximum recommended dose of certain formerly prescription antihistamines, contained in all sleeping aids and some cold or allergy medications, can slow reaction time as sharply as the amount of alcohol that would make driving illegal in many states.

■ **Drug interactions.** Without professional supervision, you're more likely to take drugs that can interact adversely. Recommended doses of the heartburn drug *Tagamet HB* can cause potentially dangerous increases in the potency of the asthma medicine theophylline (*Theo-Dur*), the blood-thinner warfarin

Heartburn: How to quench the flames

Advertising campaigns for the four heartburn drugs that have recently gone over the counter—cimetidine (*Tagamet HB*), famotidine (*Pepcid AC*), nizatidine (*Axid AR*), and ranitidine (*Zantac 75*)—have confused an already confusing situation for people trying to figure out when to stick with a traditional heartburn drug, when to choose a new one, and which particular drug to choose.

Something old, something new

Heartburn, a burning pain under the breastbone, develops when acid from the stomach backs up into the esophagus, the tube leading down from the throat. The traditional OTC remedies—antacids such as *Alka-Seltzer*, *Maalox*, *Rolaids*, and *Tums*—relieve the pain by neutralizing the acid. The new OTC drugs, called H2 blockers, fight the pain by suppressing production of the acid.

Antacids can have certain advantages over H2 blockers. They start working within a few minutes, while the blockers take at least half an hour, often longer. And while the cost per hour is usually about the same—5 to 6 cents—a single dose of an H2 blocker works for at least eight hours, a dose of an antacid for just one to three hours. So antacids are cheaper if you need relief for fewer than eight hours.

However, the longer action of H2 blockers is an advantage if you need prolonged relief. Equally important, antacids can only relieve heartburn, while blockers can prevent the pain if you take them shortly before you eat.

Blocker versus blocker

Despite what the ads say, no H2 blocker works any better than the others. Both *Pepcid AC* and *Tagamet HB*, for example, claim to relieve and prevent heartburn, while *Zantac 75* claims only to relieve it, and *Axid AR* claims only to prevent it. But those differences stem merely from differences in what the marketers thought would sell the most pills, not in what the drugs can actually do.

The makers of *Tagamet HB* have also insisted that their drug works faster than *Pepcid AC*. The initial FDA-approved directions did recommend taking *Pepcid AC* an hour before a meal, *Tagamet HB* only 30 minutes before, to prevent heartburn. But that distinction simply reflected the design of the studies originally submitted to the FDA. Since then, the makers of *Pepcid AC* have submitted new studies showing that it too can start working in just 30 minutes.

There are, however, a few potential differences in safety between *Tagamet HB* and the other H2 blockers. *Tagamet HB* is more likely to interact with the asthma drug theophylline (*Theo-Dur*), the blood-thinner warfarin (*Coumadin*), and the seizure drug phenytoin (*Dilantin*). If you're taking any of those medications along with *Tagamet HB*, your doctor should monitor blood levels of the medication. Or you could simply choose a different H2 blocker. Further, taking excessive doses of *Tagamet HB* for a long time can cause impotence or breast enlargement, although both problems disappear if you discontinue the drug.

What to do

The major advantage of H2 blockers is their ability to prevent rather than just relieve heartburn. People who often experience such pain after eating could try taking an H2 blocker 30 to 60 minutes before eating.

For relief rather than prevention, stick with a traditional antacid, unless you experience prolonged attacks and don't want to keep taking antacids every hour or two. For maximum effectiveness, you could even take both drugs at the same time—an antacid for immediate relief, an H2 blocker for relief once the antacid wears off.

Of course, if you can figure out what triggers the attacks, you may be able to avoid drugs entirely. Common dietary triggers include alcohol, caffeine, carbonated drinks, chocolate, fat, hot spices, and peppermint. Other steps that can help prevent heartburn include losing weight, eating slowly, avoiding clothes with a tight waistband, stopping smoking, and staying upright after eating, rather than lying down.

(*Coumadin*), and the seizure medicine phenytoin (*Dilantin*). Many common medications can make antihistamines even more sedating than they are when taken alone. Even food or drink can complicate the use of a drug. Acidic beverages like coffee or orange juice, for example, can interfere with the absorption of OTC nicotine gum.

■ **Overuse.** The only safeguard against excessive use of OTC drugs is the warning on the label and the package insert specifying how long you can safely use the drug without seeing a physician. People who overlook or ignore that warning on, say, naproxen, ketoprofen, or even ibuprofen can develop gastrointestinal bleeding, ulcers, increased blood pressure, or liver or kidney damage. (Prolonged aspirin use can have the same effects, though not on blood pressure; overuse of acetaminophen is even more likely to damage the liver and may harm the kidneys as well.)

Frequent, repeated use of other drugs that have switched—drugs for headaches, insomnia, nasal congestion, or eye inflammation—can lead to dependency. After the drug wears off, you develop "rebound" symptoms, even worse than the original ones. That can create a vicious cycle of increasingly frequent drug use and worsening symptoms.

■ **Overdoses.** Some people are tempted to take more than the recommended dose of an OTC drug, either because they think such readily available drugs must be harmless, or because they want the potency of a prescription dose without the bother of getting a prescription. But even moderately excessive doses, like moderately excessive use, can turn a reasonably safe remedy into a hazardous substance. The recently switched heartburn drugs, for example, can trigger headaches, lethargy, and confusion if you take too much. With a few drugs, modest overdoses can have disastrous results. Swallowing just three times more than the maximum recommended amount of phenylpropanolamine, a decongestant contained in all diet pills and some cold medicines, such as *Tavist-D*, can trigger a severe, potentially fatal rise in blood pressure.

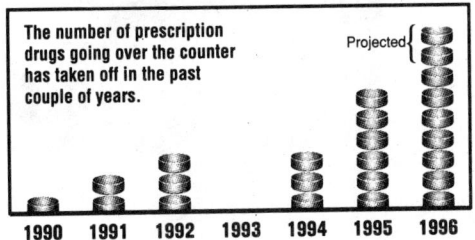

Rx-to-OTC switch hitters

The number of prescription drugs going over the counter has taken off in the past couple of years.

1990 1991 1992 1993 1994 1995 1996 (Projected)

Where to get the facts

To learn how to safely use drugs that have gone over the counter, start by reading the label and the package insert, which give certain essential directions and warnings. However, those sources may be incomplete, omitting duration of use or certain side effects, drug interactions, or reasons to avoid the drug. So seek more complete information:

■ **Ask the pharmacist.** If possible, read the insert before leaving the store. Then ask the pharmacist any questions you still have. You should know how long you can take the drug without consulting a doctor; whether there are any unlisted side effects or drug interactions; how and when to take the drug; how to store it; and, if you're older, whether you face any special risks. (Drugs tend to reach higher blood levels in older people; even at normal levels, many drugs have stronger effects on the aging body.)

If you buy all your prescription and OTC drugs at one pharmacy, have the druggist enter those medications, as well as any drug allergies you have, in the drugstore's computer. The computer will then alert the pharmacist to potential drug interactions and allergic reactions.

■ **Ask your doctor.** If the pharmacist says the medication may pose an increased risk for you, ask your physician what to do. And call the physician before starting to take an OTC drug if you have a chronic disorder, are pregnant or nursing, or have an unfamiliar symptom. It's reasonably safe to treat yourself only if you have a highly familiar symptom, such as a runny nose or a cough, or if your physician has previously diagnosed the same problem, such as acne or athlete's foot. (But it may take more than just one previous diagnosis before a woman can safely treat a vaginal yeast infection on her own.)

Tell your doctor about all the OTC preparations you're taking, including drugs, herbs, and supplements. Those products may interact with prescribed medications or skew the results of laboratory tests; they may even be the cause of your symptoms.

■ **Check the books.** Consult a drug-information book, such as "The Complete Drug Reference," published by Consumer Reports Books and available in most libraries or bookstores.

Summing up

The growing number of drugs available without a prescription places more responsibility on you to make sure you use them wisely and safely.

What to do

■ Read the label and the package insert, and ask the pharmacist for additional information.

■ If possible, have the druggist enter in the computer all your over-the-counter drugs as well as any prescription medications and drug allergies.

■ Ask your doctor about the drug if you have unfamiliar symptoms, are pregnant or nursing, or have a chronic disease.

■ Consult a reference book on drugs.

The Doctor Is On

Patients are finding a treasure trove of medical information, emotional support—and even doctors with time to talk to them—on the Internet

KATIE HAFNER

WHEN ANDY BEAVER, A 42-year-old computer specialist in Toronto, began to experience a persistent twitch in his left hand last year, his doctor sent him to a neurologist. After some tests, Beaver was told he had ALS, or Lou Gehrig's disease, and had three to five years to live. The neurologist told him to go home and put his affairs in order, then scribbled down a telephone number with a reference for a second opinion. Then he shook Beaver's hand and wished him luck. "I was in his office for a total of about three minutes," Beaver recalls. "I stumbled back to work with a Post-it note in my hand, saying 'ALS? Lou Gehrig? Three to five years?'"

So that night, Beaver logged on to the Internet. He began subscribing to an electronic mailing list—part newsletter, part online discussion group—for ALS patients. Beaver quickly found state-of-the-art medical information, an instant support group and a chance to discover just what he was in for: feeding tubes and ventilators. "It scared the bejeebers out of my wife and me," he says. But Beaver gradually came to depend on the group as a source of information and inspiration. He was reassured to find that some 15 percent of its 1,700 participants were health professionals.

Electronic mailing lists, online support forums and World Wide Web sites devoted to every conceivable disease have turned the Internet into a trove of medical information. For the newly diagnosed, and for those with chronic conditions, the information and emotional support found online can be invaluable. And the fact that cyberspace renders geography irrelevant is a boon to those with debilitating illnesses who would otherwise feel hopelessly isolated.

Perhaps the most unexpected development is that more and more doctors are coming online as volunteer consultants. Clinicians and medical researchers are taking to cyberspace to advise online support groups, get an unfiltered view of patients' experiences and do what many of them entered the medical profession for in the first place: help people. "Being online is good for physicians because they get to see what's hot before it's even in the journals," says John R. Mangiardi, chief of neurosurgery at Lenox Hill Hospital in New York City and a participant in a popular mailing list devoted to brain tumors. "It's good for patients because they get interactive information." It was certainly good for San Diegan Bob Thomas and his 12-year-old daughter, Megan. Thomas posted a question about the nature of Megan's brain tumor to the mailing list. Within a day he had heard from six different specialists.

The time saved by getting answers online can be critical when patients are faced with what can amount to life-and-death decisions. When Monica Frydman, a 42-year-old language interpreter, was diagnosed with breast cancer last June, her surgeon recommended an immediate double mastectomy within two weeks, along with an extreme course of chemotherapy and the removal of adjacent lymph nodes. Frydman and her husband found the breast-cancer mailing list. Within a day, after hearing from a doctor and a prominent radiation specialist, they sought a second opinion from a doctor who agreed with the onliners that far less extreme treatment was needed.

Many physicians "lurk," which is cyberese for reading a discussion but not participating in it. By reading what patients say to one another in online forums, doctors say, they learn things about how patients are coping with an illness that would never be disclosed during an office visit. Although patients rarely discuss cosmetics with him personally, neurosurgeon Mangiardi saw people complain to one another on the brain-tumor list about unsightly scars left in their scalp following surgery. In response, he started using tiny metal meshes to conceal the disfigurement. As a rule, Mangiardi now avoids making large incisions. "If necessary, I'll go through someone's eyebrow to take out a giant tumor," he says.

Online eavesdropping can lead to specific help as well. When Carvel Gipson, a neurologist specializing in headaches, noticed that one of the participants in a headache and migraine discussion group was taking a medication for an unusual form of migraine, he warned her against taking it. Taken for the particular migraine she suffered from, the medication could cause paralysis, a fact the physician who prescribed the drug was unaware of.

Doctors in general have been slow to adopt online communications, and when they do go online, it's rarely to talk to patients. "Some doctors have freaked out when patients want to send them e-mail, or bring in medical reports that the doctors haven't even seen yet," says Tom Ferguson, a senior associate at Harvard Medical School's Center for Clinical Computing and author of "Health Online" (Addison-Wesley). "It doesn't fit the model they were trained in." Some doctors warn that online forums can stir false hopes. Two years ago, when a few ALS patients in the Boston area began an experimental treatment with Neurontin, a drug used for epilepsy, word spread throughout the online community and ALS patients everywhere began demanding the drug from their physicians. Before long, thousands of ALS sufferers were on Neurontin, hoping to slow the deterioration of their muscle strength. In formal studies conducted so far, a positive difference has been noted, but the effect is extremely slight and tests are inconclusive.

The Neurontin episode, though harmless in the end, highlights the speed with which information both good and bad can spread online. Not surprisingly, the Internet has become ripe territory for quackery. Purveyors of magic elixirs pop up everywhere, feeding on people's desperation. But the groups with a heavy presence of health professionals guard well against fradulent claims. "My usual reply is 'That's very interesting, could you show me some data'," says Loren Buhle, a former professor of radiation oncology at the University of Pennsylvania who created OncoLink, a popular cancer-related Web site. The father of an ALS patient in Florida recently asked forum members whether his daughter should have her dental fillings removed (at $1,000 each) after hearing claims that the mercury in the fillings caused ALS. Researchers on the list gently counseled him against it.

The credibility of online information can often be gauged by who's providing it. Web sites sponsored by universities and government agencies, and those where information has obviously been pooled and reviewed by a variety of people, are usually the most reliable. While careful not to prescribe drugs or treatment for fear of liability, or offer definitive diagnoses over the Net, doctors who go on the Net say they find a particular satisfaction in doing online what they often don't have the time to do when they see patients in person: answer people's questions and help them understand what's wrong with them.

Getting Medical Help Online

FINDING THE RIGHT SPOT ON THE INTERNET FOR YOUR health concerns isn't as easy as you might think. There are more than 10,000 health-related web sites alone, and thousands more online support communities. For Web surfers, an excellent place to start is Yahoo's Health section (http://www.yahoo.com/Health), where you'll find a wealth of information on more than 2,000 sites. The Big Three commercial online service providers, America Online, CompuServe and Prodigy, are well known for their extensive health forums. Here are some other good places to go for medical information:

Web Sites
- Medaccess: http://www.medaccess.com
- OncoLink: http://www.oncolink.upenn.edu/
- National Cancer Institute: http://www.nci.nih.gov/
- HealthWorld (provides free access to MedLine): http://healthy.net/
- Psych Central: http://www.coil.com/~grohol/
- Medinfo: http://www.medinfo.org

Mailing Lists
- Breast cancer: Send the message "subscribe breast-cancer" followed by your real name to listserv@morgan.ucs.mun.ca
- Brain tumor: Send the message "subscribe braintmr" followed by your real name to listserv@mitvma.mit.edu
- ALS (Lou Gehrig's disease): Send e-mail to bro@huey.met.fsu.edu
- Depression: Send the message "subscribe walkers-in-darkness" to majordomo@world.std.com. Another list: send the message "subscribe depress" to listserv@soundprint.brandywine.american.edu

Article 45

Nature's PHARMACY

Many natural remedies are as potent as drugs, but manufacturers can't tell you how to take them. Wouldn't you like to know?

By Burkhard Bilger

An hour south of Salt Lake City, in the shadow of the 13,000-foot Wasatch Mountain Range, the largest herbal factory in the United States reclines like a contented beast, recently fed. Thirty years ago founder Tom Murdock raised this company on a single high-desert plant, chaparral, believed by some herb fanciers to treat everything from colds to cancer. Today the company takes in 450 different herbs and spits out more than 8 million capsules a day. Along the way it has evolved into an animal of a new and unpredictable kind: a drug company in herbalist's clothing.

The Murdock Madaus Schwabe factory is a naturalist's Notre Dame. Ivory walls meet vaulted ceilings; colored banners stream from the skylights, emblazoned with herbalists' slogans. But step through an air-locked door and into the belly of this particular beast, and the atmosphere changes. Seventy-gallon herb drums are stacked five stories high. Conveyor belts, looped like intestines, push boxes toward waiting trucks.

Within a matter of days the boxes will find their way into pharmacies, supermarkets, and health food stores. You may glance at the official-looking labels on the shrink-wrapped bottles and assume that some government agency has made sure the contents really work. You may even decide that supplements, being "natural," must be inherently safer than drugs. But you'd be wrong.

The truth is that despite their increasing availability and popularity, most supplements—whether herbal remedies or hormones like DHEA—haven't been proven either safe or effective.

Three years ago, when Congress passed the Dietary Supplement Health and Education Act, America's tidy well-lit drugstores began to grow as disorienting, and hazardous, as jungles. Under the act companies can sell whatever supplement they please, so long as its label makes no claim to treat a disease. That doesn't mean any given supplement is unsafe, of course, or even that it doesn't work. work. Studies in the past few years have shown impressive results from a number of these remedies. But others have taken a toll on the health of users. You're on your own as you navigate between the reliable and the risky, let alone try to figure out how much to take for what ailment.

So when you pick up a bottle of feverfew, there's nothing on the package to suggest it may be useful for migraine. Grab some melatonin and you'll have to

From *Health*, October 1997, pp. 64–72. © 1997 by Time Publishing Ventures, Inc. Reprinted by permission.

guess how much to try for insomnia. You can't even be sure you're getting what you pay for. When *Consumer Reports* tested ten ginseng products last year, one contained almost none of the active ingredient; among the others, the concentration varied by 1,000 percent.

This fall a presidential commission on dietary supplement labels is proposing a set of regulations that should help tame the jungle. But even if the Food and Drug Administration adopts the recommendations to the letter, the supplement industry may appeal them to Congress. It could be two years, in other words, before American consumers can count on the quality and efficacy of supplements they swallow.

"We're in limbo," says Varro Tyler, one of the country's foremost herb experts and author of *The Honest Herbal*. On the one hand, he says, some unethical companies are making outrageous claims for inferior products, and the law makes it difficult for the FDA to do anything about it. On the other hand, the few restrictions on the books force responsible companies to word their labels so vaguely they're useless, even misleading.

The only guarantee is confusion.

WHEN IT COMES TO the public's health, there's been a long tug-of-war between individual liberty and regulation. For most of the country's history, liberty had the upper hand. In 1937, however, a poisonous elixir killed more than 100 people, and the regulators began to gain ground. At first the FDA merely required manufacturers to prove that a drug was reasonably safe. Then a wary official in 1962 refused to approve a sedative called thalidomide. In Europe, where the drug was widely available, thousands of babies were born with terrible limb deformities after their mothers took the drug during pregnancy. Having averted disaster here, the agency went a step further and began to require large well-controlled trials to prove prescription drugs safe and effective.

The FDA also decided to reappraise all previously approved drugs to see if they worked as claimed. Of the many herbs on the list, only a handful made the cut. Most others could still be sold, but manufacturers couldn't claim they would treat a disease or condition.

That loophole left the FDA uneasy. Finally, in 1993, the agency proposed that many herbs, and any vitamins sold in dosages exceeding 150 percent of the recommended daily allowance, should be considered prescription drugs.

To many health-conscious baby boomers, it was a call to arms. In television ads Mel Gibson complained about losing the right to take vitamin C. The epicenter of the shake-up was Utah, improbable as it may seem. Mormon self-sufficiency, hospitable tax laws, and a well-educated population had been nurturing fledgling

It's true that herbs are sometimes easier on the body than the drugs derived from them. But herbal extracts can also be toxic.

herb companies. Now Utah senator Orrin Hatch helped push through the Dietary Supplement Health and Education Act. The FDA's attempt to corral supplements had ended by setting them loose.

The new law broadened the definition of *supplement* to include not just vitamins and minerals but also herbs, amino acids, and some hormones, among other things—leaving them less strictly regulated than food or drugs. There are no "good manufacturing practices" to ensure pills contain what they should. And in matters of safety, the burden of proof has shifted to the FDA, which must establish danger before pulling a worrisome product from the market.

The law's effect on Utah companies has been like a dose of growth hormone. But for the rest of us, in the short run at least, it may have done more harm than good. Says Bruce Silverglade, legal affairs director of the Center for Science in the Public Interest: "Congress opened a door, and industry drove an 18-wheeler through it."

For starters, it's not clear what exactly a supplement is. Cholestin, a natural remedy for high cholesterol, is a good example. Is it a drug or a dietary supplement? Let's see: It contains a tangy bright red yeast that's often used to coat and preserve spareribs in China. So it must be a dietary supplement, right? But along with the yeast comes a chemical it produces: a natural form of lovastatin, a prescription drug that lowers cholesterol. Okay, so Cholestin is a drug.

Actually, the FDA isn't quite sure. Last March, after a pharmacist asked the agency why lovastatin was available over the counter, investigators went to Simi Valley, California, to gather samples from the supplement's manufacturer, Pharmanex. The move provoked some maneuvering. Pharmanex filed, then dropped, a suit claiming the FDA was overstepping its bounds. In July the agency seized a shipment of Cholestin's raw material and is holding it pending further talks with the company about whether the remedy should be considered a drug. In the meantime Pharmanex continues to market Cholestin as a supplement.

Oddly enough, the law is written in such a way that Cholestin may be considered a supplement not because it's less effective or safer than a drug, but because of the kinds of claims Pharmanex is making for it. Labeling is crucial: The packaging for a drug can say the medicine will treat disease, while a supplement's label can promise nothing more than improvements in the body's workings or general well-being—its "structure and function." Cholestin's label doesn't make a drug claim, says Michael Chang, chief scientific officer at Pharmanex, because it promises to treat high cholesterol, not heart disease.

These fine points matter. Mevacor, the prescription drug that contains lovastatin, had to pass exhaustive clinical tests before Merck Pharmaceutical could say it lowers cholesterol. The assertions about Cholestin, on the other hand, are based on relatively small short-term Chinese studies, most of which used a more concentrated form of the active ingredient.

But aren't herbs and other supplements safer than drugs—milder, with fewer side effects? It's true that the chemical combinations in herbs are sometimes easier on the body than single-compound drugs. Case in point: Valerian, the herbal sleep aid, is exceptionally safe. (In Utah two years ago a woman tried to kill herself by taking about 20 times the recommended dose. She was released from the hospital a day later, undamaged.) And herb-based remedies can provide a halfway measure for people who don't want medical treatment. The lovastatin in Cholestin, for instance, is nowhere near as concentrated as that in Mevacor.

But herbal extracts can also be toxic—witness the poison strychnine. Every month dozens of reports of side effects caused by herbs make their way to the FDA. Chaparral, Murdock Madaus Schwabe's first blockbuster, may damage the liver. In June the agency proposed regulations for the stimulant ma huang, or ephedra, after it was linked to two deaths and implicated in 15 more. Amino acid and hormone supplements can pose their own risks. True, approved drugs have side effects, too, but those are spelled out on the label. "Supplements can provide real benefits," says Silverglade. "But somebody has to decide what the risks and benefits are, and that somebody can't be the supplement producer."

AT MURDOCK Madaus Schwabe, herbs such as echinacea have to pass chemical tests, microbial scans, and mold and mildew screens. The company sells many of its supplements in Europe, where herbs are regulated almost like drugs, so its quality standards are exceptionally high. Once the capsules are filled, they're checked for cracked casings, placed in bottles of recycled plastic, double-sealed, and laser-scanned.

But all this care may come to naught after the label is slapped on. "People kind of know that echinacea is for the immune system, so somebody with lupus might take it. But they shouldn't," says Neil Reay, Murdock's director of communications. Echinacea increases the activity of white blood cells, which fight invaders such as bacteria. In autoimmune diseases like multiple sclerosis and lupus, though, white blood cells attack the body. "We can't tell people that, because that would be a drug claim," he says.

In Germany echinacea labels say the herb can dispatch colds and chronic infections of the respiratory and lower urinary tracts, but warn people with systemic diseases such as MS not to use it. In the United States echinacea labels say only that the herb "promotes well-being during the cold and flu season."

Many consumers here won't be able to decode the nebulous phrases stamped on packages. Some labels on bottled feverfew, for instance, say the herb will "promote normal blood-vessel tone." From that, shoppers can hardly deduce that many herb experts consider it effective for migraine, much less that researchers at Johnson & Johnson agree; in Canada the drug company sells a feverfew medicine explicitly marketed for migraine.

But not in the United States. The FDA has priced its approval out of the market, critics claim. It costs as much as $300 million to prove a prescription remedy's safety and efficacy. No company will spend that kind of money on a plant—which, after all, can't be patented. So while well-researched, clearly labeled herbal medicines outsell prescription drugs in much of Europe, herbs remain a fringe market here.

Activists have suggested no end of remedies for our ailing regulatory system. At one extreme some public interest groups demand that the FDA return to its role of hard-nosed policeman; on the other, trade organizations insist that the free market can sort things out. Varro Tyler and most herb manufacturers stake out positions somewhere in the middle.

"If I were FDA commissioner," Tyler says, "I would take the 25 to 50 best-proven herbs in the world and approve them as over-the-counter drugs. I would set up a blue-ribbon panel of experts to review the evidence and then set about expanding the list."

Tyler models his suggestions on Germany's widely respected Commission E. In 1978 that commission began reviewing all the available literature—whether scientific or anecdotal—on more than 300 herbs, eventually approving two-thirds. The United States, he says, should adopt the German standard for sanctioning herbs as drugs: absolute proof of safety and reasonable proof of efficacy.

In June, when the presidential commission released the first draft of its recommendations, it was clearly influenced by the German system—but not enough to radically revise the law. The U.S. commission did suggest that a panel review the track records of all herbs on the market, that this panel consider whether supplements making preventive or therapeutic claims should be regulated as over-the-counter drugs, and that manufacturers be allowed to provide consumers with more information.

The commission didn't specify, though, whether the review panel would be independent or run by the supplement industry itself—"the fox guarding the henhouse," Silverglade says.

In other words, for the foreseeable future you'll have to fend for yourself. Read labels skeptically, avoid kitchen-sink herbal cocktails, and look for standardized extracts. If you have a serious condition or take prescription drugs, discuss any supplements with your doctor. (Pregnant women should be particularly careful; many supplements pose risks to the fetus.) If you buy herbs regularly, pick up a well-researched guide, or call the American Botanical Council, at 512/331-8868, to order pamphlets on specific herbs. (This fall the council is publishing an English translation of the Commission E monographs, which you can purchase for $189.) To get you started on navigating the supplement jungle, here's a primer on some of the country's most popular natural remedies.

> **While well-researched, clearly labeled herbal medicines outsell prescription drugs in Europe, herbs remain a fringe market here.**

A RELIABLE GUIDE TO TEN TOP
Natural Remedies

Supplements can be potent antidotes—to stanch your sniffles, bring a good night's sleep, maybe even keep you limber and lighthearted as the years add up. But no agency keeps watch to ensure that the pill or tincture you take is safe. A government commission is proposing regulations that should provide bewildered consumers with some help, but real change is at least a few years away. In the meantime, here's HEALTH's lowdown on some top-sellers.

Melatonin

If the supplement industry looks increasingly like the music biz—throwing a new act up the charts every few months—melatonin is its first bona fide superstar. In 1995 alone there were 20 million new melatonin users in the United States.

Secreted by the pineal gland, the hormone helps set the body's clock and may help trigger the onset of sleep. It's no wonder, therefore, that it was first promoted as a cure for jet lag (still its best-established use) and then as an all-purpose sleep aid. But melatonin scored its big hit thanks to the American fear of aging. Levels of hormones like testosterone, estrogen, melatonin, and dehydroepiandrosterone (DHEA) are age markers, endocrinologists have found: They rise through young adulthood, then taper through middle and old age. But what if people keep their levels high? Can they stave off, or even reverse, creeping pains and debility?

Studies with mice and rats suggested they could. Oncologist William Regelson of the Medical College of Virginia and Italian neuroendocrinologist Walter Pierpaoli transplanted pineal glands from young mice into middle-aged and elderly mice to boost their melatonin levels. The mice "appeared to grow young before our eyes," Regelson and Pierpaoli wrote in *The Melatonin Miracle*. The older mice lived as much as 35 percent longer than average.

Like any good tale of stardom, however, this one ends with a fall from grace. First other researchers noted that the rejuvenated mice had been melatonin-deficient at the start. Then, in October 1996, the *Journal of the American Medical Association* published an article raising a number of serious concerns: among others, that melatonin supplements may make people less fertile (and inhibit sex drive in men), and that melatonin constricts arteries in the brains of rats. Finally, in April, the National Institute on Aging launched a media campaign to dissuade people from taking antiaging hormones because of the potential risks.

Regelson is incensed. "The attempt to scare the public away is totally inappropriate," he says. To Regelson's credit, the institute doesn't refute the extravagant claims for melatonin. It only says they won't be proven or disproven for decades. Says Regelson, who turned 72 in July, "I can't afford to wait that long."

If you're equally pressed for time or simply not afraid to experiment, you can buy melatonin as powder, capsules, or tablets. If you're trying to beat insomnia, start with 1 milligram before bedtime, says melatonin researcher Al Lewy of the Oregon Health Sciences University in Portland. (You can increase the dose to as much as 3 mg if necessary.) For jet lag, the dose is .5 mg, but the regimen is more complicated. Start taking it the day before you travel—when you awake if traveling westward, in midafternoon if heading east. When you reach your destination, continue on the same pill-taking schedule according to your hometown clock. And if you hope to slow the aging process? Consult with a doctor, who can test your blood level of melatonin and decide how much would get you back up to the level typical of people in their prime. Have your level checked periodically.

DHEA

The fortunes of DHEA and melatonin have risen and fallen in near parallel. Sometimes called the mother hormone because the body converts it into estrogen and testosterone, DHEA is secreted by the adrenal gland. Fifty years of research have suggested the hormone might alleviate everything from impotence to cancer, heart disease, and the autoimmune disease lupus. Like melatonin, however, DHEA grew popular as an antiaging remedy; and as with melatonin, the most dramatic evidence comes from studies on mice. At the University of Utah School of Medicine, for instance, immunologist Raymond Daynes has seen a "clear 100 percent change" in mice given a DHEA compound, with twice as many animals on the hormone surviving two years.

William Regelson once again trumpeted the benefits of supplements, this time in his book *The Super-Hormone Promise*. Among DHEA's powers, Regelson declared, is the ability to lower the risk of cancer. But a month after the *Journal of the American Medical Association* threw cold water on the melatonin craze, a companion essay declared the verdict still out on DHEA as well; because it raises the levels of sex hormones, the journal noted, it might increase a person's odds of developing ovarian, prostate, and other kinds of cancer.

Again, the operative word is *might*: Neither the benefits nor the risks have been proven. (When it comes to more superficial concerns, however, a few are clearly grounded in fact. High doses of DHEA can increase facial hair in women.)

If you're willing to bet the glass is half full, you'll need to follow the same testing procedure as for melatonin. But don't bother with ground wild yam powder masquerading as a DHEA precursor; although the hormone is synthesized from a compound in wild yams, the powder doesn't do a thing.

Echinacea and Goldenseal

These herbs are frequently used in combination to fight off infection and speed the healing of wounds, but they have strikingly divergent records when it comes to research.

Studies of echinacea suggest it boosts the immune system by increasing the activity of certain types of white blood cells. "I use echinacea, but I wish the scientific work on it were better," says eminent herb expert Varro Tyler. "There have been about 30 studies, and practically every one of them tested a different product. Many were mixtures or different strains of the herb." All of the studies agree, at least, that echinacea almost never causes side effects.

Goldenseal is another matter. "It's okay as an antiseptic for sores in the mouth," Tyler says, "but claims that it stimulates immunity are nonsense." Moreover, the active ingredients in goldenseal can't even get past your stomach walls to do their work. And because goldenseal is scarce and expensive, it's often adulterated with other herbs.

So stick to pure echinacea if you are trying to fight off a cold, flu, or urinary tract infection. Commission E suggests six to nine milliliters of echinacea juice per day. (Most of the research has been done on EchinaGuard, from Nature's Way. Many other products use echinacea root, but the aboveground portions of the plant have been the most thoroughly researched.) Remember, echinacea increases white blood cell activity; so if you have an autoimmune disease, this herb may do more harm than good.

Saint-John's-Wort

With so many people listening to Prozac these days, it's hard for other antidepressants to get a word in edgewise. Saint-John's-wort is an exception. The herb is the most popular antidepressant in Germany: One brand alone outsells Prozac seven to one.

Last year an article in the *British Medical Journal* summarized the results of 23 studies on the herb, most performed in Germany, on 1,757 subjects in all. Fifteen of the studies compared Saint-John's-wort to a placebo; eight measured the herb against tricyclic antidepressants (the pre-Prozac variety). Saint-John's-wort outdid the placebo for mild to moderate depression and had fewer side effects than the drugs. A study not included in the analysis, involving 3,250 patients, found 80 percent felt better or free of symptoms after four weeks.

Internist Cynthia Mulrow, one of the article's authors, says she would recommend the herb as an option for people with low levels of depression. More seriously depressed people who haven't been helped by drugs could try it as well, under a doctor's supervision. Commission E suggests 2 to 4 grams of Saint-John's-wort extract, also known as hypericum, per day.

Ginkgo

The best-studied and most popular herb in Europe, ginkgo is prescribed more than 5 million times per year in Germany alone. Numerous well-controlled studies have shown it can improve blood flow in the brain and the extremities, and alleviate vertigo and ringing in the ears. In the United States it's often advertised as a smart pill. There's only one catch, according to Tyler: "If you have a normal brain, it won't improve your cognitive functions whatsoever. But if you're elderly and are suffering some memory loss, ginkgo is probably worth a try."

The evidence of its safety is solid. In a six-month study of 8,505 patients, only one in 250 suffered any side effects—generally a stomachache, headache, or rash—and these problems went away quickly even with continued use.

The dose ranges from 120 to 240 mg daily. You may have to use ginkgo for six weeks before seeing results, says Robert McCaleb, president and founder of the Herb Research Foundation and a member of the presidential commission on supplement labels. According to herb experts, the most effective ginkgo formulations are those extracted from the leaves using a strictly controlled process developed in Germany. The standardized dry extract is widely available in such products as Gingkoba, Ginkgold, and BioGinkgo.

Valerian

If worry over melatonin's long-term effects keeps you up at night, valerian may be a good alternative. The herb has been used to treat a variety of ills since the first century, when Greek physicians called it *phu*, a word that shares a root with our *phew*.

Valerian's aroma does have a certain cheesy ripeness, but its sedative impact is nothing to wrinkle your nose at. It's widely used in Europe—the French buy more than 50 tons each year—in part because it's exceptionally safe. The herb doesn't intensify the effect of alcohol, though it may increase the wallop of other sedatives. As for efficacy, much research has shown that valerian induces and improves sleep. In one randomized placebo-controlled trial, 89 percent of the subjects reported improved sleep and 44 percent reported "perfect sleep."

"They use valerian in Europe to break addictions to prescription sleep aids like benzodiazepine," says McCaleb.

Commission E recommends 2 to 3 g of the powdered root or extract, or up to one teaspoon of the tincture. The remedy should be taken before bedtime.

Cholestin

Millions of Chinese have eaten vast quantities of the yeast that is Cholestin's crucial ingredient for thousands of years, and 17 clinical trials have found no side effects other than occasional indigestion. But does the chemical produced by the yeast really lower cholesterol? In March Pharmanex, Cholestin's maker, sent U.S. pharmacists a summary of research on Cholestin, along with a cover letter by Varro Tyler. Cholestin has "an extraordinary safety record," Tyler wrote; it has been "determined beyond a doubt [to] reduce serum cholesterol by an average of 25 to 40 points" along with diet and exercise.

At the Center for Human Nutrition at the University of California at Los Angeles, internist David Heber is about to publish results from a double-blind placebo-controlled study. But he already prescribes the supplement to patients attempting to lower their cholesterol through behavioral changes. Drugs frequently aren't prescribed unless cholesterol levels top 240. But, says Heber, "many people above 200 are at risk if they have a family history of heart disease, don't exercise, or have a fatty diet."

Of course, those people should start working out and eating less fat whether or not they try this supplement. Furthermore, at $1 for four 600-mg capsules a day, a Cholestin regimen is more bothersome and expensive than, say, taking vitamin E, which studies have shown helps prevent heart disease. But in a nation where two out of five people die of heart disease, some will want to try all of the above.

Dong Quai

One of the most popular herbs in China and Japan, dong quai represents both the promise and uncertainty of traditional remedies. Chinese and Japanese women have long taken dong quai to regulate their menstrual cycles or to ease cramps. In this country it increasingly pops up as an ingredient in so-called women's supplements. Yet the herb has never been well studied. "When they sell it on the market, it's all mixed up with other things," says Kee Chang Huang, emeritus professor of pharmacology at the University of Louisville and author of *The Pharmacology of Chinese Herbs*. "Manufacturers consider their formula a secret. They will only tell you that inside is dong quai."

Dong quai is rich in vitamin B-12, Huang writes, which may stimulate the manufacture of blood cells, and contains compounds known as coumarins that help relieve cramping and regulate blood flow. But, says Tyler, studies that show the herb really works are lacking. What's more, dong quai occasionally brings on fever and excessive menstrual bleeding, and can make skin sensitive to the sun. Most pharmacologists and herb experts shy away from it.

Saw Palmetto Berry

In the past half century a number of large well-designed clinical trials have indicated that this berry is a worthwhile remedy for men with benign prostatic hypertrophy—that is, an enlarged prostate. Because about half of all men over the age of 50 have somewhat enlarged prostates, and prescription prostate drugs such as Proscar have serious side effects, the potential market for the plant is huge.

"Saw palmetto is bound to become a major herbal remedy in this country," says McCaleb of the Herb Research Foundation. "Studies show it to be more effective than conventional therapies for relief of symptoms, and considerably safer." In one clinical trial 88 percent of about 300 patients with prostate problems considered the saw palmetto therapy successful, as did their physicians.

Saw palmetto doesn't actually shrink the prostate but rather relieves symptoms of enlargement, such as the frequent urge to urinate. The herb creates no problems if taken with other drugs and causes only the rare stomachache. Commission E recommends .5 to 1 g of the dried berry or .6 to 1.5 ml of saw palmetto extract per day.

Glucosamine and Chondroitin

These two substances first pounced onto the American stage last January, with a book called *The Arthritis Cure*, by University of Arizona sports physician Jason Theodosakis. In Asia and Europe, however, the supplements have a longer history; they've been studied for almost 40 years.

The human body produces both compounds and uses them to make cartilage. In supplements glucosamine comes from crab shells, chondroitin from cow cartilage. When people with arthritis took the supplements in double-blind trials overseas, the compounds eased aches as well as standard painkillers did, though more slowly. That's not a bad trade-off, considering that ibuprofen and acetaminophen can cause stomach upset, ulcers, even kidney or liver damage, while glucosamine and chondroitin appear to have few side effects.

Should the arthritic among us rush out to buy this stuff? Well, they aren't a cure, the title of Theodosakis's book notwithstanding; no one thinks they'll prove able to restore cartilage that's been eroded down to the bone. That said, there's no reason not to give these supplements a test run, aside from the usual paucity of studies, especially on the two supplements taken together. U.S. scientists have reserved judgment on much of the research done elsewhere, compounding the uncertainty. In sum: The risks of long-term use are unclear, ideal doses haven't been determined, and the quality of supplements varies wildly. One analysis of 25 brands found that some contained neither glucosamine nor chondroitin.

A number of studies are currently under way in this country. Amal Das, an orthopedic surgeon in Hendersonville, North Carolina, is giving chondroitin and glucosamine to patients in a six-month double-blind trial. He recommends three pills a day of Cosamin DS, a product made by Nutramax, which he says reliably contains 400 mg of chondroitin and 500 mg of glucosamine.

At that dosage the remedy isn't cheap, costing more than $1.50 a day. If the supplements merely deaden pain, Das says, they'll be no big deal but still worth taking because they're relatively free of side effects. On the other hand, they may actually protect cartilage and even rebuild it somewhat. "That," he says, "would be very exciting."

Burkhard Bilger is a contributing editor.

An FDA Guide to Dietary Supplements

by Paula Kurtzweil

Set between a Chinese restaurant and a pizza and sub sandwich eatery, a Rockville health food store offers yet another brand of edible items: Bottled herbs like cat's claw, dandelion root, and blessed thistle. Vitamins and minerals in varying doses. Herbal and nutrient concoctions whose labels carry claims about relieving pain, "energizing" and "detoxifying" the body, or providing "guaranteed results."

This store sells dietary supplements, some of the hottest selling items on the market today. Surveys show that more than half of the U.S. adult population uses these products. In 1996 alone, consumers spent more than $6.5 billion on dietary supplements, according to Packaged Facts Inc., a market research firm in New York City.

But even with all the business they generate, consumers still ask questions about dietary supplements: Can their claims be trusted? Are they safe? Does the Food and Drug Administration approve them?

Many of these questions come in the wake of the 1994 Dietary Supplement Health and Education Act, or DSHEA, which set up a new framework for FDA regulation of dietary supplements. It also created an office in the National Institutes of Health to coordinate research on dietary supplements, and it called on President Clinton to set up an independent dietary supplement commission to report on the use of claims in dietary supplement labeling.

In passing DSHEA, Congress recognized first, that many people believe dietary supplements offer health benefits and second, that consumers want a greater opportunity to determine whether supplements may help them. The law essentially gives dietary supplement manufacturers freedom to market more products as dietary supplements and provide information about their products' benefits—for example, in product labeling.

The Council for Responsible Nutrition, an organization of manufacturers of dietary supplements and their suppliers, welcomes the change. "Our philosophy has been ... to maintain consumer access to products and access to information [so that consumers can] make informed choices," says John Cordaro, the group's

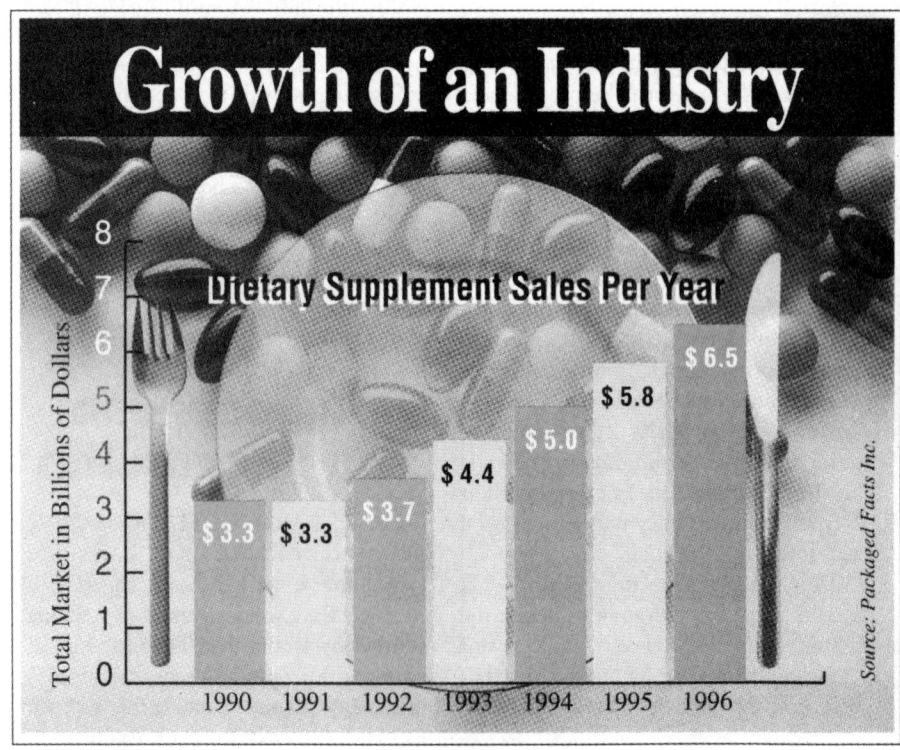

president and chief executive officer.

But in choosing whether to use dietary supplements, FDA answers consumers' questions by noting that under DSHEA, FDA's requirement for premarket review of dietary supplements is less than that over other products it regulates, such as drugs and many additives used in conventional foods.

This means that consumers *and* manufacturers also have responsibility for checking the safety of dietary supplements and determining the truthfulness of label claims.

What Is a Dietary Supplement?

Traditionally, dietary supplements referred to products made of one or more of the essential nutrients, such as vitamins, minerals, and protein. But DSHEA broadens the definition to include, with some exceptions, any product intended for ingestion as a supplement to the diet. This includes vitamins; minerals; herbs, botanicals, and other plant-derived substances; and amino acids (the individual building blocks of protein) and concentrates, metabolites, constituents and extracts of these substances.

It's easy to spot a supplement because DSHEA requires manufacturers to include the words "dietary supplement" on product labels. Also, starting in March 1999, a "Supplement Facts" panel will be required on the labels of most dietary supplements.

Dietary supplements come in many forms, including tablets, capsules, powders, softgels, gelcaps, and liquids. Though commonly associated with health food stores, dietary supplements also are sold in grocery, drug and national discount chain stores, as well as through mail-order catalogs, TV programs, the Internet, and direct sales.

FDA oversees safety, manufacturing and product information, such as claims, in a product's labeling, package inserts, and accompanying literature. The Federal Trade Commission regulates the advertising of dietary supplements.

One thing dietary supplements are not is drugs. A drug, which sometimes can be derived from plants used as traditional medicines, is an article that, among other things, is intended to diagnose, cure, mitigate, treat, or prevent diseases. Before marketing, drugs must undergo clinical studies to determine their effectiveness, safety, possible interactions with other substances, and appropriate dosages, and FDA must review these data and authorize the drugs' use before they are marketed. FDA does not authorize or test dietary supplements.

A product sold as a dietary supplement and touted in its labeling as a new treatment or cure for a specific disease or condition would be considered an unauthorized—and thus illegal—drug. Labeling changes consistent with the provisions in DSHEA would be required to maintain the product's status as a dietary supplement.

Another thing dietary supplements are not are replacements for conventional diets, nutritionists say. Supplements do not provide all the known—and perhaps unknown—nutritional benefits of conventional food.

Monitoring for Safety

As with food, federal law requires manufacturers of dietary supplements to ensure that the products they put on the market are safe. But supplement manufacturers do not have to provide information to FDA to get a product on the market, unlike the food additive process often required of new food ingredients. FDA review and approval of supplement ingredients and products is not required before marketing.

Food additives not generally recognized as safe must undergo FDA's premarket approval process for new food ingredients. This requires manufacturers to conduct safety studies and submit the results to FDA for review before the ingredient can be used in marketed products. Based on its review, FDA either authorizes or rejects the food additive.

> **Structure-function claims can be easy to spot because, on the label, they must be accompanied with the disclaimer "This statement has not been evaluated by the Food and Drug Administration. This product is not intended to diagnose, treat, cure, or prevent any disease."**

In contrast, dietary supplement manufacturers that wish to market a new ingredient (that is, an ingredient not marketed in the United States before 1994) have two options. The first involves submitting to FDA, at least 75 days before the product is expected to go on the market, information that supports their conclusion that a new ingredient can reasonably be expected to be safe. Safe means that the new ingredient does not present a significant or unreasonable risk of illness or injury under conditions of use recommended in the product's labeling.

The information the manufacturer submits becomes publicly available 90 days after FDA receives it.

Another option for manufacturers is to petition FDA, asking the agency to establish the conditions under which the new dietary ingredient would reasonably be expected to be safe. To date, FDA's Center for Food Safety and Applied Nutrition has received no such petitions.

Under DSHEA, once a dietary supplement is marketed, FDA has the responsibility for showing that a dietary supplement is unsafe before it can take action to restrict the product's use. This was the case when, in June 1997, FDA proposed, among other things, to limit the amount of ephedrine alkaloids in dietary supplements (marketed as ephedra, Ma huang, Chinese ephedra, and epitonin, for example) and provide warnings to consumers about hazards associated with use of dietary supplements containing the ingredients. The hazards ranged from nervousness, dizziness, and changes in blood pressure and heart rate to chest pain, heart attack, hepatitis, stroke, seizures, psychosis, and death. The proposal stemmed from FDA's review of adverse event reports it had received,

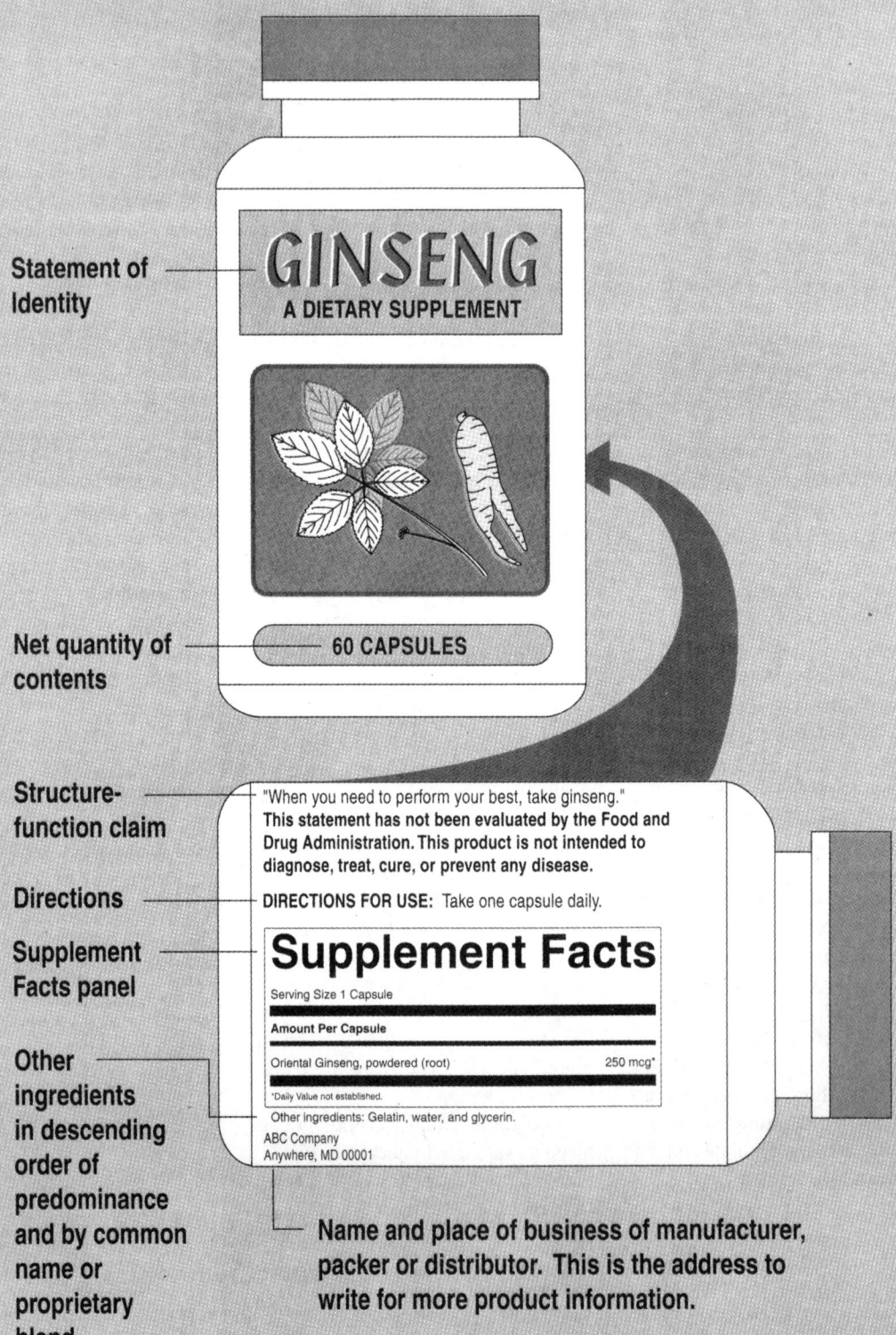

scientific literature, and public comments. FDA has received many comments on the 1997 proposal and was reviewing them at press time.

Also in 1997, FDA identified contamination of the herbal ingredient plantain with the harmful herb *Digitalis lanata* after receiving a report of a complete heart block in a young woman. FDA traced all use of the contaminated ingredient and asked manufacturers and retailers to withdraw these products from the market.

DSHEA also gives FDA authority to establish good manufacturing practices, or GMPs, for dietary supplements. In a February 1997 advance notice of proposed rulemaking, the agency said it would establish dietary supplement GMPs if, after public comment, it determined that GMPs for conventional food are not adequate to cover dietary supplements, as well. GMPs, the agency said, would ensure that dietary supplements are made under conditions that would result in safe and properly labeled products. At press time, FDA was reviewing comments on the 1997 notice.

Some supplement makers may already voluntarily follow GMPs devised, for example, by trade groups.

Besides FDA, individual states can take steps to restrict or stop the sale of potentially harmful dietary supplements within their jurisdictions. For example, Florida has already banned all ephedra-containing products, and other states have said they are considering similar action.

Also, the industry strives to regulate itself, the Council for Responsible Nutrition's Cordaro says. He cites the GMPs that his trade group and others developed for their member companies. FDA is reviewing these GMPs as it considers whether to pursue mandatory industry-wide GMPs. Another example of self-regulation, Cordaro says, is the voluntary use of a warning about ephedra products that his organization drafted. He says that about 90 percent of U.S. manufacturers of products containing ephedra alkaloids now use this warning label.

Understanding Claims

Claims that tout a supplement's healthful benefits have always been a controversial feature of dietary supplements. Manufacturers often rely on them to sell their products. But consumers often wonder whether they can trust them.

Under DSHEA and previous food labeling laws, supplement manufacturers are allowed to use, when appropriate, three types of claims: nutrient-content claims, disease claims, and nutrition support claims, which include "structure-function claims."

Nutrient-content claims describe the level of a nutrient in a food or dietary supplement. For example, a supplement containing at least 200 milligrams of calcium per serving could carry the claim "high in calcium." A supplement with at least 12 mg per serving of vitamin C could state on its label, "Excellent source of vitamin C."

Disease claims show a link between a food or substance and a disease or health-related condition. FDA authorizes these claims based on a review of the scientific evidence. Or, after the agency is notified, the claims may be based on an authoritative statement from certain scientific bodies, such as the National Academy of Sciences, that shows or describes a well-established diet-to-health link. As of this writing, certain dietary supplements may be eligible to carry disease claims, such as claims that show a link between:
- the vitamin folic acid and a decreased risk of neural tube defect-affected pregnancy, if the supplement contains sufficient amounts of folic acid
- calcium and a lower risk of osteoporosis, if the supplement contains sufficient amounts of calcium
- psyllium seed husk (as part of a diet low in cholesterol and saturated fat) and coronary heart disease, if the supplement contains sufficient amounts of psyllium seed husk.

Nutrition support claims can describe a link between a nutrient and the deficiency disease that can result if the nutrient is lacking in the diet. For example, the label of a vitamin C supplement could state that vitamin C prevents scurvy. When these types of claims are used, the label must mention the prevalence of the nutrient-deficiency disease in the United States.

These claims also can refer to the supplement's effect on the body's structure or function, including its overall

Supplement Your Knowledge

Some sources for additional information on dietary supplements are:

Federal Agencies

Food and Drug Administration:

Office of Consumer Affairs
HFE-88
Rockville, MD 20857

Food Information Line
1-800-FDA-4010
(202) 205-4314 in the Washington, D.C., area

FDA Website
www.cfsan.fda.gov/~dms/supplmnt.html

Federal Trade Commission
Public Reference Branch
Room 130
Washington, DC 20580
www.ftc.gov

National Institute on Aging
NIA Information Center
P.O. Box 8057
Gaithersburg, MD 20898-8057
1-800-222-2225
TTY: 1-800-222-4225
http://128.231.160.11/nia/health/pubpub/hormrev.htm

Health Professional Organizations

American Dietetic Association
216 W. Jackson Blvd.
Chicago, IL 60606-6995
1-800-366-1655 (recorded messages)
1-900-225-5267 (to talk to a registered dietitian)
www.eatright.org

9 ❖ CONSUMER HEALTH

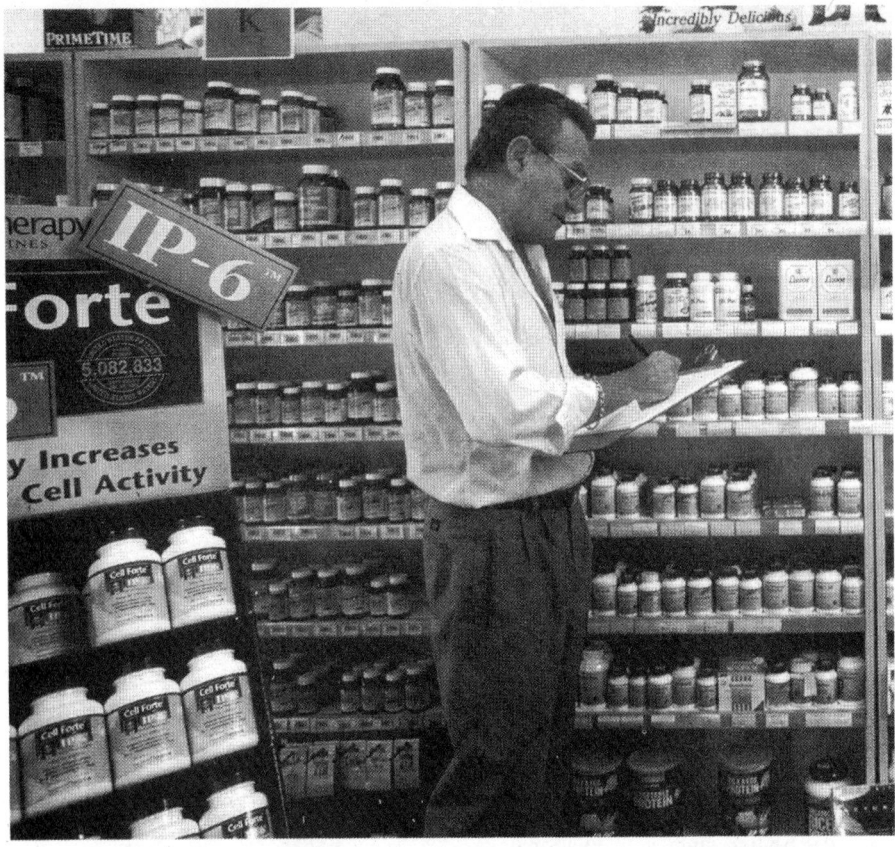

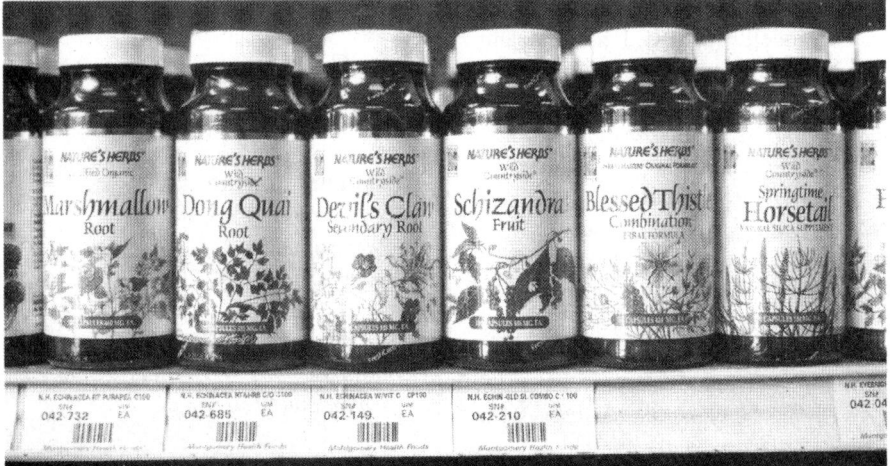

Carlo Scarzella, owner of Montgomery Health Foods in Rockville, Md., checks inventory (top photo). Like many health food stores, his carries an array of herbal products.

PHOTOGRAPHS BY NORMAN WATKINS

effect on a person's well-being. These are known as structure-function claims.

Examples of structure-function claims are:
- Calcium builds strong bones.
- Antioxidants maintain cell integrity.
- Fiber maintains bowel regularity.

Manufacturers can use structure-function claims without FDA authorization. They base their claims on their review and interpretation of the scientific literature. Like all label claims, structure-function claims must be true and not misleading.

Structure-function claims can be easy to spot because, on the label, they must be accompanied with the disclaimer *"This statement has not been evaluated by the Food and Drug Administration. This product is not intended to diagnose, treat, cure, or prevent any disease."*

Manufacturers who plan to use a structure-function claim on a particular product must inform FDA of the use of the claim no later than 30 days after the product is first marketed. While the manufacturer must be able to substantiate its claim, it does not have to share the substantiation with FDA or make it publicly available.

If the submitted claims promote the products as drugs instead of supplements, FDA can advise the manufacturer to change or delete the claim.

Because there often is a fine line between disease claims and structure-function claims, FDA in April proposed regulations that would establish criteria under which a label claim would or would not qualify as a disease claim. Among label factors FDA proposed for consideration are:
- the naming of a specific disease or class of diseases
- the use of scientific or lay terminology to describe the product's effect on one or more signs or symptoms recognized by health-care professionals and consumers as characteristic of a specific disease or a number of different specific diseases
- product name
- statements about product formulation
- citations or references that refer to disease
- use of the words "disease" or "diseased"
- art, such as symbols and pictures
- statements that the product can substitute for an approved therapy (for example, a drug).

46. FDA Guide to Dietary Supplements

FDA's proposal is consistent with the guidance on the distinction between structure-function and disease claims provided in the 1997 report by the President's Commission on Dietary Supplement Labels.

If shoppers find dietary supplements whose labels state or imply that the product can help diagnose, treat, cure, or prevent a disease (for example, "cures cancer" or "treats arthritis"), they should realize that the product is being marketed illegally as a drug and as such has not been evaluated for safety or effectiveness.

FTC regulates claims made in the advertising of dietary supplements, and in recent years, that agency has taken a number of enforcement actions against companies whose advertisements contained false and misleading information. The actions targeted, for example, erroneous claims that chromium picolinate was a treatment for weight loss and high blood cholesterol. An action in 1997 targeted ads for an ephedrine alkaloid supplement because they understated the degree of the product's risk and featured a man falsely described as a doctor.

Fraudulent Products

Consumers need to be on the lookout for fraudulent products. These are products that don't do what they say they can or don't contain what they say they contain. At the very least, they waste consumers' money, and they may cause physical harm.

Fraudulent products often can be identified by the types of claims made in their labeling, advertising and promotional literature. Some possible indicators of fraud, says Stephen Barrett, M.D., a board member of the National Council Against Health Fraud, are:

- Claims that the product is a secret cure and use of such terms as "breakthrough," "magical," "miracle cure," and "new discovery." If the product were a cure for a serious disease, it would be widely reported in the media and used by health-care professionals, he says.
- "Pseudomedical" jargon, such as "detoxify," "purify" and "energize" to describe a product's effects. These claims are vague and hard to measure, Barrett says. So, they make it easier for success to be claimed "even though nothing has actually been accomplished," he says.
- Claims that the product can cure a wide range of unrelated diseases. No product can do that, he says.
- Claims that a product is backed by scientific studies, but with no list of references or references that are inadequate. For instance, if a list of references is provided, the citations cannot be traced, or if they are traceable, the studies are out-of-date, irrelevant, or poorly designed.
- Claims that the supplement has only benefits—and no side effects. A product "potent enough to help people will be potent enough to cause side effects," Barrett says.
- Accusations that the medical profession, drug companies and the government are suppressing information about a particular treatment. It would be illogical, Barrett says, for large numbers of people to withhold information about potential medical therapies when they or their families and friends might one day benefit from them.

Though often more difficult to do, consumers also can protect themselves from economic fraud, a practice in which the manufacturer substitutes part or all of a product with an inferior, cheaper ingredient and then passes off the fake product as the real thing but at a lower cost. Varro Tyler, Ph.D., Sc.D., a distinguished professor emeritus of pharmacognosy (the study of medicinal products in their crude, or unprepared, form) at Purdue University in West LaFayette, Ind., advises consumers to avoid products sold for considerably less money than competing brands. "If it's too cheap, the product is probably not what it's supposed to be," he says.

Quality Products

Poor manufacturing practices are not unique to dietary supplements, but the growing market for supplements in a less restrictive regulatory environment creates the potential for supplements to be prone to quality-control problems. For example, FDA has identified several problems where some manufacturers were buying herbs, plants and other ingredients without first adequately testing them to determine whether the product they ordered was actually what they received or whether the ingredients were free from contaminants.

To help protect themselves, consumers should:

- Look for ingredients in products with the U.S.P. notation, which indicates the manufacturer followed standards established by the U.S. Pharmacopoeia.
- Realize that the label term "natural" doesn't guarantee that a product is safe. "Think of poisonous mushrooms," says Elizabeth Yetley, Ph.D., director of FDA's Office of Special Nutritionals. "They're natural."
- Consider the name of the manufacturer

Expert Advice

Before starting a dietary supplement, it's always wise to check with a medical doctor. It is especially important for people who are:

- pregnant or breastfeeding
- chronically ill
- elderly
- under 18
- taking prescription or over-the-counter medicines. Certain supplements can boost blood levels of certain drugs to dangerous levels.

Varro Tyler, Ph.D., Sc.D., distinguished professor emeritus of pharmacognosy at Purdue University, cites as examples garlic and the supplement ginkgo biloba. Both can thin the blood, which can be hazardous, he says, for people taking prescription medicines that also thin the blood.

In addition to medical doctors, other health-care professionals, such as registered pharmacists, registered dietitians and nutritionists, also can be sources of information about dietary supplements. ∎

—P.K.

9 ❖ CONSUMER HEALTH

Supplements Associated

NAME	POSSIBLE HEALTH HAZARDS
Herbal Ingredients	
Chaparral (a traditional American Indian medicine)	liver disease, possibly irreversible
Comfrey	obstruction of blood flow to liver, possibly leading to death
Slimming/dieter's teas	nausea, diarrhea, vomiting, stomach cramps, chronic constipation, fainting, possibly death (see "Dieter's Brews Make Tea Time a Dangerous Affair" in the July-August 1997 *FDA Consumer*)
Ephedra (also known as Ma huang, Chinese Ephedra and epitonin)	ranges from high blood pressure, irregular heartbeat, nerve damage, injury, insomnia, tremors, and headaches to seizures, heart attack, stroke, and death
Germander	liver disease, possibly leading to death
Lobelia (also known as Indian tobacco)	range from breathing problems at low doses to sweating, rapid heartbeat, low blood pressure, and possibly coma and death at higher doses
Magnolia-Stephania preparation	kidney disease, possibly leading to permanent kidney failure
Willow bark	Reye syndrome, a potentially fatal disease associated with aspirin intake in children with chickenpox or flu symptoms; allergic reaction in adults. (Willow bark is marketed as an aspirin-free product, although it actually contains an ingredient that converts to the same active ingredient in aspirin.)
Wormwood	neurological symptoms, characterized by numbness of legs and arms, loss of intellect, delirium, and paralysis

or distributor. Supplements made by a nationally known food and drug manufacturer, for example, have likely been made under tight controls because these companies already have in place manufacturing standards for their other products.
• Write to the supplement manufacturer for more information. Ask the company about the conditions under which its products were made.

Reading and Reporting

Consumers who use dietary supplements should always read product labels, follow directions, and heed all warnings.

Supplement users who suffer a serious harmful effect or illness that they think is related to supplement use should call a doctor or other health-care provider. He or she in turn can report it to FDA MedWatch by calling 1-800-FDA-1088 or going to *www.fda.gov/medwatch/report/hcp.htm* on the MedWatch Website. Patients' names are kept confidential.

Consumers also may call the toll-free MedWatch number or go to *www.fda.gov/medwatch/report/consumer/consumer.htm* on the MedWatch Website to report an adverse reaction. To file a report, consumers will be asked to provide:

• name, address and telephone number of the person who became ill
• name and address of the doctor or hospital providing medical treatment
• description of the problem
• name of the product and store where it was bought.

Consumers also should report the problem to the manufacturer or distributor listed on the product's label and to the store where the product was bought.

Today's Dietary Supplements

The report of the President's Commission on Dietary Supplement Labels, released in

46. FDA Guide to Dietary Supplements

With Illnesses And Injuries

NAME	POSSIBLE HEALTH HAZARDS
Vitamins and Essential Minerals	
Vitamin A in doses of 25,000 or more International Units a day	birth defects, bone abnormalities, and severe liver disease
Vitamin B_6 in doses above 100 milligrams a day	balance difficulties, nerve injury causing changes in touch sensation
Niacin in slow-released doses of 500 mg or more a day or immediate-release doses of 750 mg or more a day	range from stomach pain, vomiting, bloating, nausea, cramping, and diarrhea to liver disease, muscle disease, eye damage, and heart injury
Selenium in doses of about 800 micrograms to 1,000 mcg a day	tissue damage
Other Supplements	
Germanium (a nonessential mineral)	kidney damage, possibly death
L-tryptophan (an amino acid)	eosinophilia myalgia syndrome, a potentially fatal blood disorder that can cause high fever, muscle and joint pain, weakness, skin rash, and swelling of the arms and legs

(Source: FDA Statement before Senate Committee on Labor and Human Resources, Oct. 21, 1993)

November 1997, provides a look at the future of dietary supplements. It encourages researchers to find out whether consumers want and can use the information allowed in dietary supplement labeling under DSHEA. It encourages studies to identify more clearly the relationships between dietary supplements and health maintenance and disease prevention. It urges FDA to take enforcement action when questions about a product's safety arise. And it suggests that FDA and the industry work together to develop guidelines on the use of warning statements on dietary supplement labels.

FDA generally concurred with the commission's recommendations in the agency's 1998 proposed rule on dietary supplement claims.

While much remains unknown about many dietary supplements—their health benefits and potential risks, for example—there's one thing consumers can count on: the availability of a wide range of such products. But consumers who decide to take advantage of the expanding market should do so with care, making sure they have the necessary information and consulting with their doctors and other health professionals as needed.

"The majority of supplement manufacturers are responsible and careful," FDA's Yetley says. "But, as with all products on the market, consumers need to be discriminating. FDA and industry have important roles to play, but consumers must take responsibility, too."

Paula Kurtzweil is a member of FDA's public affairs staff.

Unit 10

Unit Selections

47. **Quiz: Are You Ready for the Sun?** Cynthia Moekle Pigott
48. **Germ Crazy,** Deborah Franklin
49. **The Frog Solution,** Josie Glausiusz
50. **Prevent Sexually Transmitted Diseases,** Lauren Picker
51. **Irradiation: A Safe Measure for Safer Food,** John Henkel
52. **Why Is Date Rape So Hard to Prove?** Sheila Weller

Key Points to Consider

❖ What do you consider to be our greatest environmental health hazard today?

❖ Are you concerned about the damaging effects of UV radiation on your skin? What steps are you taking to prevent such damage?

❖ Do you use antibacterial products such as antibacterial soap? Would you use it if you knew that doing so would lead to the same kind of bacterial resistance that we have observed with antibiotics?

❖ How do feel about using irradiation to safeguard our food? Would you buy food products that you knew had been irradiated?

❖ What could the government do to help combat the spread of STDs? What are you personally doing to reduce your risk of contracting them?

❖ What safety measures can you take to reduce your chances of being a victim of date rape or some other form of violent crime?

❖ Do our laws governing violent acts need to be changed? Explain.

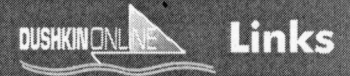 **Links** www.dushkin.com/online/

33. **Centers for Disease Control and Prevention**
    http://www.cdc.gov
34. **Sexual Assault Information Page**
    http://www.cs.utk.edu/~bartley/saInfoPage.html

These sites are annotated on pages 4 and 5.

Contemporary Health Hazards

This unit examines a variety of health hazards that Americans must face on a daily basis and includes topics ranging from environmental health issues to infectious illness to acts of violence.

Over the past 25 years, Americans have been inundated with health warnings about toxic substances in the air, water, and food. While some improvements have been observed in the areas of air and water pollution, much remains to be done, and new areas of concern continue to surface.

Of all the environmental health issues, atmospheric pollution by chlorofluorocarbon compounds (CFCs) and carbon dioxide seems to have generated the most concern worldwide. CFCs are synthetic products that have achieved worldwide acceptance as components of refrigerants, propellants, and solvents. These compounds, when released into the atmosphere, destroy the ozone layer that shields Earth from ultraviolet (UV) radiation. This protective layer appears to be undergoing a rapid depletion; consequently, there has been a steady rise in the amount of UV radiation to which we are exposed. Most experts agree that we will witness significant increases in the incidence of skin cancer because of this depletion. To protect against the damaging effects of this form of radiation, medical authorities have encouraged us to apply liberal amounts of sunscreen to our skin. But do sunscreens really work? Cynthia Moekle Pigott, in her article "Quiz: Are You Ready for the Sun?" addresses the issue of sunscreens and cancer through a self-test and provides useful tips for protecting oneself from the damaging effects of ultraviolet radiation.

According to the Centers for Disease Control and Prevention in Atlanta, the spectrum of infectious diseases is growing, and many infectious diseases once thought to be under control are becoming increasingly resistant to standard antibiotic interventions. Ironically, many of the antibiotic-resistant bacteria found today probably had their origins in our hospitals, where massive amounts of antibiotics were being used. "Germ Crazy" by Deborah Franklin discusses the growing concern among scientists that our overuse of antibacterial consumer products such as antibacterial soap may result in the same kind of resistance to these products that we have observed with antibiotics. Amid all this gloom and doom regarding infectious illnesses there is one bright spot worth noting, and that is the discovery of "peptide antibiotics." Peptide antibiotics are small strings of amino acids that display the same disease-fighting ability as traditional antibiotics. What is different about them is that they originate from an animal's own immune system, and their mode of action against pathogens is different from standard antibiotics in a way that makes it much more difficult for resistance to develop. "The Frog Solution," by Josie Glausiusz explains what "peptide antibiotics" are, and discusses how their use may revolutionize our treatment of infectious illnesses.

The infectious illness that consistently gets media coverage is AIDS. AIDS is, however, just one of a number of sexually transmitted diseases (STDs). While AIDS has clearly received the most publicity, other STDs, such as chlamydia, human papilloma virus (HPV), genital herpes, gonorrhea, and hepatitis B, are infecting Americans at the rate of 12 million new cases a year, with 66 percent of the new cases affecting people under the age of 25. Based on current statistics, the infection rate of these STDs is 10 times that of AIDS, and individuals infected with these diseases are more susceptible to contracting AIDS should they be exposed to the HIV virus. It should also be noted here that AIDS is not the only STD for which there is no cure. HPV, Hepatitis B, and genital herpes are also viral infections and are currently incurable. When most people think of STDs other than AIDS, they generally regard them as embarrassing infections rather than the serious health threat that they are. It has often been said that STDs do not discriminate with regard to whom they infect, but current findings suggest otherwise. Women appear to be much more likely to become infected (through sexual intercourse) than men, and the health consequences of such infections are greater for them as well. Just how serious a health hazard are the STDs? Consider this: It is estimated that by age 30, over 50 percent of all Americans will have been infected at least once. The essay "Prevent Sexually Transmitted Diseases" explains why the public needs to become more aware of STDs and presents the reader with a short discussion of the six most common STDs.

Still another example of a health hazard attributable to microorganisms is food-borne illnesses. Despite the numerous safety precautions taken by the food industry, there may be as many as 80 million cases of "food poisoning" annually in the United States with a death toll in excess of 9,000. Due to the widespread occurrence of these illnesses, irradiation of food products is becoming an increasingly popular idea within the food industry. Irradiation has been found to be a safe and effective way to destroy both disease-causing microorganisms and insects, which can lead to spoilage and food-borne infections. Just how safe is irradiated food and will consumers accept it are questions addressed in the article, "Irradiation: A Safe Measure for Safer Food."

Another health hazard that warrants inclusion in this unit is violence. Sexual assault or rape is one of the most violent acts. It has become so common on college campuses that it frequently surpasses theft as the foremost security issue. Sheila Weller's article "Why Is Date Rape So Hard to Prove?" addresses the issue of why it is difficult to make the rape charge stick.

Article 47

Quiz: Are You Ready for the Sun?

May is National Skin Cancer Detection and Prevention Month, so it's a good time to test your knowledge about the subject. Answer true or false to the following questions.

___ **1.** About 70,000 Americans develop skin cancer each year.

___ **2.** Basal cell carcinoma is the most dangerous type of skin cancer.

___ **3.** You should do a self-exam for skin cancer every six to eight weeks.

___ **4.** A mole that is wider than the diameter of a pinhead may be a sign of malignant melanoma.

___ **5.** Skin cancer is most often caused by exposure to ultraviolet (UV) rays.

___ **6.** Fair-skinned people are at greater risk of developing all types of skin cancer than are darker-skinned people.

___ **7.** One or more blistering sunburns during childhood or adolescence can double one's risk of developing malignant melanoma.

___ **8.** People who spend time in the sun only on weekends are at greater risk of developing malignant melanoma than those who are in the sun every day.

___ **9.** Since the sun's rays are strongest between 10 a.m. and 3 p.m., there's no need to take precautions at other times.

___ **10.** Unlike ultraviolet B (UVB) rays, ultraviolet A (UVA) rays are harmless.

___ **11.** If you burn without protection after 10 minutes in the sun, wearing a sunscreen with an SPF of eight would allow you to stay in the sun eight times longer (80 minutes) before you'd burn.

___ **12.** You should wear a sunscreen even on overcast days, since 80% of the sun's rays pass through clouds.

___ **13.** A sunscreen with an SPF of 50 is 67% more effective than one with an SPF of 30.

___ **14.** You should apply sunscreen 15 to 30 minutes before going outside.

___ **15.** A UV index reading of 15 is very high.

___ **16.** The sun can penetrate some types of clothing.

___ **17.** You can get a sunburn even sitting under an umbrella at the beach.

___ **18.** The UV rays in tanning booths are safe.

___ **19.** It's okay to use a sunscreen that's been sitting in your medicine chest for a few years.

___ **20.** In addition to sunscreen, a baseball cap provides good protection for your face.

ANSWERS

1. *False.* Every year, more than 800,000 Americans develop skin cancer, and some 9,300 die from it.

2. *False.* Basal cell carcinoma is the most *common* form of skin cancer, affecting some 560,000 Americans each year. BCC's usually take the form of translucent nodules and are frequently found on the face (especially the nose), neck, hands and torso. Rarely deadly, BCC's grow slowly and usually don't spread to other organs; if treated early, they can be cured in at least 95% of cases.

Squamous cell carcinoma is the second most prevalent skin cancer, affecting about 150,000 people every year. SCC's are red or pink scaly nodules or wart-like growths that ulcerate in the center; they're typically found on the face (especially the lips), the ears, the hands and other sun-exposed parts of the body. SCC's can be deadly, grow-

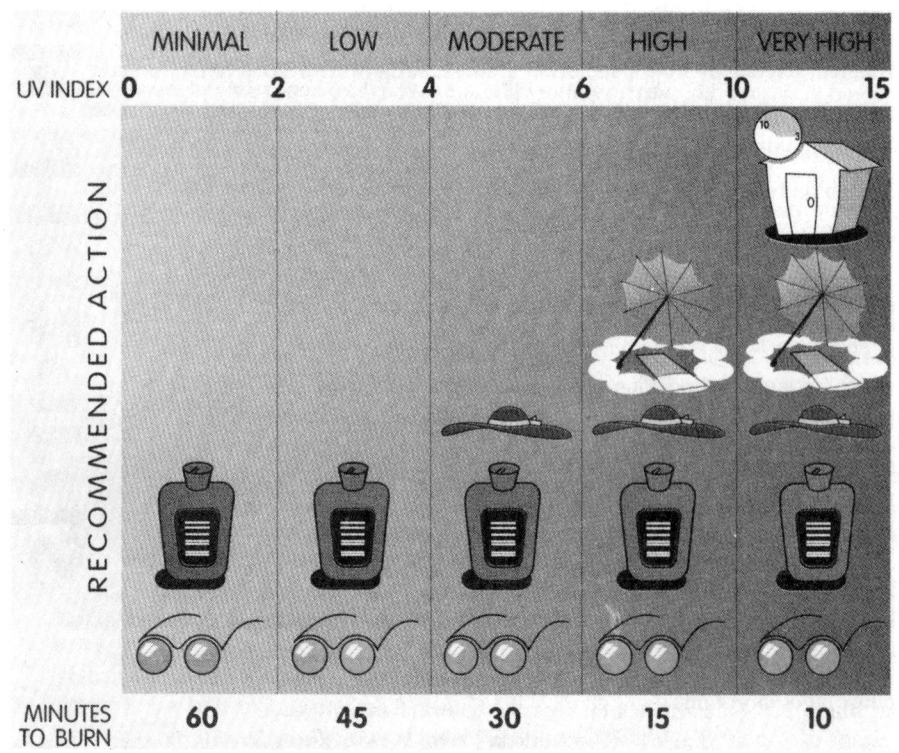

THIS CHART SHOWS THE LEVELS OF THE UV INDEX, HOW LONG IT TAKES TO BURN IN THE SUN *WITHOUT* SUNSCREEN AND WHAT YOU CAN DO TO PROTECT YOURSELF.

ing quickly and spreading to other organs. But if treated early, SCC's also have a 95% cure rate.

Malignant melanoma is the least common skin cancer—about 32,000 cases each year—but it is the most dangerous form, accounting for 75% of skin cancer deaths. Melanomas are cancerous moles that most frequently appear on the upper back, torso, lower legs, head and neck. Melanoma is likelier than other skin cancers to spread to other parts of the body, making it more difficult to cure.

3. *True.* Use a full-length and a hand mirror to look for any new skin discolorations or growths and any changes in the shape, size or color of moles, birthmarks and freckles. Don't forget to check your palms, soles and scalp and the spaces between your fingers and toes. If you notice anything unusual, see your primary-care doctor or a dermatologist right away. And fair-haired people especially should have an all-body exam by a doctor every year.

4. *False.* A mole that is wider than the diameter of a pencil eraser (a quarter-inch) may be a sign of melanoma. To distinguish normal moles from pigmentations that could be melanoma, use the "ABCD" guideline:

Asymmetry. Does one half look different from the other?

Border irregularity. Are the edges of the mole ragged, notched or blurred?

Color. Does the color vary within the mole, including shades of tan, brown or black and sometimes patches of white, red or blue?

Diameter. Is the mole wider than the diameter of a pencil eraser?

5. *True.* In one recent study, melanoma incidence was 68% to 97% lower in people or body sites (such as the buttocks) with little or no sun exposure.

6. *True.* Fair-skinned people, especially those with blond or red hair, have less melanin, a pigment in skin cells that helps prevent burning and long-term skin damage.

7. *True.*

8. *True.*

9. *False.* The sun is still strong enough to cause damage at other times of day.

10. *False.* Two types of UV light reach the Earth: UVA rays, which primarily cause premature wrinkling, and UVB rays, which primarily cause burning. Researchers now believe that both UVA and UVB light cause cancer. For this reason, a "broad-spectrum" sunscreen, which protects against both UVA and UVB rays, is the best choice. (Note: A sunscreen's SPF refers only to UVB, not UVA, rays.)

11. *True.* To figure out how long a sunscreen will allow you to stay in the sun, multiply the amount of time it takes you to burn without protection by the sunscreen's SPF.

12. *True.*

13. *False.* A sunscreen with an SPF of 50 is actually only 1% to 2% more effective than one with an SPF of 30. "After SPF 30, you tend to reach a point of diminishing returns," explains microbiologist Jeanne Rippere of the office of over-the-counter drugs at the FDA. For this reason, the agency plans to limit sunscreen ratings to SPF 30.

14. *True.*

15. *True.* Many newspapers and local TV stations now report the day's UV index, a measurement of the sun's intensity for a particular region. Developed by the Environmental Protection Agency, the National Weather Service and the Centers for Disease Control and Prevention, the index rates UV levels from 0, or "minimal," to 15, or "very high." For each number, consumers are advised on the best actions to take to protect themselves from harmful rays (see chart).

16. *True.* Fabrics that are loosely woven, such as crepe or knit, allow UV rays to penetrate. (A rule of thumb: If you can see through the fabric, it won't protect you.) Opt for silk or denim, fabrics with dark colors or special sun-protective clothing, such as the Sun Precautions Solumbra line (800-882-7860). And keep in mind that clothes of any kind are less protective when wet.

17. *True.* Sand, like pavement and snow, reflects UV rays.

18. *False.* The UV rays emitted by tanning booths and sun lamps can cause burning, skin aging and cancer.

19. *False.* A sunscreen's active ingredients are effective for only about two years. And any sunscreen you buy may have been sitting on the store shelf for a long time. So it's a good idea to replace your sunscreen every year.

20. *False.* A broad-brimmed hat is better, since it protects the cheeks as well as the nose.

—CYNTHIA MOEKLE PIGOTT

Germ Crazy

ANTIBACTERIAL PRODUCTS FROM SOAPS TO KITTY LITTER ARE FLOODING THE MARKET. DO THEY KEEP YOU HEALTHIER—OR JUST MAKE THE BUGS MEANER?

By **Deborah Franklin**

We hooted at Howard Hughes's obsessive cleanliness; we scoffed at his nutso ways. If the once-dashing film mogul and millionaire wanted to autoclave his clothes in the 1930s or scrub the fingernails of Hollywood beauties in the 1940s, well, didn't that just prove what we always knew: that money not only corrupts the soul but rots the mind?

So, these many years later, what's our excuse?

As we prepare to wash our hands of the 20th century, America's gone germ crazy. In 1996 more than 120 new products laced with antibacterial agents came on the market, and that's only a fraction of those for sale today. You can now buy Brillo pads with a patented "microbe shield"; you can get bacteria-fighting hand lotion, cutting boards, kitty litter, and bathtub toys. The message is clear: It's a wicked, wicked world out there, and if we don't stay hypervigilant and scrub ourselves silly, They'll Get Us.

There's good reason we feel under siege. In the 1950s, if Beaver Cleaver stayed home from school with an upset stomach, nobody suggested he might have swallowed lethal germs with his lunch. If he skinned a knee, June didn't fret over flesh-eating bacteria. And in an era when tonsillectomies were almost a childhood rite of passage, most everyone considered a hospital the cleanest, safest place to recover.

Times have changed, and not just for the Beaver. Each year millions of children and adults fall ill with food poisoning, and at least 9,000 die of it. The Centers for Disease Control and Prevention estimates that every year another 80,000 die from an infection with one or another vicious superbug they first encountered while in the hospital.

Granted, one reason the number of recorded cases of salmonella poisoning, for instance, has doubled in 20 years is simply because we're keeping better track of what makes us sick. Still, there's no question that our modern ways have made us more vulnerable. In the Leave-It-to-Beaver 1950s much of what we ate was poured from cans that had been flash-heated and vacuum-sealed seasons before—limp, lifeless, but relatively free of bacteria. Today we insist on fresh produce year-round. We want it tasty and we want it now, which means we're eating more takeout and buying more produce grown continents away. Before it gets to your fork, nearly every morsel you swallow has traveled more miles, been handled by more people, and had more chances to sit out a little too long on some counter than at any time in history.

And it's not just our food that's getting around more. Every time you climb aboard a DC-10, you and 300 or so fellow passengers share not only recirculated air but germs. Start counting connecting flights and you'll soon see why a killer flu in Hong Kong threatens salesmen in Des Moines. Even nontravelers today get exposed to germs from a greater number of people. More toddlers are in day care, where they swap colds faster than you can say Slobber-Me-Elmo. They sniffle all the way home; and once Mom and Dad get sick, their coworkers aren't far behind.

Is a germ-killing toilet seat beginning to sound pretty good? There's more: Even as lifestyle changes have facilitated germ transmission, microbes themselves have been getting craftier.

Among bacteria, as in every other corner of the biological world, evolution is a patient, if mindless, cardplayer. It shuffles and deals genes in new combinations with new mutations until an organism arises that has some competitive edge. Juice companies were shocked in 1996 when *Escherichia coli* 0157:H7, a deadly version of the common stomach bug, showed up in unpasteurized apple juice. "The dogma had always been that E. coli can't survive in something as acidic as fruit juice," says Dean Cliver, a microbiologist and food safety specialist at the University of California at Davis. "But guess again. This strain does."

E. coli can reproduce—and hence get a new deal of the genetic hand—every 20 minutes or so. Plus, the germs trade small loops of genetic material, called plasmids, just as frequently. So in hindsight, Cliver says, it makes sense that a version of killer E. coli with a tougher membrane eventually popped up.

Similar genetic reshuffling can also give rise to microbes that shrug off powerful drugs. One of the scariest turns of events in the past 40 years has been the emergence of bacteria impervious to nearly every antibiotic in a hospital's pharmacy. Frightening, but predictable: Scientists now know that genes for antibiotic resistance often cluster together on the same plasmid, like recipes for disaster bound in the same cookbook.

Most bacteria readily exchange those cookbooks even with unrelated neighbors. And keep in mind that theirs is a neighborhood of cheek-by-jowl tenements. Your gut is crowded with many more bacteria than there are people on earth. Most of those 400 species are benign, some even crucial to your health. But a problem can develop if a noxious strain of salmonella, say, makes it into your intestine and meets up with a harmless resident microbe armed with a gene for antibiotic resistance. A bit of recipe swapping and bingo: The drugs are rendered less effective or even useless against that organism. Add a little sloppy hygiene to the mix and the superbug spreads from person to person.

What's more, some common antibiotics actually seem to increase the likelihood that bacteria will exchange genes, says Abigail Salyers, a microbiologist at the University of Illinois. "Tetracycline is like an aphrodisiac for them," she says.

Faced with all that bad news, it's tempting to rush home and amass an arsenal of germ fighters. But listen to the experts. The solution *isn't* to try to create a microbe-free world, they say. Indeed, some researchers worry that too liberal a hand with bacteria busters could hurt our health in the long run. So which is it: Are these products effective weapons, or are they more likely to shoot you in the foot? Read on.

Do antibacterials help prevent disease?

SOME DO, and scientific data prove it. A number of others have common sense on their side. But health officials warn that makers of many products billed as antibacterial are skating on the thin edge of the law with claims that seem absurd.

Antibacterial skin cleansers generally contain chemicals that in high concentrations are known to kill bacteria. The lower concentrations found in the new products slow bacterial growth, enough that it sometimes makes a dent in disease transmission. In a hospital nursery several years ago, for example, *Staphylococcus aureus* sickened 22 newborns over the course of seven weeks, despite control measures. The problem was squelched only after the staff started using antibacterial hand soap—of the same strength as versions found in the supermarket—to wash their hands and bathe the babies.

Another household staple, heavy-duty kitchen and bathroom disinfectants, for years have been promoted as fighting germs. And they do, if used properly. Spray these on the bathroom floor (windows open; the fumes can be dangerous) and they can put the kibosh on the fungus that causes athlete's foot. Squirt them on doorknobs and wipe off bacteria left by unwashed hands—bacteria that could otherwise hitch a ride on *your* hands into your mouth, giving rise to so-called stomach flu or food poisoning.

On the other hand, there's no evidence that plastic items advertised as antibacterial, such as cutting boards and children's toys, reduce illness from infections.

THE Fine Print

On anything designed to clean objects, as opposed to people, look for an Environmental Protection Agency registration number, which shows the manufacturer has proved the product does what its label promises. Look as well for two words that signal power:

A **disinfectant** contains a chemical that has been EPA-certified to "destroy or irreversibly inactivate infectious fungi and bacteria." That's the strongest germ-fighting designation on home cleansers. If you want the cleanser to cut through grease and grime—so that disinfecting chemicals can reach their microbial targets—make sure it contains a **detergent**, too.

Labels on skin cleansers are harder to evaluate. The Food and Drug Administration, which regulates these products, has not yet set standards for cleaning power. According to the Soap and Detergent Association, povidone-iodine and ethyl alcohol are the "most aggressive" germ-stopping ingredients used in such products—that is, the toughest on germs *and* your skin. Two other common ingredients, triclosan and chloroxylenol, are slightly milder but still slow bacterial growth.

As you scrutinize labels, make sure you really want what you're paying for. Several companies have had run-ins with the EPA over antibacterial claims made for products. Playskool responded by slapping a new blurb on its packaging that is technically accurate but easy to misinterpret. ANTIBACTERIAL PROTECTION, the label screams in bold red letters. INHIBITS THE GROWTH OF BACTERIA! Sandwiched between those two phrases, the real point—BUILT IN TO PROTECT THE TOY!—is easy to overlook. —*D.F.*

The Cleanup Crew

The antimicrobial products crowding store shelves are not all alike. Some really can help prevent disease, while others are unlikely to make a difference to your health. Here's a rundown, from the good to the goofy.

Household Cleansers

These are the big guns, loaded with chlorine, ammonia, or other corrosive substances.

Given the chance, they'll maim you as well as the germs. But when used as directed—with rubber gloves in a well-ventilated room—they're your best tools against the bacteria, viruses, and fungi that flourish on kitchen and bathroom fixtures, counters, and the drain grates in sinks.

According to germ buster Chuck Gerba of the University of Arizona, regularly disinfecting these "hot zones" curbs the chance that one person's cold, stomach flu, or athlete's foot will spread to the rest of the family.

"Manufacturers have gotten a lot better at putting this stuff in spray bottles that are easy to use," Gerba says. "A bucket of water mixed with a half cup of bleach gives you the same effect, but it's not as convenient." Besides, point-and-spray application helps limit the amount of noxious chemicals going down the drain and into groundwater.

A few cautions: No cleanser will disinfect a surface that's caked with grime; so scrub first, then spray. Since few substances kill germs "on contact," you need to let the solution stand for whatever time the label urges. And remember: These products are caustic, so use with care.

Hand Soaps

A 20-second scrub with plain old-fashioned soap and water will send about 96 percent of the troublesome viruses and bacteria on your grubby paws down the drain. Antibacterial soaps seem to provide a very slight edge. Unlike plain soap, they leave a persistent chemical residue that slows bacterial growth and so wipes out maybe another 1 percent of the potentially harmful bugs.

The active ingredient in about 90 percent of these products is triclosan, a chemical that fights a broad range of bacteria and has been used in underarm deodorants and deodorant soaps for 30 years.

At the high concentrations used in most hospital soaps, triclosan quickly kills bacteria by punching holes in their membrane coating. At the lower concentrations found in household soaps, deodorants, and toothpastes, the chemical interferes with the organisms' ability to absorb nutrients. While that won't kill the critters, it effectively keeps their numbers down between washings.

One caveat: Antibacterial soaps can be more drying to your skin than regular soap. You may need to try a few to find one you can live with.

"I don't care how great a soap is at killing germs. If it's too harsh, you won't use it," says microbiologist Dean Cliver of the University of California at Davis. "And to keep from getting sick or passing your illness on to someone else, what's most important is that you wash your hands with some kind of soap frequently."

Dishwashing Liquids

Many dishwashing liquids now have the word

Is it possible to be too clean?

THE FRENCH certainly think so. Lynn Payer, author of *Medicine and Culture*, says the prevailing view in the land of delectably moldy cheese is that forcing your body to grapple with germs—in moderation—can bolster your immune system. A grimier lifestyle, some French doctors argue, offers a natural form of vaccination for children, exposing them to illnesses, such as hepatitis A, that are milder when contracted in childhood.

Most U.S. health officials call that philosophy dangerously outdated. Today's America, they say, is plenty germy enough to provide children with the exposure needed to rev the immune system. And while hepatitis A may be easier on children than grown-ups, other viruses that don't generally harm adults can trigger fatal diarrhea in small children.

However, there is one risk to germ phobia that infection experts have not antibacterial splashed across their labels. But don't read too much into that claim.

Such products, which contain triclosan or another active ingredient with the same effect, have been shown to curb germs on hands. However, there's no evidence—or reason to think—that they are any better than milder dish soaps at reducing germs on dishes, cutlery, clothes, or other inanimate objects.

Water-Free Hand Gels

These products, which are only slightly less drying than rubbing alcohol, are designed for those diaper-changes-by the-side-of-the-road moments when there's no soap or water with which to scrub.

Studies of food industry workers showed such gels achieved a reassuring 99.9 percent kill rate against viruses and bacteria. Harried parents, as well as politicians, pastors, day care workers, and others who press the flesh for a living, might well appreciate the gels' efficacy and convenience. Be aware that they won't cut through dirt, though. And you may find them too harsh for frequent use.

Sponges and Dishcloths

Scientists who track the spread of germs call the kitchen dishcloth or sponge the strongest link in the chain: a moist, inviting spa where microbes meet, mingle, and multiply before moving on to hands and countertops.

"Self-disinfecting" sponges grow significantly fewer disease-causing bacteria than untreated ones, according to Gerba, and so may limit the transfer of bacteria from sponge to fingers. Still, you shouldn't sop up raw chicken juice with an antibacterial dishcloth, then use it to wash your fork. In short, it's not clear how much extra protection these products offer.

Last spring the Environmental Protection Agency fined two companies for claiming their sponges or cloths could stop germs. They were ordered to tone it down; hence today's labels limply read, "Kills odor-causing bacteria in the sponge."

Whatever sponge you choose, Gerba says, you'd do well to boil it, run it through a dishwasher, or zap it (while moist) in the microwave for two minutes, ideally once a day. Replace it every couple of weeks. And when cleaning up juice from meat, poultry, or other especially germy spills, disposable is best: Use a soapy paper towel.

Cutting Boards, Toys, Furniture

These days a slew of plastic products are impregnated with antibacterial chemicals. But they don't qualify as guardians of your health.

In the past year infuriated EPA officials have chastised Hasbro, Joyce Chen, and a number of other manufacturers for implying that the germicide embedded in their plastic products could check the spread of disease-producing germs. "If that evidence exists, we haven't seen it," says Brenda Mosley, a microbiologist at the EPA.

Triclosan and other such chemicals may retard the growth of bacteria and mildew that can rot plastic. But to suggest a dash of antibactérial substance locked in plastic could neutralize germy slobber on a high chair or meat juices splashed across a cutting board goes beyond the pale.

"Our main concern is that people will think they're protected and be less careful about cleaning these products," Mosley says.

The bottom line: In day care centers vigilant hand washing, along with a daily soapy scrub of communal toys—"antibacterial" or not—is the best way to curb transmission of colds and flus.

As for cutting boards, Cliver's latest studies show that while wood and plastic boards are equally easy to keep clean when new, wood resists germs slightly better under heavy use. But both types should be scrubbed with soap after each use, Gerba says, and periodically wiped down with a solution of a tablespoon of bleach in a quart of water. The bleach mixture is also a good idea after the board has come into contact with raw meat.—D.F.

---

entirely dismissed. America's penchant for all things antiseptic, some fear, could speed the rate at which bacteria learn to thwart antibiotics. Stuart Levy, a microbiologist at Tufts University who specializes in antibiotic resistance, has been among the most vocal worriers. "How do we know that this massive attempt to rid our environment of microbes isn't of massive consequence in our ability to treat infections?" he asks.

What makes Levy nervous is the discovery that some plasmids (those genetic cookbooks that bacteria like to swap) contain genes conferring antibiotic resistance as well as genes conferring disinfectant resistance. This suggests the two types of resistance genes can travel together. Indeed, in laboratory studies scientists have used hospital disinfectants to nudge microbes into developing resistance to the cleansers and found that the organisms had simultaneously become less vulnerable to a range of antibiotics.

No one knows how frequently this sort of thing happens in the real world, says Levy. But it's possible that flooding the world with low-level germ fighters could ratchet up the rate at which our mightiest antibiotics lose their strength.

At a meeting of an advisory committee to the Food and Drug Administration last year, several scientists argued that such a link is strictly theoretical. The scientists pointed out that the zealous use of antibacterial soaps hasn't made them any less effective—even in hospitals, where they're used much more intensively than in homes.

"I see this as a *potential* problem," Levy says. "It hasn't been studied enough and needs to be." The FDA apparently agrees. At last year's meeting the committee said researchers should keep an eye on the situation.

Who needs these germ fighters?

IF YOU'RE AN ADULT blessed with a healthy immune system, whatever extra protection antibacterial soaps provide is probably unnecessary. What's important is that you use soap—any kind—and that you wash frequently, particularly after using the bathroom and before you eat.

But some people are especially vulnerable. Forty percent of all serious cases of food poisoning linked to salmonella occur in children under the age of five. Adults over 60 are also more susceptible, as are nursing home residents, pregnant women, and anybody whose immune system has been weakened by illness or medication. For these people, says microbiologist Chuck Gerba of the University of Arizona, a small boost in protection from bacteria might spell the difference between fending off an infection and succumbing.

Even people in the pink may have chinks in their immune armor. Someone who regularly downs antacids, for example, is less protected against microbes that cause food poisoning because the same stomach acid that stirs up heartburn also inhibits the growth of bacteria. And though it may seem counterintuitive, anyone on antibiotics will have weaker defenses, too. "Antibiotics tend to wipe out the natural flora in your gut," Cliver says. "So any bad bug you swallow can more easily take over and make you ill."

Levy sees the value of antibacterial soaps for these vulnerable groups or to help keep a truly virulent infection from spreading. But, he says, that's all the more reason for the rest of us to lay off the extrapotent cleansers until they're needed. "If you've got somebody coming home from the hospital, then by all means break out the antibacterial soap if you want to," he says. "Otherwise, we've got to get over the idea that it would be desirable to sterilize our environment, even if we could."

After all, microbiologist Salyers says, bacteria have nurtured us for millennia, even as they colonized our every crevice. Microbial gut residents add to our stores of vitamin K, for instance. And without the digestive assistance of intestinal bacteria, we'd miss out on perhaps 7 percent of the energy we get from food.

Staying healthy is not so much a matter of destroying microbes as it is of keeping them in balance, says Salyers. In practical terms this may translate to: Wash your hands, wash your hands, wash your hands; keep cold foods very cold and hot foods very hot; and if you are laid low by what seems to be a run-of-the-mill bug, stay home, drink plenty of fluids, and call the doctor if your fever lingers after a week or so. If the infection is viral, don't push for antibiotics; the drugs are useless against viruses and might pave the way for a more serious contagion.

And if you're tempted in your snuffling misery to surround yourself with store-bought germ slayers, remember Howard Hughes and choose appropriately. At his autopsy in 1976, an examination of the tycoon's brain showed his ultimate madness was likely caused by syphilis—a bacterial infection, all right, but one better prevented with a condom than with soap, no matter how strong.

Deborah Franklin is a senior editor.

The Frog Solution

By Josie Glausiusz

Scientists are hunting for the next generation of antibiotics in frog skin and pig gut, in silk moths and salamanders, in snakes, sharks, and honeybees.

AT MAGAININ PHARMACEUTICALS, in leafy Plymouth Meeting, Pennsylvania, amphibians abound. A plastic toad guards the entrance, startling strangers with a mournful mechanical croak. A beanbag frog sits atop the desk of Magainin's founder, Michael Zasloff. And in a tank that Zasloff keeps in his lab swim a clutch of African clawed frogs, *Xenopus laevis*. The fun begins when he lifts one out. Grasping the squirming frog firmly in his hand, Zasloff sprinkles a dried form of the hormone adrenaline on its back and rubs it in. Within seconds, hundreds of tiny white spots dot the frog's skin, then slowly merge into a creamy sheen. Zasloff calls the white film "a beautiful bandage" because it's filled with bacteria-killing antibiotic peptides—small strings of amino acids, which are the building blocks of all proteins.

The discovery of one of these peptides, which Zasloff named magainin after the Hebrew word *magain*, or "shield," inspired him to found the company of the same name 11 years ago. He wasn't looking for unconventional antibiotics at the time. As a physician and molecular biologist researching gene expression at the National Institutes of Health, he was harvesting immature eggs from *Xenopus* ovaries. Although he operated on the frogs in nonsterile conditions and then returned them to microbe-infested water tanks, their wounds never became infected or even showed signs of inflammation. Zasloff concluded that something in the frogs' skin was protecting them from bacterial attack. So he took a piece of skin, ground it up, and extracted its protective component, which turned out to

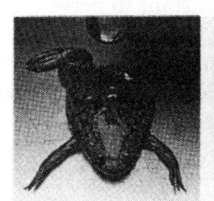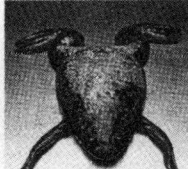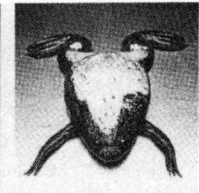

DRIED ADRENALINE is sprinkled on a frog's back. Within seconds, tiny spots appear and merge into a film filled with bacteria-killing agents.

Photographs by Brian Smale

be a peptide. Magainin, he found, is discharged onto the frog's skin in response to adrenaline, which is released when pain receptors in the skin send the brain a message that an injury has occurred.

Since that early find, Zasloff has discovered peptide antibiotics in all manner of places: the airway and tongue of a cow, the gut of a pig, the stomach of the spiny dogfish shark. Other researchers are in on the hunt, too, and they have found peptide antibiotics in a witches' brew of beasts: in silk moths, fruit flies, honeybees, and budworms; in salamanders, snakes, and horseshoe crabs; in the white blood cells of pigs and cows and humans; in our skin; and in fish, birds, and even plants. "They are now recognized in every species of life, from the smallest to the biggest, from things that fly or swim or just sit around on rocks to human beings—all defend themselves with antimicrobial peptides," says microbiologist Bob Hancock of the University of British Columbia in Vancouver. "And they're a very large proportion of what protects us daily from infection."

Hancock and Zasloff are among a handful of pioneers who are turning these peptides into antibiotic drugs in hopes of someday providing an alternative or an adjunct to currently available antibiotics. The need for new antibiotics is becoming increasingly urgent as misuse and overuse of conventional antibiotics has bred resistance in many common disease-causing bacteria. And so the possibility of new antibiotics with novel modes of action that may be immune to resistance is exciting news. Some of them are even active against some disease-causing protozoans, fungi, and viruses such as *Herpes simplex* and HIV. Still, it must be stressed that although some of these new peptides are undergoing clinical trials, none have yet emerged into general use, and many problems in their manufacture remain.

WHAT MAKES THESE NEW peptide antibiotics different from penicillin and its kin is that they stem from animals' own immune defenses rather than from other microbes. That means they have spent millions of years in an evolutionary battle with invasive bacteria and have emerged victorious time and again. Moreover, their mechanism of action is entirely different from that of most conventional antibiotics. Instead of disabling a vital bacterial enzyme, as penicillin does, antimicrobial peptides appear to punch holes in bacterial cell membranes, making them porous and leaky. To develop resistance to conventional antibiotics, bacteria need only remodel an enzyme or two, changing them so that they still perform their function but no longer bind to the antibiotic. It's far more complicated for a bacterium to completely remodel its membrane in response to pore-forming peptides.

"To make bacteria resistant to peptides," says Hancock, "you need to change the entire composition of the membrane," which means altering dozens of interrelated proteins. "So it's very difficult." For these reasons, advocates of peptide antibiotics believe that bacteria are far less likely to become resistant to them.

Peptide antibiotics are the first particles to protect us from the constant onslaught of invasive bacteria that we breathe in or swallow, or which simply land on our skin. They line every surface of the body—eyes, skin, lungs, tongue, and intestinal tract. They are found in the kidneys and in macrophages and neutrophils, white blood cells that use them to destroy engulfed bacteria. Peptide antibiotics are the rapid response troops that kill bacteria within minutes of encounter—far faster than antibodies or T cells, which can take a week or more to recruit and which do not exist in more primitive animals like insects. And most eukaryotic organisms—that is, every organism but bacteria and viruses—are immune to attack by these peptides because of a quirk in the makeup of their cell membranes. Eukaryotic cell membranes, which consist of fats and cholesterol, carry only a very low electric charge. But bacterial cell membranes, which are made up of a mixture of fats and sugars, carry a much stronger, negative charge. Because peptide antibiotics are positively charged, they are able to bind quickly to bacteria.

That's when the killing begins. The interior of a bacterium is even more negatively charged than its exterior, and the strong attraction pulls the peptides into the cell membrane. There they adopt a helical form and gather into barrel-like clusters, each peptide acting as one stave in the barrel, with a hole in the middle of the cluster. The cell's cytoplasm can now leak out through the holes, causing the bacterium to collapse. Furthermore, the holes can form entry points for conventional antibiotics, thus enhancing their action.

Unfortunately, not many peptide antibiotics are on their way to the clinic, and even those currently undergoing testing would have only limited use. One reason for the slow pace is the cost of bringing a drug to market, which has been estimated to cost about $300 million, including clinical trials. Another major expense is producing peptide antimicrobials in the first place. Grinding up frogs to extract magainin is clearly not an option, which leaves chemical synthesis—stringing together the relevant amino acids—or some form of recombinant production using genetically engineered bacteria. But there are problems with both approaches.

"When we started, the only techniques out there for production of therapeutic peptides were archaic chemical techniques," recalls Zasloff. "This would lead to a cost for the peptide of about $1,000 to $2,000 a gram." Improvements in chemical synthesis have brought the

> **Peptide antibiotics are rapid response troops, killing bacteria within minutes of encounter. They line every body surface— eyes, skin, lungs, tongue, intestinal tract.**

cost of magainin down to $100 a gram, but that's still pricey. On the other hand, splicing a gene for the peptide into a bacterium that will be killed by its product doesn't make sense either. Magainin Pharmaceuticals says it has bypassed the problem by fusing its peptide to a protein that renders it unable to attack bacteria until the protein is removed.

Despite the difficulties, some peptides are beginning the arduous trek to market. One of the most promising is a compound called BPI (for "bactericidal/permeability-increasing" protein), originally derived from human neutrophils and developed for clinical use by a small Berkeley, California, company called Xoma. In November 1997, Xoma published the results of a clinical trial of BPI for the treatment of meningococcemia, a virulent infection that affects nearly 3,000 children a year in the United States. This condition can progress from flulike symptoms to death within one or two days. The trial showed that BPI could significantly reduce the death rate from the disease, which is caused by a bacterium called *Neisseria meningitidis*. This bug releases a poison called endotoxin into the bloodstream. Endotoxin triggers a massive reaction, called a sepsis cascade, that in turn can cause severe inflammation and collapse of the circulatory system. The beauty of BPI is that it not only kills bacteria but binds to endotoxin, stopping the sepsis cascade. The endotoxin is then broken down by the liver and excreted.

ANOTHER PEPTIDE ANTIBIOTIC that's winding through clinical trials—and should be available for use, if approved, in the fall of 1999—is a magainin derivative called pexiganan, an antibiotic cream for the treatment of infected diabetic foot ulcers. Untreated diabetic foot ulcers can lead to bone infections and ultimately amputation. Tests showed pexiganan to be effective in curing infection, and without the side effects—diarrhea and insomnia—that are common to the currently favored oral antibiotic.

There are other peptide antibiotics at similarly early phases, all being developed by small companies funded by venture capital. For example, the Vancouver-based Micrologix Biotech (a company with which Hancock is affiliated) produces peptides called bactolysins, originally derived from insects, which it claims can kill resistant strains of *Staphylococcus aureus*—in mice, anyway. IntraBiotics Pharmaceuticals, a company in Mountain View, California, is running human safety trials of peptides called protegrins, derived from ones originally discovered in the white blood cells of pigs, for the treatment of oral mucositis, a painful mouth infection often brought on by cancer chemotherapy. And Robert Lehrer, a UCLA physician also affiliated with IntraBiotics, is developing a protegrin-containing vaginal microbicide that could be used by women to prevent sexually transmitted diseases.

Obstacles remain. One is that peptide antibiotics given orally would be digested by intestinal enzymes, which are designed to pounce on proteins. That means that the antibiotics' use would have to be restricted to injection or topical application. But even this hurdle can be overcome, says peptide chemist Bruce Merrifield of Rockefeller University in New York. A few years ago he synthesized a "mirror image" version of a peptide called cecropin, which is derived from the silk moth *Hyalophora cecropia*.

> "Bacteria have been around for more than 3 billion years, and they've developed pretty good ways of figuring out how to overcome just about anything."

The mirror-image peptide uses amino acids that are backward versions of those found in nature, which make it invulnerable to intestinal enzyme attack. But it can still kill bacteria, says Merrifield, including some in the same family as the bacteria that cause tuberculosis.

Another sticky issue is toxicity. "The antibiotic peptides are charged, which causes them to exhibit certain toxicities as the dose is increased," cautions Zasloff. "I think they begin to irritate parts of the nervous system"—whose cells are also electrically charged—"so the therapeutic window is not as broad. That can be dealt with by chemical manipulation, and we are dealing with it."

THEN THERE'S THE TOUCHY TOPIC of resistance. Most peptide researchers say that the potential for disease-causing bacteria to develop resistance to the peptides is small—and that try as they might, they can't induce resistance in their target bacteria. Though Hancock concedes that a few species of bacteria are naturally resistant because their cell membranes lack a strong negative charge, they are not, he insists, of major clinical significance. It's a view not shared by microbiologist Eduardo Groisman of the Howard Hughes Medical Institute and Washington University School of Medicine in St. Louis, who works on *Salmonella typhimurium*. "*Salmonella* has been isolated from a hundred different animal species," says Groisman. "You name an animal—elephants, yes; camels, yes; cockroaches, yes. Who was isolating it from cockroaches or lizards, don't ask me, but people have reported in reputable journals that *Salmonella* is there. Now, many animals that it infects have been shown to produce antimicrobial peptides against invading pathogens. So our rationale was this: since *Salmonella* has been isolated from many different animal species, it must have evolved ways to deal with these peptides."

In fact, Groisman has found one strain of *Salmonella*—originally isolated from a cow it had killed—that can comfortably survive a dose of magainin. He claims that most peptide researchers who can't find resistance aren't culturing their bacteria under the right conditions and adds that *Salmonella* only expresses resistance when it needs it—that is, when conditions are similar to those it experiences inside the cells it infects. Those cells are macrophages, or scavenger cells, and the small, saclike organs in which they envelop *Salmonella* seem to be low in magnesium. Grow *Salmonella* in magnesium-deficient culture and they will survive peptide attack, says Groisman. Although he doesn't know how *Salmonella* becomes resistant, he suspects that it may reduce its negative charge by modifying its membrane. Alternatively, it may secrete an enzyme that can chop magainin in two before the peptide can attack.

Despite his disturbing results, Groisman doesn't believe that antimicrobial peptides should be dismissed lightly. For one thing, manufacturing them in mirror image, though expensive, may render them immune to resistance. And the supply of effective antibiotics is rapidly running out. "We really need new classes of antibiotics," says Groisman, "and I think we should give them a chance."

But could they ever replace the antibiotics to which so many bacteria have become resistant? Zasloff thinks they can as a last resort; however, he thinks it equally likely that they'll be used to complement existing antibiotics, since the damage they do to bacterial membranes can open the door to other drugs. Clinical microbiologist Fred Tenover of the Centers for Disease Control and Prevention in Atlanta, who specializes in the molecular biology of antimicrobial resistance, paints a darker picture. "Every year there's a meeting called ICAAC—the Interscience Conference on Antimicrobial Agents and Chemotherapy—and we see poster after poster of new drugs, some totally synthetic, some natural products, that inhibit wide ranges of bacteria at very low concentrations," he says. "But three years later they're never heard of again because they're either too toxic or cause significant side effects, or trigger an immune response. So it's hard to look into the crystal ball and say these really are the future of antibiotic therapy until we see how they do in well-controlled clinical trials."

Nonetheless, Tenover remains hopeful. "We're always looking for new ways to inhibit emerging infectious diseases," he says. "Of course, one of our favorite ways is to prevent them in the first place with vaccines. But given that you can't have a vaccine to everything, what do you do with the bacteria that remain that cause infections? And as many new things as we could have to throw at the bacteria are going to be helpful, because it's our feeling that use eventually leads to resistance. Bacteria have been around for more than 3 billion years, and they've developed pretty good ways of figuring out how to overcome just about anything. So we're happy to see lots of new things coming down the road."

Prevent SEXUALLY TRANSMITTED DISEASES

Lauren Picker

Shortly after graduating from college in 1988, Sara Lewis* noticed a constellation of small red bumps on her vagina. She assumed they'd go away by themselves, but instead they became larger and more plentiful. She finally went to her gynecologist, who diagnosed a sexually transmitted disease (STD)—in her case, genital warts.

"I just lay there crying in the stirrups," recalls Lewis. At 21, she'd had few sexual partners and she had never seriously considered the risks of sex beyond an unwanted pregnancy. "This shouldn't happen to me—I'm a 'good girl,' " she remembers thinking. It's an attitude that's all too common.

"Most people think of STD's as something that happens to the other guy, but they're really everybody's problem," says Dr. H. Hunter Handsfield, director of the STD control program at the Seattle–King County (Wash.) Department of Public Health. "It's a fair bet that half of us acquire an STD at least once by age 30."

AIDS is the STD that receives the most attention. This lethal and incurable disease is caused by a virus, HIV, that currently has infected more than 1.2 million Americans, killing more than 220,000 of them. But the AIDS plague has overshadowed other important STD's that are spreading at a rate of 12 million new infections per year in the U.S., with two-thirds of new cases affecting people under 25.

*Name has been changed.

The most worrisome of these are, like AIDS, caused by viruses and are incurable. These viral STD's can have devastating health impacts and can even prove fatal. Genital warts, for example, are caused by the human papilloma virus, the most common STD. HPV is now believed responsible as well for most cases of cervical cancer, a disease that kills more than 4,000 American women each year. Add in cases of herpes and hepatitis B, and the proportion of Americans infected with an incurable viral STD other than HIV may approach 50%. For just one STD, genital herpes, "we know that about a quarter of all Americans become infected by age 35," says Handsfield.

Unfortunately, someone with almost any STD runs a much greater risk of contracting AIDS through sex with an HIV-infected partner. Herpes and syphilis cause sores or ulcers that facilitate HIV's entry into the body, but even nonulcerative STD's such as chlamydia and gonorrhea promote HIV infection, presumably because they allow the virus to enter the body through the microscopic lesions they cause. In fact, these much more common diseases, says Handsfield, "may contribute more to HIV transmission than do the ulcerative STD's." Preventing and controlling them, he adds, "is emerging as one of the most important but least appreciated ways of preventing the transmission and spread of AIDS."

STD's are blatantly discriminatory. Not only are women likelier than men to become infected (through sex with an

CONTEMPORARY HEALTH HAZARDS

HALF OF ALL AMERICANS WILL ACQUIRE AN STD AT LEAST ONCE BY AGE 30

infected partner), but the consequences of those infections for women are also much more severe.

A woman has a greater susceptibility than a man to almost all STD's, including AIDS, for two reasons: She has a larger genital surface area that can be breached by microbes; and during sex, the man's secretions are deposited directly into the woman's body. In a single act of unprotected heterosexual intercourse with an infected partner, for example, a woman has a 50% or greater chance of contracting chlamydia, while a man runs only a 20% to 40% chance of being infected by a woman with the disease.

Once infection occurs, effective treatment for women is often delayed, partly because early symptoms of STD's are usually more subtle in women, so they don't seek treatment as promptly as men do. And when a woman does seek medical attention, the diagnostic tests don't work as well as they do for men, so an infection can persist for months or even years and cause extensive damage, particularly to reproductive organs, before being detected and treated.

"Women *far* more than men have serious long-term consequences from STD's," says Handsfield, who lists as examples infertility, life-threatening tubal pregnancies, sick infants and cervical cancer. "Unfortunately, women can't assume that their sexual partners will assume responsibility for the woman's sexual health."

Not all the news about STD's is bleak. Some bright spots:
● STD's are preventable by using latex or polyurethane condoms. The first male polyurethane condom, Avanti, is now available west of the Rockies and will be nationally distributed this fall. The FDA approved these "plastic" condoms so that people allergic to latex could have a way to prevent STD's, as well as pregnancy. Because testing has been limited, however, product labels state that "the risks of pregnancy and STD's ... are not known for this condom." Polyurethane condoms are thinner than latex and therefore provide greater sensitivity and heat transfer between partners. The new male condoms cost $1 to $1.50 each, or about twice the cost of a latex condom. Reality, the female condom, also made of polyurethane, has been available since 1994.
● While rates of viral STD's (genital herpes, hepatitis B, genital warts) are rising or showing no signs of decline, rates of some key *bacterial* STD's (syphilis, gonorrhea and possibly chlamydia) have fallen significantly in recent years, due to behavioral changes as well as public health efforts to educate people about prevention and screen them for infection. Another reason for the falling rates is that bacterial STD's can be cured with antibiotics once they're detected.

● A new detection test is available for chlamydia, and another one should be widely available soon. The new tests require just a urine specimen and will encourage many more people to be screened.
● Several vaccines for preventing genital herpes are being tested in clinical trials. Experts predict that a herpes vaccine will receive federal approval within a few years.
● A very effective vaccine for hepatitis B has been available since 1982, though it is vastly underused.

Here's a guide to some of the most important STD's.

CHLAMYDIA

During her senior year of college in 1984, Nancy Hartman* was stricken with such severe abdominal pain she could barely walk. She didn't connect her agony to a brief fling several weeks earlier. Then the campus doctor told Hartman that her pain was due to pelvic inflammatory disease caused by a chlamydial infection.

Chlamydia, a bacterial infection, strikes more often each year—about 4 million cases in the U.S.—than any other bacterial STD. The infections respond readily to antibiotics, but if they persist, they can cause devastating complications, especially for women.

"I was lucky the pain got severe," says Hartman, who was promptly treated and cured with antibiotics. Actually, she was lucky to have felt any discomfort at all. As many as 75% of women and 25% of men with chlamydia have no idea they're infected, a situation that can lead to unwitting spread of the microbe as well as to serious complications.

For many women, the first sign of a chlamydial infection is an inability to get pregnant. An examination may then reveal chronic tubal inflammation, a sign the infection has festered in the genital tract and scarred the fallopian tubes. Chlamydial infections account for up to 40% of all cases of female

5 tips for foiling STD's

1. **Be selective in choosing sex partners.** "Meeting people in bars as opposed to being introduced by a friend increases your risk for sexually transmitted diseases," says Dr. H. Hunter Handsfield, director of the STD control program at the Seattle–King County (Wash.) Department of Public Health.

2. **Use condoms.** "Condoms work, and the noise out there that they don't is flat-out false," says Handsfield. "Consistent use of latex condoms markedly reduces the risk of transmission of a variety of STD's." Recent studies show that no more than 2% of condoms break during intercourse.

3. **Be aware of subtle symptoms.** "Things that many of us might tend to disregard can be terribly important in indicating an infection that requires medical attention, to protect both your health and that of your partner," says Handsfield. For women, such symptoms may include increased vaginal discharge or an abnormal odor in the genital area; for men, a small amount of cloudy discharge from the penis; for both sexes, tiny painless sores in the genital area.

4. **Be in a mutually monogamous relationship.** Some data suggest that the person at highest risk for contracting STD's is someone who is monogamous (one partner at a time) in a relationship with someone who has many partners. The monogamous person, usually a woman, assumes her partner is also monogamous and takes no precautions.

5. **Get screened periodically.** Go to your doctor, a family-planning clinic or a public STD clinic and ask to be tested for the common STD's. Remember, it's not the infection itself that's so bad but rather the complications that can occur if an STD persists undetected and untreated.

infertility and also increase the risk for ectopic pregnancy (when the embryo develops in one of the fallopian tubes rather than in the uterus).

For the one in four infected women who experience them, symptoms generally appear one to three weeks after exposure and may include an abnormal vaginal discharge, a burning sensation while urinating, abdominal pain or pain during intercourse. Men may notice a discharge from the penis or burning when urinating.

Since symptoms so often are absent, all sexually active women should have a chlamydia test as part of a yearly pelvic exam and whenever suspicious symptoms appear. Experts also recommend frequent testing for men and women under 25 who have more than one partner.

Until recently, doctors tested for chlamydia by culturing genital secretions, an accurate but time-consuming (up to one week) procedure that is uncomfortable for men. The two tests recently developed for chlamydia can detect the microbes in a couple of days. Treatment of chlamydia has also improved, with just a single dose of the antibiotic azithromycin able to cure most infections.

GENITAL WARTS/HPV

HPV, the infection that caused Lewis's genital warts, is the most prevalent viral STD. As many as 40 million Americans have it, and up to a million more contract it each year. A 1991 study found that 46% of the women who used a health clinic at the University of California at Berkeley were infected with this highly contagious virus: If someone is infected with HPV, there is at least a 70% chance that his or her partner is also infected.

Genital warts generally appear as fleshy, cauliflower-like growths on the genitals or around the anus. Warts tend to surface within three months of exposure, but they sometimes don't appear until several years later. Although the warts HPV causes sometimes clear up on their own, more typically, people have them removed, because they often itch and are unattractive.

Treatments to remove warts include liquid nitrogen (freezing), electrocautery (burning), podophyllin (a caustic liquid) and, when warts are widespread, surgical or laser excision. The immune compound alpha interferon, which is injected into warts, has also received FDA approval, but it can cause flu-like symptoms. Unfortunately, getting rid of visible warts may not get rid of the virus particles, which are much more extensive, and so many patients who have warts removed need repeat treatments for new ones.

The main danger from HPV infection is not warts but cervical cancer. In a recent international study, more than 85% of women with cervical cancer were found to be infected with HPV. Ironically, an HPV infection expressed as warts is relatively good news. "As a rule, warts don't turn into cancer," notes Dr. Mark Schiffman, a medical epidemiologist at the National Cancer Institute and an expert on HPV.

Of some 70 types of HPV that have been identified, the two mainly responsible for genital warts, types six and 11, are only rarely implicated in cervical cancer. At least 10 other types of HPV cause cervical lesions that may ultimately develop into cancer.

These precancerous lesions usually don't cause symptoms, and the first sign of infection is often an abnormal Pap test. "I thought if I contracted something there would be some form of warning," says Alisa Spitler, a 32-year-old woman from Oakman, Ga., who was stunned to learn she had HPV after a Pap test detected abnormal cells.

Fortunately, regular Pap tests can detect cervical cell abnormalities, or dysplasia, well before the condition progresses to cancer. Mild dysplasias often go away on their own, without treatment. But if lesions persist or worsen, physicians can remove them, greatly reducing the risk of cancer without impairing a woman's ability to bear children.

HEPATITIS B

In 1982 Joe Brown* went to his university health center complaining of dizziness and fatigue and assuming he had mononucleosis. But a blood test revealed that his problem was hepatitis B, a viral infection that damages the liver.

Few people think of hepatitis B as an STD, but more than half of the 200,000 new infections each year are contracted through sex. This highly contagious virus, which is much hardier than HIV, can also spread through casual contacts such as sharing a toothbrush or razor blade. Like Brown, half of people newly infected with hepatitis B become acutely ill (about 5,000 of them die from it each year). The rest of those infected show no symptoms (or trivial ones perhaps mistaken for a cold) and don't realize they're infected.

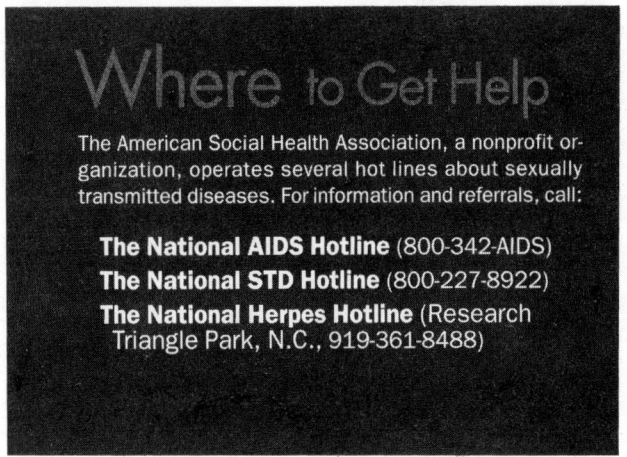

Where to Get Help

The American Social Health Association, a nonprofit organization, operates several hot lines about sexually transmitted diseases. For information and referrals, call:

The National AIDS Hotline (800-342-AIDS)
The National STD Hotline (800-227-8922)
The National Herpes Hotline (Research Triangle Park, N.C., 919-361-8488)

Whether they get sick or not, the great majority of infected people manage to lick the disease completely. But 5% to 10% of infected adults can't shake the virus and become hepatitis B carriers; they not only can transmit the infection to others but also may develop chronic hepatitis, a progressive disease that kills an additional 5,000 people each year, mostly from cirrhosis (scarring of the liver), but also from liver cancer.

Brown, who went on to become a carrier, was upset to learn there is a vaccine that could have prevented his infection. In fact, the safe and highly effective hepatitis B vaccine has been available from family doctors and many public health clinics since 1981, but it hasn't been widely used.

Those who could benefit most from the vaccine are sexually active young adults, both straight and gay, since three-fourths of all cases affect people between 18 and 39. Yet only 1% of Americans in this age group have been vaccinated against hepatitis B. In an effort to protect young adults, the American Academy of Pediatrics recommends that all adolescents be routinely immunized against hepatitis B. The Centers for Disease Control and Prevention takes things a step further by recommending that all infants be vaccinated.

The Major STD's

CHLAMYDIA
Estimated New Cases Yearly: 4 million.
Who's at Risk: People with multiple sexual partners; most prevalent among young people; cuts across all socioeconomic groups.
Symptoms: None in most infected women and up to half of infected men, but abnormal genital discharge or burning during urination (in both sexes); abdominal pain or pain during intercourse (women); testicular pain or swelling (men).
Consequences: For untreated women, pelvic inflammatory disease, which can lead to chronic pelvic pain, ectopic pregnancy or infertility; for untreated men, may lead in rare cases to sterility. Increased risk of HIV infection if a person with chlamydia is exposed to the virus.
Treatment: Antibiotics (azithromycin, doxycycline, ofloxacin).
Prevention: Condoms; probably some protection from spermicides.

GENITAL WARTS/HUMAN PAPILLOMA VIRUS
Estimated New Cases Yearly: 500,000 to 1 million.
Who's at Risk: People with multiple sexual partners; most prevalent among young people.
Symptoms: Fleshy, cauliflower-like growths or warts on and inside the genitals and anus; may appear on the throat when acquired through oral sex; abnormal Pap test.
Consequences: Some strains of HPV believed to cause cervical cancer; HPV also linked to vulvar, vaginal, penile and anal cancers.
Treatment: Warts removed by freezing with liquid nitrogen, burning with electrocautery, applying caustic liquids or by surgical or laser excision for cases where warts are widespread. The precancerous lesions caused by HPV can also be removed.
Prevention: Condoms, though they offer no protection against uncovered lesions.

GONORRHEA
Estimated New Cases Yearly: 500,000.
Who's at Risk: People with multiple sexual partners; most common among teens and young adults in poor inner city areas and in rural southeastern U.S.
Symptoms: None in many cases, but discharge from the vagina, penis or rectum; burning or itching during urination; low abdominal pain (women).
Consequences: Same as with chlamydia.
Treatment: Antibiotics; some strains are resistant to penicillin, but alternatives (such as cefixime and ceftriaxone) are available.
Prevention: Condoms; probably some protection from spermicides. Vaccine in development.

HEPATITIS B
Estimated New Cases Yearly: 200,000, with slightly more than half of them sexually transmitted.
Who's at Risk: (sexually transmitted cases only): gay men; people with multiple sexual partners.
Symptoms: None in about one-third of those infected, but fever, muscle aches and fatigue and, as the disease progresses, dark urine and jaundice in the skin and eyes.
Consequences: For the chronically infected, possibly cirrhosis of the liver or liver cancer.
Treatment: No effective one.
Prevention: Condoms; hepatitis vaccine.

GENITAL HERPES
Estimated New Cases Yearly: 200,000 to 500,000.
Who's at Risk: People with multiple sexual partners.
Symptoms: Recurring blisters or sores usually in the genital area; fever, nausea and genital pain often occur during the first episode; in two-thirds of those infected, herpes symptoms are so mild they don't realize they have the virus.
Consequences: Increased risk of HIV infection if a person with herpes is exposed to the virus.
Treatment: Acyclovir to reduce symptoms and outbreaks.
Prevention: Condoms, though they offer no protection against uncovered sores. A vaccine could be available by 1998.

SYPHILIS
Estimated New Cases Yearly: 120,000.
Who's at Risk: People with multiple sexual partners; most commonly occurs in poor urban communities.
Symptoms: Syphilis sores, or chancres, in the primary stage of the disease; can appear anywhere on the body but are often hidden from view.
Consequences: If untreated, can lead to mental illness, blindness, heart disease and death. Increased risk of HIV infection if exposed to the virus.
Treatment: Penicillin.
Prevention: Condoms, though they offer no protection against uncovered sores.

Sources: Centers for Disease Control and Prevention and the Alan Guttmacher Institute

---

GENITAL HERPES

In a 1982 cover story, *Time* magazine proclaimed herpes "today's scarlet letter." Though AIDS soon pushed herpes out of the headlines, the ranks of herpes sufferers continue to swell. Today about 60 million Americans, or one in four, are believed to be infected with herpes simplex type 2, the virus that causes genital herpes. In 1992 Megan Smith* contracted the disease from her boyfriend.

"We always used a condom, but somehow I got it," says Smith, 29. Her symptoms: swollen glands and a lesion so tiny that "I practically had to use a magnifying glass to see it," she says.

Herpes symptoms usually show up two to 21 days after exposure and can vary enormously in severity from one person to the next. Many people associate genital herpes with recurring bouts of blisters or sores in the genital area, accompanied by pain, fever and nausea. But it's now clear that most people with herpes are not seriously affected.

Some two-thirds of herpes cases are so mild that people don't even know they're infected. Although herpes is most contagious during an outbreak, when sores are visible, it can also be passed by asymptomatic shedding of viruses from someone who feels perfectly fine, a fact that helps explain why up to half a million new infections occur each year.

The oral drug acyclovir, available since 1985, can reduce the frequency, duration and severity of outbreaks. A vaccine against genital herpes is now in clinical trials and could be available by 1998.

GONORRHEA

Although gonorrhea is waning, it still causes more than half a million new infections each year, primarily in impoverished urban areas and in rural southeastern communities, where nearly one in ten 15- to 19-year-olds may have it. Women have a 50% chance of contracting gonorrhea in a single act of unprotected intercourse with an infected partner.

Symptoms of gonorrhea, which is caused by gonococcus bacteria, mirror those caused by chlamydia and usually surface two to five days after infection. In fact, the two infections are virtually indistinguishable without a microscopic exam of genital discharge (for men) or a culture of cervical secretions (for women).

Untreated, gonorrhea can lead to fever, pain and, in women, pelvic inflammatory disease, which can cause infertility. Infectious disease experts are concerned about the growing number of gonorrhea cases that are resistant to one or more antibiotics. The antibiotics penicillin and tetracycline have historically been used to cure the infection, but cases resistant to these drugs have risen rapidly, from fewer than 1% of infections in the U.S. in 1980 to 10% at present. Work on a gonorrhea vaccine is under way.

SYPHILIS

The introduction of penicillin in the 1940s sharply curtailed syphilis as a public health problem. But from 1970 to 1985, syphilis surged among gay men, and in the late 1980s cases soared once again, to their highest level in 40 years, due to the practice among crack addicts of trading sex for drugs. Syphilis cases are now declining rapidly again in most of the country. But they remain prevalent among blacks in lower socioeconomic groups, who have an infection rate more than 60 times higher than whites. The good news about syphilis: A course of penicillin can still cure the disease.

Article 51
IRRAD

by John Henkel

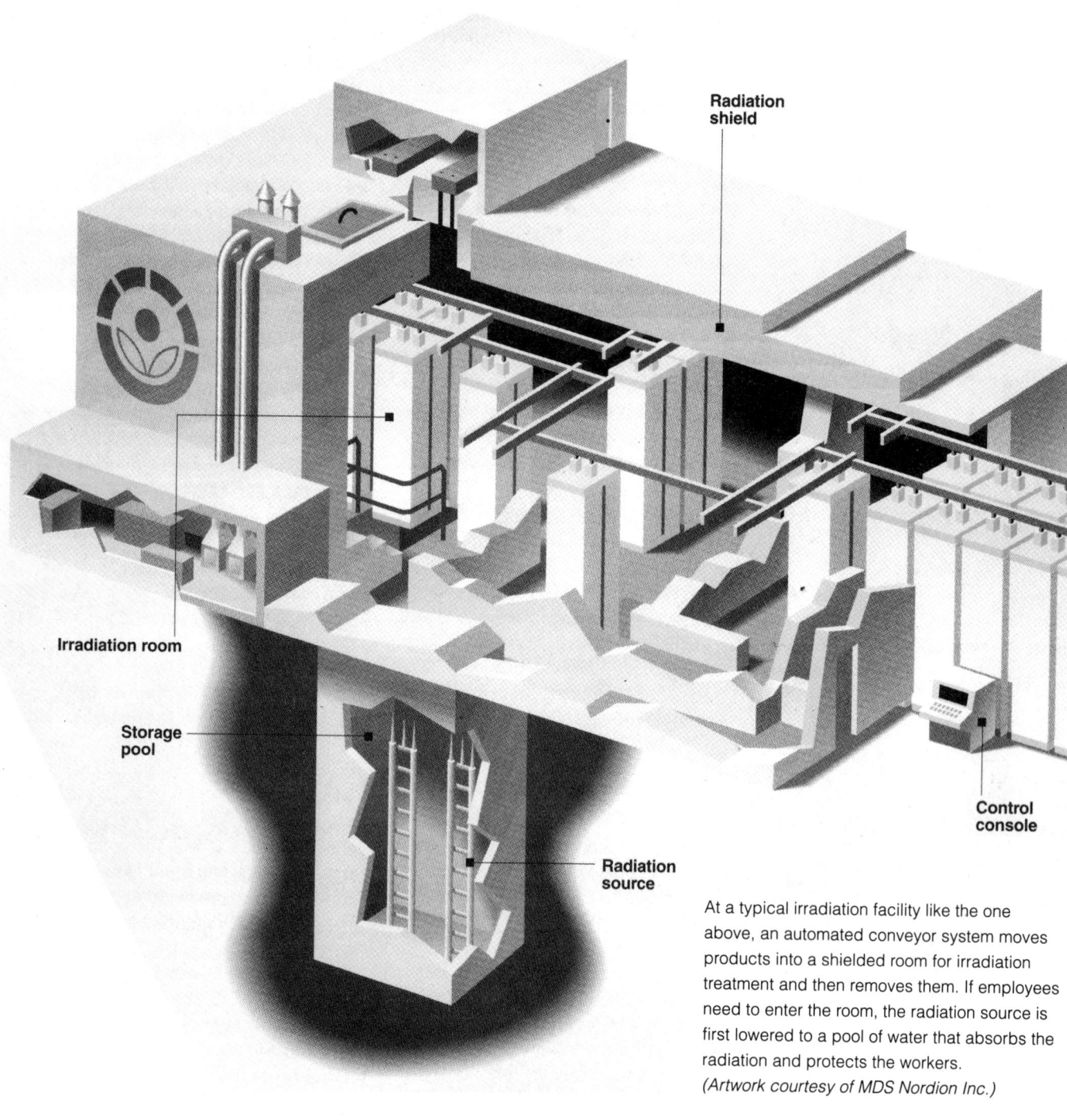

At a typical irradiation facility like the one above, an automated conveyor system moves products into a shielded room for irradiation treatment and then removes them. If employees need to enter the room, the radiation source is first lowered to a pool of water that absorbs the radiation and protects the workers.
(Artwork courtesy of MDS Nordion Inc.)

51. Irradiation

ATION

A Safe Measure For Safer Food

BEEF is one of the U.S. food industry's hottest sellers—to the tune of 8 billion pounds a year, according to trade figures. Whether at a fast-food meal, a dinner on the town, or a backyard barbecue, beef is often front and center on America's tables.

But in recent years, beef, especially ground beef, has shown a dark side: It can harbor the bacterium *E. coli* O157:H7, a pathogen that threatens the safety of the domestic food supply. If not properly prepared, beef tainted with *E. coli* O157:H7 can make people ill, and in rare instances, kill them. In 1993, *E. coli* O157:H7-contaminated hamburgers sold by a fast-food chain were linked to the deaths of four children and hundreds of illnesses in the Pacific Northwest.

In 1997, the potential extent of *E. coli* O157:H7 contamination came to light when Arkansas-based Hudson Foods Inc. voluntarily recalled 25 million pounds of hamburger suspected of containing *E. coli* O157:H7. It was the largest recall of meat products in U.S. history.

Nationally, *E. coli* O157:H7 causes about 20,000 illnesses and 500 deaths a year, according to the federal Centers for

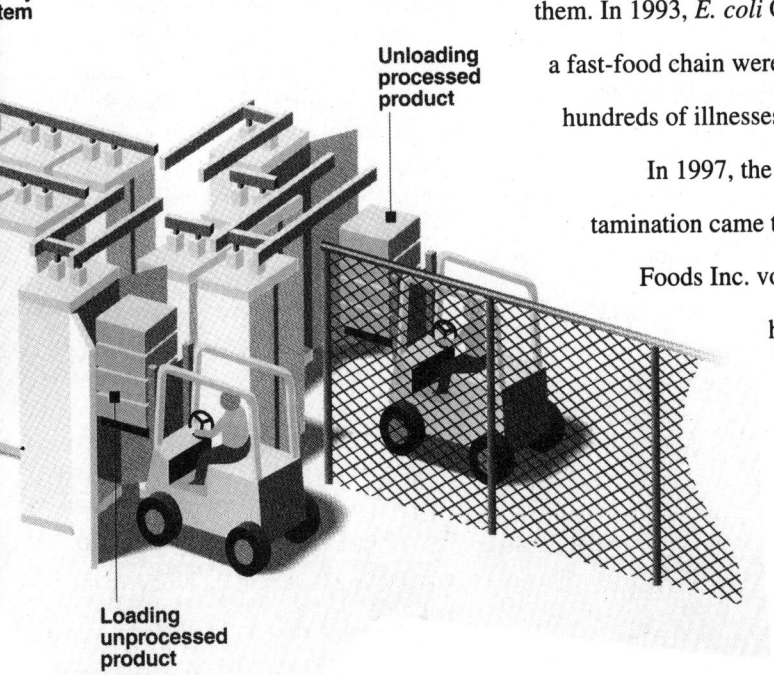

INFOGRAPHIC BY SAM WARD

FDA's approval of red meat irradiation adds to a lengthy list of foods approved for the process, including poultry, fresh fruits and vegetables, and dry spices.

Disease Control and Prevention. Scientists have only known since 1982 that this form of *E. coli* causes human illness.

To help combat this public health problem, the Food and Drug Administration last December approved treating red meat products with a measured dose of radiation. This process, commonly called irradiation, has drawn praise from many food industry and health organizations because it can control *E. coli* O157:H7 and several other disease-causing microorganisms. As with other regulations governing meat and poultry products, irradiation will be authorized when the U.S. Department of Agriculture completes its implementing regulations.

Though irradiation is the latest step toward curbing food-borne illness, the federal government also is implementing other measures, which include developing new technologies and expanding the use of current technologies.

A Long Safety Record

FDA's red meat approval added another product category to the already lengthy list of foods the agency has approved for irradiation since 1963. These include poultry, fresh fruits and vegetables, dry spices, seasonings, and enzymes.

As part of its approval, FDA requires that irradiated foods include labeling with either the statement "treated with radiation" or "treated by irradiation" and the international symbol for irradiation, the radura (pictured above). Irradiation labeling requirements apply only to foods sold in stores. For example, irradiated spices or fresh strawberries should be labeled. When used as ingredients in other foods, however, the label of the other food does not need to describe these ingredients as irradiated. Irradiation labeling also does not apply to restaurant foods.

FDA has evaluated irradiation safety for 40 years and found the process safe and effective for many foods. Before approving red meat irradiation, the agency reviewed numerous scientific studies conducted worldwide. These included research on the chemical effects of radiation on meat, the impact the process has on nutrient content, and potential toxicity concerns.

In this most recent review and in previous reviews of the irradiation process, FDA scientists concluded that irradiation reduces or eliminates pathogenic bacteria, insects and parasites. It reduces spoilage, and in certain fruits and vegetables, it inhibits sprouting and delays the ripening process. Also, it does not make food radioactive, compromise nutritional quality, or noticeably change food taste, texture or appearance as long as it's applied properly to a suitable product.

Health experts say that in addition to reducing *E. coli* O157:H7 contamination, irradiation can help control the potentially harmful bacteria *Salmonella* and *Campylobacter*, two chief causes of food-borne illness. The Centers for Disease Control and Prevention estimates that *Salmonella*—commonly found in poultry, eggs, meat, and milk— sickens as many as 4 million and kills 1,000 per year nationwide. *Campylobacter*, found mostly in poultry, is responsible for 6 million illnesses and 75 deaths per year in the United States. A May 1997 presidential report, "Food Safety from Farm to Table," estimates that "millions" of Americans are stricken by food-borne illness each year and some 9,000, mostly the very young and elderly, die as a result.

FDA officials emphasize that though irradiation is a useful tool for reducing food-borne disease risk, it complements, but doesn't replace, proper food handling practices by producers, processors and consumers.

Limited Success So Far

Though irradiation would appear to

Many spices are irradiated, which eliminates the need for chemical fumigation to control pests.

have much going for it, retail outlets have been slow to carry irradiated foods. This, experts say, is partially because many store owners and food producers fear consumers won't buy the products based on misgivings about radiation in general.

But some stores have plunged in anyway—with limited success. Carrot Top, a Chicago-area grocery market, was one of the first to carry irradiated fruits (see "Berry Successful Irradiation"). Owner Jim Corrigan says the products have been selling steadily since 1992. Other stores—mostly small, independent markets—have followed suit, offering irradiated vegetables, fruits and poultry to a modest, but loyal, group of irradiation-savvy customers.

Because irradiated red meat is not yet on the market, it remains to be seen if consumers will buy products such as irradiated ground beef—or if large food processors will even offer it. Irradiated products sold to date have cost slightly more than their untreated counterparts because of the extra step irradiation adds to food processing. But in the future, these costs could be offset by improved shelf life and increased consumer demand, according to food trade groups.

Major food companies such as poultry processors, meat packers, and grocery chains have yet to embrace irradiation, not only because of perceived consumer attitudes, but also due to logistics. Food Technology Service Inc., in Mulberry, Fla., is the only irradiating facility dedicated solely to treating agricultural products. More than 40 other facilities nationwide primarily handle sterilization of medical supplies, though these plants also can irradiate food products. In fact, it was a New Jersey-based medical irradiation company, Isomedix Inc., that petitioned FDA to approve red meat irradiation.

Beyond physical distances and lack of facilities, sheer product volume makes it unlikely that irradiation will be wide-

Berry Successful Irradiation

The huge sign hanging over the rows of boxed strawberries left little doubt for Chicago-area grocery shoppers that the produce before them was something new and unusual.

Not that the berries looked any different. But the massive poster above them bore a message in mammoth letters that might as well have been neon: "Treated by irradiation for freshness and health." To the store owner's surprise, patrons flocked to the new product, buying nine times more of it than of standard strawberries.

That scene took place in 1992 at Carrot Top, one of the first retail stores to venture into the then-uncharted realm of irradiated foods. The decision to stock radiation-treated berries in the store, however, came slowly. Owner Jim Corrigan spent about a year reading up on the irradiation process and passing details to his regular customers through periodic newsletters. He says informing customers before the store actually stocked the new products helped allay possible fears.

When the Florida-grown strawberries finally arrived, along with irradiated oranges and grapefruits, shoppers were well acquainted with the process and responded with sales.

Today, Corrigan remains enthusiastic. He says irradiation ensures that strawberries will be free of insects and will keep longer—in some cases, up to three weeks, versus three to five days for conventional berries.

"One of our ways of rating the freshness of strawberries is to examine the small hairs that grow by the seed," he says. "If they are standing up and plentiful, the strawberries are still fresh. [With irradiated strawberries] we see a lot of that after three weeks."

The products remain steady sellers, and Corrigan has since added irradiated onions and papayas to his stock. ■

—J.H.

CONTEMPORARY HEALTH HAZARDS

Irradiating food is similar to passing luggage through an airport scanner.

spread anytime soon. The domestic poultry trade, for instance, processes about 25 billion pounds per year, according to industry figures. Says Kenneth May, spokesman for the National Broiler Council, which represents poultry producers: "We think [irradiation is] a process that will work. But for practical purposes, we just don't see anything happening with it in the near future." He adds, however, that if the public really wants an irradiated product, the poultry industry will find a way to deliver it.

Will Consumers Accept It?

Before irradiation can really take off, the public must "warm up" to a method associated with nuclear energy, a source that carries its share of negative perceptions. George Pauli, Ph.D., FDA's food irradiation safety coordinator, compares irradiation to milk pasteurization, another decontaminating process that dramatically curbed disease but took decades before achieving public acceptance. "When the public finally sees a need for irradiation and realizes its value, I think people will accept it, maybe even demand it," Pauli says. "But you have to give them time."

A Louis Harris poll released in 1986 found that 76 percent of Americans considered irradiated food a hazard. But later studies have shown that consumer attitudes can be changed through education.

In 1995, researchers at the University of Georgia reported that 87.5 percent of consumers had heard of irradiation but knew little about it. So the university set up a "simulated supermarket setting" and labeled irradiated products, put posters at the point of sale, and developed a slide show explaining irradiation. "Our goal was to see which one of those techniques was most effective in changing people's attitudes," says Kay McWatters, agricultural research scientist and one of the study authors.

The study found that any kind of education helps convey the benefits of irradiation, McWatters says. "But the one that turned out most effective was the slide show, because visual images and [narration] are much more attention-getting than just a static label or poster."

After the study's education strategy, about 84 percent of participating consumers said irradiation is "somewhat necessary" or "very necessary." Fifty-eight percent said they would always buy irradiated chicken if available, and 27 percent said they would buy it sometimes.

Another study in 1997 by the Food Marketing Institute had similar results. After receiving education about the process, 60 percent of those in the study said they would buy irradiated foods.

Approved Uses of Irradiation

FDA approved the first use of irradiation on a food product in 1963 when it allowed radiation-treated wheat and wheat flour to be marketed. In approving a use of radiation, FDA sets the maximum radiation dose the product can be exposed to, measured in units called kiloGray (kGy). The following is a list of all approved uses of radiation on foods to date, the purpose for irradiating them, and the radiation dose allowed.

Food	Approved Use	Dose
Spices and dry vegetable seasoning	decontaminates and controls insects and microorganisms	30 kGy
Dry or dehydrated enzyme preparations	controls insects and microorganisms	10 kGy
All foods	controls insects	1 kGy
Fresh foods	delays maturation	1 kGy
Poultry	controls disease-causing microorganisms	3 kGy
Red meat (such as beef, lamb and pork)	controls spoilage and disease-causing microorganisms	4.5 kGy (fresh) 7 kGy (frozen)

Carrot Top owner Corrigan also discovered this on a small scale after sending his regular customers information about irradiation in periodic newsletters.

Luggage and Milk

Other studies, however, show that many consumers still question if irradiation is safe. They wonder if the process transfers radiation to the product or if it causes chemical changes in the food that might be hazardous. Even the word "irradiation" is scary to some, carrying images of atomic explosions or nuclear reactor accidents.

Radiolytic products, formed when food is irradiated, are similar to those formed by cooking food. FDA has found them to be safe.

But as long as radiation is applied to foods in approved doses, it's safe, says FDA's Pauli. Similar to sending luggage through an airport scanner, the process passes food quickly through a radiation field—typically gamma rays produced from radioactive cobalt-60. That amount of energy is not strong enough to add any radioactive material to the food. The same irradiation process is used to sterilize medical products such as bandages, contact lens solutions, and hospital supplies such as gloves, sutures and gowns. Many spices sold in this country also are irradiated, which eliminates the need for chemical fumigation to control pests. American astronauts have eaten irradiated foods since 1972.

Irradiation is a "cold" process that gives off little heat, so foods can be irradiated within their packaging and remain protected against contamination until opened by users. Because a few bacteria can survive the process in poultry and meats, it's important, Pauli says, to keep products refrigerated and to cook them properly.

Irradiation interferes with bacterial genetics, so the contaminating organism can no longer survive or multiply. Although chemicals called radiolytic products are created when food is irradiated, FDA has found them to pose no health hazard. In fact, the same kinds of products are formed when food is cooked.

Praises and Protests

Though irradiation has its share of detractors, many prestigious organizations endorse it, including the World Health Organization, the International Atomic Energy Agency, the American Medical Association, and the American Dietetic Association. Trade groups such as the National Meat Association, the Grocery Manufacturers of America, and the National Food Processors Association also support irradiation.

However, some groups have given irradiation a thumbs down. Consumer activist Jeremy Rifkin, president of the Pure Food Campaign, says more attention should be placed on raising healthier livestock, which he says would reduce pathogens and make irradiation unnecessary. The Center for Science in the Public Interest calls irradiation "expensive" and "an end-of-the-line solution to contamination problems that can and should be addressed earlier."

But with so many influential organizations backing irradiation, along with concerns about rising numbers of disease cases, the stage is set for the process to pick up momentum, despite negative sentiments, supporters say. First, however, says FDA's Pauli, the food industry needs to get more irradiated products into the marketplace. "Most people in this country haven't even seen an irradiated food," he says. "When products start appearing, then the public can make up its mind."

John Henkel is a staff writer for FDA Consumer.

Radiation's Positive Side

Scientists first studied radiation as a way to improve food products in the 1930s, but research didn't begin in earnest until just after World War II. At that time, the U.S. Army was seeking a means to lessen dependence on refrigeration and replace K rations and other preserved products that troops used in the field.

In the early 1950s, the Atomic Energy Commission (now part of the U.S. Department of Energy) explored food irradiation as part of President Eisenhower's "Atoms for Peace" program. This research differed from the Army's in that it examined the effects smaller radiation doses had on certain fruits and vegetables. The end result was not a sterile product but one where insects would be killed or sterilized. Because this produce still could spoil, refrigeration was needed. But at least potentially harmful insects would not cross state or national borders.

Such research, augmented by studies from other countries, established that the most important benefit from irradiation could be the control of disease-causing pathogens and that the maximum practical and effective dose depended on the food and the purpose for irradiating. ■

—J.H.

Why Is Date Rape So Hard to Prove?

SHEILA WELLER

Sheila Weller is the author of Marrying the Hangman, *recently published by Random House.*

WITH ACQUAINTANCE RAPE cases now a TV spectator sport, lots of women I know are having some variation of this black-humored fantasy: You're on the witness stand, watching an expensively suited defense attorney pace around as he spits out accusations: What about those one-night stands six years ago? Your taste for double margaritas? Is it true that you met this man at a nightclub? And weren't you wearing a lace camisole under your blouse? That's the last straw. You stand up, rip the fuzzy blue dot off your face and say, "I give up! Let the bastard walk. It's not worth this trying to convict him."

After the past year's parade of well-publicized rape cases, such fantasy seems all too black and none too humorous. First there was the William Kennedy Smith case, during which the *New York Times* implied that rape complainant Patricia Bowman's speeding tickets bolstered a schoolmate's claim of her "little wild streak." More recently, when a young Manhattan architect accused three New York Mets of rape, her ex-boyfriend, Mets pitcher David Cone, reportedly told her that no one would believe her and her reputation would be ruined. He turned out to be right on both scores. The *New York Post* trumpeted the headline: "Mets accuser was 'No Vestal Virgin.'" And in early April, the Florida state attorney, pointing to a lack of physical evidence, decided to drop the case. The message to women has been clear: Many of us would not make believable accusers.

Not that a woman who says she's been raped shouldn't be scrutinized. After all, what about the reputation of the accused?

There's no getting around the fact that acquaintance rape is a crime in which the victim and the sole eyewitness are often one and the same. Both sides admit they had intercourse. The only issue is consent. When it's her word against his, it's only fair that her credibility and ulterior motives be questioned.

But that doesn't mean the woman is the one who should go on trial. All too often the legitimate question "Did this woman consent to intercourse?" leaps dangerously to "Was she leading him on?" In another recent case, a group of young men from prominent Tampa families admitted to drugging a woman and then raping her. The defense argued that by willingly accompanying the men after a night of drinking, she invited the ensuing events. The men were acquitted.

No wonder so few women actually report being raped. A new study by the National Victim Center estimates that one in eight women in the United States has been raped, in most cases by someone she knew, but that only about 16 percent of the rapes were reported. Of those cases that are reported, the majority are dropped by the prosecutor, according to Gary LaFree, a sociologist at the University of New Mexico and author of *Rape and Criminal Justice*. Only the rare resilient case, roughly one to 5 percent of all rapes, actually reaches the courtroom.

The road into and out of that courtroom can be so treacherous that even some rape counselors question whether it's worth it. "When I first started working here," says Colleen Leyrer of the Washington, D.C., Rape Crisis Center, "I was uncomfortable not encouraging a woman to prosecute. Now, after seeing victims go through a second trauma as a result of prosecuting, I urge the woman to decide for herself."

It's a tough decision—one that a woman should make with both eyes open. "If it's likely the case will end in acquittal, and if the woman's wavering, then I probably wouldn't recommend prosecution," says Andrea Parrot, a rape expert and psychologist at Cornell University.

But how does a woman know whether her case is likely to end in acquittal? How can she know if it will even make it to the courtroom? The people who deal with acquaintance rape cases daily—prosecutors, judges, defense attorneys—know firsthand why so few of them end in conviction. Here's what they say makes acquaintance rape so hard to prove.

UNLESS THE WOMAN IS A GIRL SCOUT OR VIRGIN, THE JURY WILL GIVE MORE WEIGHT TO HER CHARACTER THAN TO THE EVIDENCE.

EVEN THE MIKE TYSON conviction seemed to confirm this theory: Wasn't Desiree Washington a naive, churchgoing teenager? "A woman who has a good reputation, does not dress suggestively, has a nine-to-five job, and goes home after work will be looked on more favorably by a jury," says Brooks Leach, sex crimes prosecutor in Columbiana, Alabama.

In a study of 880 rape cases, sociologist Gary LaFree found that a complainant's "questionable" character was the best predictor of a defendant's acquittal. "We found that juries were most swayed by things like whether she had been drinking or even if she had birth control pills in her pocket," says LaFree. Juries find it more important that a woman frequents bars than that the man had a gun; more important that she had sex outside of marriage than that she was physically injured in the rape; more important that she was a "party girl" than that her clothes were torn that evening.

But you don't have to be a wanton woman for your morality to be suspect. Anyone who's had multiple sexual partners or an abortion is vulnerable. Even though 40 states now have "rape shield" laws making details of an accuser's past sexual life inadmissable in trials, such legislation is hardly foolproof. "There's an insidious way to get around the law," says sociologist Susan Caringella-McDonald. "Defense attorneys question the woman about her past sexual activity; the prosecutor objects; the judge sustains the objection—but the jury's already heard it so the damage is done."

Many well-off defendants hire private investigators to scout for information on accusers that can either be "leaked" at the trial or used to derail a case before it reaches the courtroom. "We'll do a surveillance of a rape complainant to find out: Does she go to parties and bars? Leave with somebody? Come home drunk?" says attorney Marshall Stern of Bangor, Maine. "You can't use these findings on the stand, but it's a bargaining tool with the prosecutor. If you say, 'See, she smoked dope here . . . ,' he may not think he has the winning case he once had."

Even a woman who's been sexually abused in the past might be considered less credible if that comes out in court, says Nancy Hollander, president of the National Association of Criminal Defense Attorneys: "If she has a history of abuse, we can use it to suggest that it's left her misunderstanding signals and thinking she was raped when she wasn't."

JURIES DON'T HAVE MUCH
....
SYMPATHY FOR A WOMAN
....
WHO WAS A WILLING
....
PARTICIPANT UP TO THE TIME
....
OF THE ALLEGED RAPE.
....

THE MORE ROMANTIC contact the woman had with the man, the tougher her case is to win. "You can almost diagram it," says Nancy Diehl, assistant prosecuting attorney for Detroit's Wayne County. "Fair to good is: The woman was in her or his house with him voluntarily, but she didn't have a previous relationship with him, it wasn't late at night, and she didn't kiss him. The more of those conditions that change from negative to positive, the harder it gets to win the case."

Patricia Bowman's case, for instance, was crippled by the lateness and the kissing. "When a woman has been acting in a way that juries see as encouraging a sexual encounter, they tend to say, 'Lady, you can't act like that and then change your mind,'" says Rock Harmon, deputy district attorney in Oakland, California. One of the most outrageous examples of this kind of bias occurred in the Tampa case. A defendant (later acquitted) explained at the trial that the complainant used profanity, smoked cigarettes, and dressed in green stretch pants: "She was not commanding as much respect from the guys as we would normally give other, more ladylike females."

Women jurors can often be hardest on women, perhaps because they want to deny that they too could be victims. Larry Donoghue, head of one of the sex crimes units of the Los Angeles district attorney's office, finds that female jurors are especially biased against assertive, ambitious women. Men are often surprisingly empathetic. "Fathers and grandfathers seem to take a protective attitude toward the victim," says Des Moines–based trial consultant Hale Starr. "But religious homemakers are the worst jurors for the victim. Their attitude is, 'I would never have gone to that room with that man . . .' They're unforgiving."

Still, there are some surprising exceptions. In a recent Detroit case, jurors convicted a man for the rape of a topless go-go dancer who had accepted a ride from him, changed into her street clothes in the back of his van, and driven with him in search of cocaine. Nancy Diehl says an eyewitness's testimony and strong physical evidence pushed the jurors past the tendency to believe that the woman "got what she deserved."

UNLESS THERE'S PHYSICAL
....
EVIDENCE, IT'S HER WORD
....
AGAINST HIS.
....

RARELY ARE THERE broken bones with acquaintance rape, but that doesn't mean there's no physical evidence. Even if a woman is uncertain whether she wants to pursue a complaint, she should go immediately to a doctor's office or the hospital for an examination. Forcible as opposed to consensual sex *is* often medically verifiable, even in long-sexually-active women. "When a woman is having consensual sex with a man, she needs to do what is referred to as a 'pelvic tilt' to accommodate his penis," says D.A. Donoghue. "In forcible sex, the last thing that she wants is to accommodate him. His force can lead to anything from reddening to bruises to lacerations. If it's just reddening, you've got to identify it fast, or it fades. It's not perfect evidence, but it can make the difference between winning and losing."

Immediate report of the assault also makes a rape victim appear more genuine. "Juries look for an immediate outcry. They want to see that she wasted no time telling the authorities," says Barry Levin, a defense attorney in the St. John's College case in which seven men were charged with gang-raping a black woman student. Levin, who plea-bargained his client down from a felony to a misdemeanor, says he got his biggest boost from the complainant, who waited a month before reporting the rape. The same holds true for the woman who accused the three Mets players a year after the rape. The prosecutor said her long delay and the resulting lack of physical evidence meant she didn't have a case.

"If you delay, the defense is going to say, 'See? She made it up to get back at the guy,' and the jury will believe it," says D.A. Nancy Diehl. "My advice always is: Report first, *then* decide. If you choose not to pursue the complaint, you can always back out of it."

EMOTIONAL OR CONFLICTING
....
TESTIMONY CAN DESTROY
....
A WOMAN'S CREDIBILITY.
....

THE ACCUSER should be calm but not robotic, testifying with feeling but not appearing overly emotional. Despite the harrowing experience she's endured, a victim who cries may be viewed as unstable. A calm but concerned woman, able to summon up the trauma without relapsing into it—like Desiree Washington—appeals more to juries.

Believability is crippled when the accuser tells a story that contains even a few loose threads, which defense attorneys use to unravel her entire story. Many prosecutors say that this is what most damaged Patricia Bowman's case: Her story was inconsistent and prosecutor Moira Lasch did her no favor by letting those inconsistencies reach the courtroom. "I did not find Bowman's story credible, and Lasch did not confront this before trial," says Karyn Sinunu, head of the sexual assault division of the Santa Clara County, California, district attorney's office. "I listened to Bowman say that she kissed him 'but it wasn't sexual' and I thought, 'You can kiss a husband of twenty years good-bye in the morning and it isn't sexual, but you don't kiss someone you've just met and it isn't sexual.' When you try to make your story sound better, the jury ends up seeing through it."

Even when a prosecutor catches all evasions well before the trial, they can come back to haunt the complainant and end up destroying her case. D.A. Donoghue tried a case in which a very credible woman had initially told police she was forced into the rapist's car: "She was too embarrassed to admit she had misjudged the man's motives when he offered her a ride home and had gotten into the car voluntarily." Though she corrected her story by trial time, the original falsification was bandied about by the defense attorney: If she had lied about that, then she could have lied about the whole thing. The defendant walked.

A skilled prosecutor plays devil's advocate early on, gently pushing the woman past her urge to apply face-saving spin control to her memory of the ordeal. "The woman needs to convince me that she was raped," says D.A. Nancy Diehl. "I say, 'Look, I need the whole truth. No matter how bad you think it looks, if you tell me, I'll be able to explain it to the jury.'"

These days, with Desiree Washington's success as inspiration, prosecutors say more women are deciding to press charges on a crime that has mostly been endured in silence and shame. But individual women can't be expected to live their day-in-and-day-out lives as political symbols, or as statistics in a war against apathy. In the end, the decision to pursue prosecution is deeply personal. "Victims and psychiatrists tell me it's therapeutic to prosecute," says Donoghue. Wanda Jones, who became a victims' service officer in Birmingham, Alabama, after she was raped by seven men, says the experience of seeing her rapists brought to justice was empowering. Says sociologist Andrea Parrot: "Some women, even understanding the likelihood of the man's acquittal, need to go through with prosecution to feel whole and vindicated. In those cases, I'd say go ahead."

Index

A

acceptance, sense of, 31
acetominophen, 97, 179, 180, 189
acquaintance rape, 222–224
aerobic exercise. *See* exercise
aerobic fitness test, 76
aflatoxin, 26
ageism, 156
AIDS, 33, 102, 103, 114, 115, 145, 155, 211; treatment of, 148–151
air pollution, 146
Alar, 24, 26
alcohol, 23, 99–100, 137, 144, 146
allergies, 179
ALS, 182
alternative therapies, 162
Alzheimer's disease, 128
American Dietetic Association, 61
American Pharmaceutical Association, 98
aminotriazole, 26
anesthesia, preparing for, 159
animal studies, 177
anorexia nervosa, 92
antibacterial products, 202–206
antibiotics, 154, 159; peptide, 207–210
antibodies, 32
anti-CD3, 151
antidepressants, 96, 124, 164
antihistamines, 98, 124
antioxidants, 14, 62, 63
anxiety, 93, 129
arrythmia, 42, 43
Arthritis Cure, The, (Theodosakis), 189
aspirin, 15, 97, 136–137, 180
asthma, 129, 146

B

bactolysins, 209
bad moods, 48–49
balance test, 78
barrier methods, 110, 113
basal cell carcinoma (BCC), 200
basic research, 14
beta-carotene, 14, 67, 174, 178
billing errors, hospital, 73
binge-eating disorder, 92–93
biofeedback, 43
birth control pill, 110–111, 112, 145; triphasic, 111
body-fat distribution, heart disease in women and, 135–136
body-mass index (BMI), 83
BPI (bactericidal/permeability-increasing protein), 209
breast cancer, 57, 144, 145, 146; alcohol and, 99–100
brown bread, 54
bulimia nervosa, 92

C

calcium, 174, 193
Campylobacter, 218
cancer, 16, 23, 57, 62, 76, 102, 103, 128, 142–147, 174. *See also* specific type of cancer
carbohydrates, 85
cardiac rehabilitation programs, progessive, 43
cardiovascular disease. *See* heart disease
cardiovascular system, 31, 32
case control studies, 15
cataracts, 176
catecholamines, 32, 33
cervical cancer, 117, 142, 143, 145, 211, 212, 213
cesarian sections, increase in, 156
change, stages of, and health, 19–21
Chaparral, 196
"character disorders," 155
chemotherapy, 102, 103, 124
childbirth, 30, 32
chiropractic, 163, 164
chlamydia, 118, 119, 213, 214, 216
Chlamydia pneumoniae, 132, 133, 134
cholesterol, 64, 131, 133, 138–141, 179; AIDS treatment and, 150–151; exercise and, 74–75; fat and, 60
Cholestin, 185–186, 188–189
chondroitin, 189
chronic obstructive pulmonary disease (COPD), 106
clemastine fumarate, 98
clinical trials, 14, 17
Clinton, Bill, 101
codeine, 97
cognitive behavior therapy, for binge-eating disorder, 93
cognitive restructuring, 34, 44
cognitive therapy, 40
cohort studies, 15
cold remedies, 96–98
colds, 173
colon cancer, 144
colonoscopy, 143
colorectal cancer, 142, 143
Comfrey, 196
condoms, 113, 145, 212; female 112, 116, 124, 212; sexually transmitted diseases and, 114–116, 121
confiding, 32
confounding, 15
constipation, 62, 63
contact lenses, 173
control, loss of, 33
coronary heart disease. *See* heart disease
cortisol, 30, 38
cough suppressants, 97
cyclamates, 26
cystic fibrosis, 128
cytomegalovirus, 132, 133, 134

D

Daily Values, Percent (DV), 65
dairy foods, 53
date rape, 222–224
decongestants, oral, 96, 97
dehydroepiandrosterone (DHEA), 187
Delaney clause, 26
Delaney, James, 216
Depo Provera, 112
depression, 42, 93, 129, 164
dexfenfluramine, 84
diabetes, 16, 62, 63, 76, 92, 128, 135; fat and, 60; Type II, 129, 135
Dietary Supplement Health and Education Act (DSHEA), 184, 190–191, 193
dietary supplements, 190–197
dieter's teas, 196
digitalis, 168, 193
disease, versus illness, 31
dishcloths, 205
dishwashing liquids, 204–205
diverticulosis, 62
Doctors, Patients, and Placebos (Spiro), 164
dong quai, 189
douching, 123
drug interactions, 160

E

"eating disorder otherwise unspecified," 90–91
eating disorders, 90–91, 92–93
echinacea, 188; colds and, 98; lupus and, 186
endometrial cancer, 145, 146
emphysema, 106
environment, versus genetic origins of disease, 23
ephedrine, 191, 193, 196
epidemiological studies, 15, 16, 17–18, 177
epididymitis, 119
epilepsy, 102
epinephrine, 30
Espstein-Barr virus, 145
Escherichia coli 0157:H7, 52, 203, 217–218
estrogen replacement therapy, 124, 174. *See also* hormone replacement therapy
estrogen(s), 62, 124, 146, 187
exercise, 16, 20, 60, 72–75, 83–84, 129; aerobic, 34, 74–75, 144, 146, 185

F

family trees, 130
fast food industry, pressure to eat and, 87
fat(s), 57–60, 144; AIDS treatment and metabolism of, 150; animal, 146; heart disease and, 57, 59–60, 133; low-, diets, 53–54, 84–85
Fauci, Anthony, 151
female condom, 112, 116, 124, 212
fenfluramine, 84
fen-phen, 84

feverfew, migraines and, 186
fiber, 61–65, 133
fish, 174
flexibility, test for, 77–78
folic acid, 67–68, 131, 132, 141, 144, 193
Food and Drug Administration (FDA), 102, 163, 164, 179, 185, 186; dietary supplements and, 190–191, 193, 194–195
food industry, pressure to eat and, 86–87, 89
forgiveness, mind-body connection and, 45–47
Freud, Sigmund, 155
frogs, peptide antibiotics and, 208
frontiers, 156
fungiform papillae, 56

G

gargling, 97
genes, 128, 142
genetic factors, in disease, 23, 129
genetic testing, 128
genital herpes. *See* herpes simplex virus
germander, 196
germanium, 197
Germany, 32, 186, 188
ginkgo, 188
glaucoma, 102, 103, 129
glucosamine, 189
goldenseal herb, 188
gonorrhea, 117, 119, 211, 212, 214, 215
good manufacturing practices (GMPs), dietary supplements and, 193
group therapy, for binge-eating disorder, 93
guaifenesin, 97

H

HAART (highly active anti-retroviral therapy), 148–151
hand gels, water-free, 205
hand soaps, antibacterial, 204
Handbook of Nonprescription Drugs (American Pharmaceutical Association), 98
hardiness, AIDS survival and, 33
HDL (high-density lipoprotein) cholesterol, 74–75, 131, 133, 135, 139, 140, 179
health care costs, 156
health priorities, as inverted, 22–27
heart attacks, 31–32, 37–41, 42, 61
heart disease, 16, 42, 43, 53, 62, 76, 129, 131–134; alcohol and, 99, 100; B vitamins and, 67–68, 103, 131, 176; cholesterol and, 131, 133, 138–141; fat and, 57, 59–60; vitamin E and, 69; women and, 135–137
Heidelberg Appeal, 27
Helicobacter pylori, 145
hemophilia, 128

hepatitis B, 117, 119, 211, 212, 213, 214; hepatocellular carcinoma and, 145; vaccinations for, 142, 145, 213
herbal remedies, 162, 163, 165, 167–169, 174–189
hereditary disease, 128–130
herpes simplex virus, 117, 119, 125, 211; Type II, 214
high blood pressure. *See* hypertension
high responders, 38
histamines, 98
HIV, 114, 115, 117, 145, 211
Ho, David, 151
homocysteine, 131–132, 133, 140
hope, 163–165
hormone replacement therapy, heart disease and, 136. *See also* estrogen replacement therapy
hospital billing errors, 73
hospitals, surviving stays at, 158–161
hot dogs, 17
household cleaners, 204
H2 blockers, 180
human clinical trials, 177–178
human growth hormone, 102
human papilloma virus, 117, 119, 125, 145, 211, 213, 214
hypercholesterolemia, 128
hypertension, 76, 93, 129, 132, 133, 135, 175, 180
hysterectomies, 124

I

ibuprofen, 75, 97, 179, 180, 189
immune system, 31, 34, 165
impotence, 175
infertility, 155, 213
insulin resistance, fat and, 60
insurance, 164
Internet, 182–183
intervention trials, population-based, 18
intrauterine devices (IUDs), 110
irradiation, 216–221

J

Joint Commission on Accreditation of Healthcare Organizations (JCAHO), 160

K

ketoprofen, 102, 179, 180
"killer flu," 9

L

lactobacilli, 122
lactose intolerance, 53
LDL (low-density lipoprotein) cholesterol, 61, 64, 131, 133, 139, 140, 174
LDL pattern, 140–141

life events, illness and critical, 30–36
Life Extension (Pearson and Shaw), 163
lipoprotein(a), 139–140
"Live Better, Live Longer" quiz, 8–13
lobelia, 196
Lou Gehrig's disease, 182
lovastatin, 185, 186
low birth weight, heart disease and, 133
L-tryptophan, 197
lung cancer, 106–107

M

magainin, 207–209
Magnolia-Stephania preparation, 196
marijuana, medical, 101–103
massage therapy, 165
McCaffrey, Barry, 101, 103
meaning, survival and, 32
meat, 53; ground, 176
Medicaid, 157
meditation, 43, 163
melanoma, 146, 201
melatonin, 187
mental illness, 155
Meridia, 84
mind-body approaches, 43; forgiveness and, 45–47
mini-pill, 112–113
monounsaturated fat, 58
morphine, postoperative, 159
multiple sclerosis (MS), 102, 103

N

naproxen sodium, 179, 180
nasal sprays, 97
National Institutes of Health, 162
niacin, 197
norepinephrine, 30, 32, 38
Norplant, 111
nuclear power accidents, 30, 33
nuts, 53, 175

O

oats, 61
obesity, 16, 76, 92, 129, 144; pressure to eat and, 86–89
obsession, with foods, 90–91
Office of Alternative Medicine, 162
oils, 85
omega-3 fatty acids, 58, 175
optimism, 165, 166
Origin of Everyday Moods, The (Thayer), 49
orlistat, 84
Orudis KT, 179
osteoarthritis, 75
osteoporosis, 124, 129, 174
ovarian cancer, 145, 146
over-the-counter medications, 179–181

P

pain medication, self-administered, 159, 160
Palmer, B. J., 163
Pap tests, 124, 143, 145, 213
Partnership for a Drug-Free America, 101
patient advocates, 159
Patient's Bill of Rights, 159
Pauling, Linus, 163
pausing, binge-eating disorder and, 93
Pearson, Durk, 163
PC-SPES, 168–169
pelvic inflammatory disease (PID), 110, 119
peptide antibiotics, 207–210
pesticides, 23
pexiganan, 209
phentermine, 84
phenylpropanolamine, 97, 181
phlebitis, 159
phytochemicals, 62
pill. *See* birth control pill
placebo effect, 164, 166
placebos, 164–165
Pneumocystis carinii, 34
pneumonia, postoperative, 159
pollution, 146
polyunsaturated fat, 58
porphyromonas gingivalis, 132, 133, 134
postnasal drip, 97
prayer, 163
pregnancy, 30, 32, 110, 186
productive cough, 97
Proposition 200, in Arizona, 101
Proposition 215, in California, 101
prostate cancer, 144, 168–169
prostate, enlarged, 189
protease inhibitors, 148–149, 150
"protease paunch," 150
protegrins, 209
proteins, 85
psychoneuroimmunology (PNI), 30, 34
psyllium seed husk, 193

R

rationing, of heath care, 156–157
rebound symptons, 180
Redux, 84
Regelson, William, 187
Reich, Wilhelm, 155
relaxation therapy, 40
resistance: antibiotic, 203, 205, 209–210; drug, and AIDS treatment, 149
rhinovirus, transmission of, 98

S

saccharine, 24, 26
Saint-John's-wort, 165, 188
Salmonella, 202, 206, 209–210, 218
Sarason, I. G., 31
saturated fat, 58
saw palmetto berry, 189
schedule I drugs, 102
schizophrenia, 129, 155
science, politically correct, 25
sedentary lifestyle, 79–82, 87
selenium, 197
Selye, Hans, 30
sexually transmitted diseases (STDs), 110, 113, 117–121; condoms and, 114–116, 121; conservative approach to preventing, 118–119, 120; liberal approach to preventing, 119–120
Shaw, Sandy, 163
sibutramine, 84
sickle-cell anemia, 128
sigmoidoscopy, 143
sit-ups, 176
6-n-propylthiouracil, 55
skin cancer, 200–201
sleep apnea, 176
smoking, 16, 17, 23, 64–65, 104–107, 129, 142, 143–144, 174
snoring, 176
sodium, hypertension and, 175
sore throat, 97
sponges, 205
Spiro, Howard, 164
sprains, 175
squamous cell carcinoma (SCC), 200–201
stomach cancer, 145
strawberries, irradiation of, 219
strength tests, 77–78
strength training, 74, 83
stress, 93, 165
strokes, 23, 173
Sudafed, 97, 179
sugar, 174
sulfonamides, 154
sunscreens, 146, 201
Superfund, 23
Super-Hormone Promise, The (Regelson), 187
supertasters, vegetables and, 55–56
supplements, dietary, 145
surgery, 158, 159, 164
Sustiva, 150
sympathetic-adrenal medullary system, 31
"syndrome X," 136
syphilis, 117, 119, 155, 211, 212, 214, 78

T

Tai chi, 78
tamoxifen, 146
taste buds, 56
taxes, on tobacco products, 143
T-cells, AIDS treatment and, 151
teeth, 174, 175
testosterone, 32, 102, 187
thalidomide, 185
Thayer, Robert E., 49
Theodosakis, Jason, 189
throat sprays, 97
timed-release pills, 98
tobacco industry, 25
trans fat, 58
trichomoniasis, 117, 119, 128
triclosan, 204
triglycerides, 138, 140; AIDS therapy and, 150–151
tubal ligations, 112, 146
Type A personality, 38, 41
Type H personality, 38, 41

U

ulcers, 180
ultraviolet light, skin cancer and, 201
urethritis, 119
urinary tract infections, 159

V

vaginal infections, 123–124
vaginismus, 124
Valerian, 188
vegetables, 52–53; canned and frozen, versus fresh, 175; supertasters and, 55–56
vitamin A, 67, 197
vitamin B-6, 67–68, 131, 132, 141, 197
vitamin B-12, 67, 68, 131, 132, 141
vitamin C, 14, 67, 98, 163, 173, 174, 193
Vitamin C and the Common Cold (Pauling), 163
vitamin D, 67, 68–69, 174
vitamin E, 14, 67, 69, 163, 174, 178, 189
vitamin K, 67, 76

W

walking, 76
water, bottled vs. tap, 54
water-free hand gels, 205
weight loss, 83–85
weight training, 74, 83
whole wheat bread, 54
willow bark, 196
willpower, 19
women, heart disease and, 135–137
wormwood, 196
worriers, 42, 102

X

Xalatan, 102
Xenical, 84

Y

yeast infections, 125
yoga, 44, 78

Z

zinc lozenges, 98

AE Article Review Form

We encourage you to photocopy and use this page as a tool to assess how the articles in **Annual Editions** expand on the information in your textbook. By reflecting on the articles you will gain enhanced text information. You can also access this useful form on a product's book support Web site at **http://www.dushkin.com/online/.**

NAME: DATE:

TITLE AND NUMBER OF ARTICLE:

BRIEFLY STATE THE MAIN IDEA OF THIS ARTICLE:

LIST THREE IMPORTANT FACTS THAT THE AUTHOR USES TO SUPPORT THE MAIN IDEA:

WHAT INFORMATION OR IDEAS DISCUSSED IN THIS ARTICLE ARE ALSO DISCUSSED IN YOUR TEXTBOOK OR OTHER READINGS THAT YOU HAVE DONE? LIST THE TEXTBOOK CHAPTERS AND PAGE NUMBERS:

LIST ANY EXAMPLES OF BIAS OR FAULTY REASONING THAT YOU FOUND IN THE ARTICLE:

LIST ANY NEW TERMS/CONCEPTS THAT WERE DISCUSSED IN THE ARTICLE, AND WRITE A SHORT DEFINITION:

We Want Your Advice

ANNUAL EDITIONS revisions depend on two major opinion sources: one is our Advisory Board, listed in the front of this volume, which works with us in scanning the thousands of articles published in the public press each year; the other is you—the person actually using the book. Please help us and the users of the next edition by completing the prepaid article rating form on this page and returning it to us. Thank you for your help!

ANNUAL EDITIONS: Health 99/00

ARTICLE RATING FORM

Here is an opportunity for you to have direct input into the next revision of this volume. We would like you to rate each of the 52 articles listed below, using the following scale:

1. **Excellent: should definitely be retained**
2. **Above average: should probably be retained**
3. **Below average: should probably be deleted**
4. **Poor: should definitely be deleted**

Your ratings will play a vital part in the next revision. So please mail this prepaid form to us just as soon as you complete it. Thanks for your help!

RATING	ARTICLE
	1. How Does Your Life Measure Up?
	2. Why Do Those #&*?@! "Experts" Keep Changing Their Minds?
	3. Yet Another Study—Should You Pay Attention?
	4. "Just Do It" Isn't Enough: Change Comes in Stages
	5. Challenging America's Inverted Health Priorities
	6. Critical Life Events and the Onset of Illness
	7. The Talking Cure for Stress
	8. Using Your Mind to Heal Your Body
	9. Forgiveness
	10. Bad Mood Rising
	11. Tall Tales from the Table
	12. The Bitter Truth
	13. Are You Getting Enough Fat?
	14. Bulking Up Fiber's Healthful Reputation
	15. The Vitamin Revolution: B D E
	16. How Fitness Savvy Are You?
	17. How Fit Are You?
	18. Rebel against a Sedentary Life
	19. The Skinny on Weight Loss
	20. The Pressure to Eat
	21. Does Food Control You?
	22. Binge-Eating That Plagues Adults Now Recognized as a Disorder
	23. The Postmodern Guide to Cold Relief
	24. Alcohol and Health: Straight Talk on the Medical Headlines
	25. The War over Weed
	26. Will You Pay for Your Past as a Smoker?
	27. Rethinking Birth Control

RATING	ARTICLE
	28. Condoms: Barriers to Bad News
	29. America: Awash in STDs
	30. Your Sexual Landscape
	31. Family History: What You Don't Know Can Kill You
	32. The Heart Attackers
	33. Heart Disease in Women: Special Symptoms, Special Risks
	34. Beyond Cholesterol
	35. Strategies for Minimizing Cancer Risk
	36. AIDS, after the 'Cure': Amid Setbacks, Search for New Hope
	37. Health Unlimited
	38. Your Hospital Stay: A Guide to Survival
	39. Choose Treatments You Believe In
	40. Alternative Medicine—The Risks of Untested and Unregulated Remedies
	41. How Health Savvy Are You?
	42. Nutrition in the News: What the Headlines Don't Tell You
	43. The Switch to OTC: No Prescription, No Protection?
	44. The Doctor Is On
	45. Nature's Pharmacy
	46. An FDA Guide to Dietary Supplements
	47. Quiz: Are You Ready for the Sun?
	48. Germ Crazy
	49. The Frog Solution
	50. Prevent Sexually Transmitted Diseases
	51. Irradiation: A Safe Measure for Safer Food
	52. Why Is Date Rape So Hard to Prove?

(Continued on next page)

ANNUAL EDITIONS: HEALTH 99/00

BUSINESS REPLY MAIL
FIRST-CLASS MAIL PERMIT NO. 84 GUILFORD CT
POSTAGE WILL BE PAID BY ADDRESSEE

Dushkin/McGraw-Hill
Sluice Dock
Guilford, CT 06437-9989

NO POSTAGE NECESSARY IF MAILED IN THE UNITED STATES

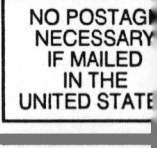

ABOUT YOU

Name _____ Date _____

Are you a teacher? ☐   A student? ☐
Your school's name _____

Department _____

Address _____ City _____ State _____ Zip _____

School telephone # _____

YOUR COMMENTS ARE IMPORTANT TO US!

Please fill in the following information:
For which course did you use this book? _____

Did you use a text with this *ANNUAL EDITION*? ☐ yes ☐ no
What was the title of the text? _____

What are your general reactions to the *Annual Editions* concept? _____

Have you read any particular articles recently that you think should be included in the next edition? _____

Are there any articles you feel should be replaced in the next edition? Why? _____

Are there any World Wide Web sites you feel should be included in the next edition? Please annotate. _____

May we contact you for editorial input? ☐ yes ☐ no
May we quote your comments? ☐ yes ☐ no